Infections Related to Biologics

Editors

DORA Y. HO
ARUNA K. SUBRAMANIAN

INFECTIOUS DISEASE CLINICS
OF NORTH AMERICA

www.id.theclinics.com

Consulting Editor
HELEN W. BOUCHER

June 2020 • Volume 34 • Number 2

ELSEVIER

1600 John F. Kennedy Boulevard • Suite 1800 • Philadelphia, Pennsylvania, 19103-2899.

http://www.theclinics.com

INFECTIOUS DISEASE CLINICS OF NORTH AMERICA Volume 34, Number 2
June 2020 ISSN 0891–5520, ISBN-13: 978-0-323-73320-5

Editor: Kerry Holland
Developmental Editor: Donald Mumford

Infectious Disease Clinics of North America (ISSN 0891–5520) is published in March, June, September, and December by Elsevier Inc., 360 Park Avenue South, New York, NY 10010-1710. Periodicals postage paid at New York, NY and additional mailing offices. Subscription prices are $340.00 per year for US individuals, $703.00 per year for US institutions, $100.00 per year for US students, $396.00 per year for Canadian individuals, $878.00 per year for Canadian institutions, $432.00 per year for international individuals, $878.00 per year for international institutions, $100.00 per year for Canadian students, and $200.00 per year for international students. To receive student rate, orders must be accompanied by name of affiliated institution, date of term, and the *signature* of program/residency coordinator on institution letterhead. Orders will be billed at individual rate until proof of status is received. Foreign air speed delivery is included in all *Clinics* subscription prices. All prices are subject to change without notice. **POSTMASTER**: Send address changes to *Infectious Disease Clinics of North America,* Elsevier Health Sciences Division, Subcription Customer Service, 3251 Riverport Lane, Maryland Heights, MO 63043. **Customer Service: 1-800-654-2452 (US). From outside of the US and Canada, call 1-314-447-8871. Fax: 1-314-447-8029. E-mail: JournalsCustomerService-usa@elsevier.com (print support) or JournalsOnlineSupport-usa@elsevier.com (online support).**

Infectious Disease Clinics of North America is also published in Spanish by Editorial Inter-Médica, Junin 917, 1er A 1113, Buenos Aires, Argentina.

Reprints. For copies of 100 or more, of articles in this publication, please contact the Commercial Reprints Department, Elsevier Inc., 360 Park Avenue South, New York, New York 10010-1710. Tel. 212-633-3874, Fax: 212-633-3820, E-mail: reprints@elsevier.com.

Infectious Disease Clinics of North America is covered in *MEDLINE/PubMed (Index Medicus), Current Contents/ Clinical Medicine, Science Citation Alert, SCISEARCH,* and *Research Alert.*

Contributors

CONSULTING EDITOR

HELEN W. BOUCHER, MD, FIDSA, FACP
Director, Infectious Diseases Fellowship Program, Division of Geographic Medicine and Infectious Diseases, Tufts Medical Center, Associate Professor of Medicine, Tufts University School of Medicine, Boston, Massachusetts, USA

EDITORS

DORA Y. HO, MD, PhD
Clinical Associate Professor, Division of Infectious Diseases and Geographic Medicine, Department of Medicine, Stanford University School of Medicine, Stanford, California, USA

ARUNA K. SUBRAMANIAN, MD
Clinical Professor of Medicine, Division of Infectious Diseases and Geographic Medicine, Department of Medicine, Stanford University School of Medicine, Stanford, California, USA

AUTHORS

MICHAEL S. ABERS, MD
Clinical Fellow, Fungal Pathogenesis Section, Laboratory of Clinical Immunology and Microbiology (LCIM), National Institute of Allergy and Infectious Diseases (NIAID), National Institutes of Health (NIH), Bethesda, Maryland, USA

JOSÉ MARÍA AGUADO, MD, PhD
Unit of Infectious Diseases, Hospital Universitario "12 de Octubre," Instituto de Investigación Sanitaria Hospital "12 de Octubre" (imas12), Spanish Network for Research in Infectious Diseases (REIPI RD16/0016/0002), Instituto de Salud Carlos III, School of Medicine, Universidad Complutense, Madrid, Spain

JUAN AGUILAR-COMPANY, MD
Infectious Diseases Department, Oncology Department, Vall d'Hebron University Hospital, Barcelona, Spain

ESTHER BENAMU, MD
Assistant Professor of Medicine, Transplant Infectious Diseases, Division of Infectious Diseases, University of Colorado Anschutz Medical Campus, Aurora, Colorado, USA

CASSANDRA CALABRESE, DO
Associate Staff, Department of Rheumatologic and Immunologic Disease, Cleveland Clinic Foundation, Cleveland, Ohio, USA

MATTHEW R. DAVIS, PharmD
Department of Pharmacy, University of California, Los Angeles Ronald Reagan Medical Center, Los Angeles, California, USA

KYLE ENRIQUEZ, MS
Stanford University, Stanford, California, USA

MARIO FERNÁNDEZ-RUIZ, MD, PhD
Unit of Infectious Diseases, Hospital Universitario "12 de Octubre," Instituto de
Investigación Sanitaria Hospital "12 de Octubre" (imas12), Spanish Network for Research
in Infectious Diseases (REIPI RD16/0016/0002), Instituto de Salud Carlos III, Madrid,
Spain

DORA Y. HO, MD, PhD
Clinical Associate Professor, Division of Infectious Diseases and Geographic Medicine,
Department of Medicine, Stanford University School of Medicine, Stanford, California,
USA

BETTY HSIAO, MD
Section of Rheumatology, Department of Internal Medicine, Yale School of Medicine,
New Haven, Connecticut, USA

INSOO KANG, MD
Section of Rheumatology, Department of Internal Medicine, Yale School of Medicine,
New Haven, Connecticut, USA

AISHA KHAN, MD
Department of Internal Medicine, Griffin Hospital, Derby, Connecticut,
USA

ANDREW KIN, MD
Assistant Professor, Department of Oncology, Wayne State University School of
Medicine, Karmanos Cancer Institute, Detroit, Michigan, USA

MARIA J. LEANDRO, MD, PhD
Centre for Rheumatology and Bloomsbury Rheumatology Unit, Division of Medicine,
University College London, London, United Kingdom

MICHAIL S. LIONAKIS, MD, ScD
Senior Investigator, Fungal Pathogenesis Section, Laboratory of Clinical
Immunology and Microbiology (LCIM), National Institute of Allergy and
Infectious Diseases (NIAID), National Institutes of Health (NIH), Bethesda,
Maryland, USA

ANNE Y. LIU, MD
Clinical Associate Professor, Division of Infectious Diseases, Department of Medicine,
Division of Allergy/Immunology/Rheumatology, Department of Pediatrics, Stanford
University School of Medicine, Stanford, California, USA

ASHRIT MULTANI, MD
Clinical Instructor, Division of Infectious Diseases, Department of Medicine, David Geffen
School of Medicine at UCLA, Los Angeles, California, USA

MINDIE H. NGUYEN, MD, MAS
Division of Gastroenterology and Hepatology, Department of Medicine, Stanford
University Medical Center, Palo Alto, California, USA

EIICHI OGAWA, MD, PhD
Department of General Internal Medicine, Kyushu University Hospital, Fukuoka,
Japan

THOMAS F. PATTERSON, MD
Division of Infectious Diseases, Department of Medicine, The University of Texas Health Science Center at San Antonio, South Texas Veterans Health Care System, San Antonio, Texas, USA

ISABEL RUIZ-CAMPS, MD, PhD
Infectious Diseases Department, Vall d'Hebron University Hospital, Barcelona, Spain

CHARLES A. SCHIFFER, MD
Professor of Medicine and Oncology, Joseph Dresner Chair for Hematologic Malignancies, Chief, Multidisciplinary Leukemia/Lymphoma Group, Wayne State University School of Medicine, Karmanos Cancer Institute, Detroit, Michigan, USA

STANFORD SHOOR, MD
Clinical Professor of Immunology and Rheumatology, Stanford University, Palo Alto, California, USA

GEORGE R. THOMPSON III, MD
Division of Infectious Diseases, Departments of Internal Medicine, and Medical Microbiology and Immunology, University of California Davis Health, Sacramento, California, USA

MIKE T. WEI, MD
Division of Gastroenterology and Hepatology, Department of Medicine, Stanford University Medical Center, Palo Alto, California, USA

KEVIN L. WINTHROP, MD, MPH
Professor, Division of Infectious Diseases, Schools of Medicine and Public Health, Oregon Health & Science University, Portland, Oregon, USA

Contents

> B cells are an essential component of the adaptive immune system. Since the late 1990s biologic drugs targeting B cells have been used to treat not only lymphoproliferative diseases of B-cell lineage cells but also autoimmune diseases, in particular, those associated with autoantibody production. Although some of these agents are relatively safe, they have been associated with serious infections including opportunistic infections. To what extent the infectious complications reported are directly related to the use of the B-cell targeting agent or to previous and/or concomitant immunosuppressive therapies and/or the specific disease being treated is often difficult to ascertain. A comprehensive knowledge of infectious risks associated with B-cell targeting agents in general and with each individual drug and of the measures available to decrease these risks are important for patient education and for early diagnosis and adequate treatment of infectious complications. Adaptation of general prevention guidelines in response to endemic conditions and local guidelines should be considered when appropriate.

> Co-stimulatory T-cell inhibitors are used in the treatment of rheumatoid arthritis and to prevent rejection of renal transplants. Inhibitors of the interleukin (IL)-17 cytokine are indicated for psoriasis, psoriatic arthritis and ankylosing spondylitis and anti- IL-23 drugs for psoriasis. Serious infections occur in 4.2% to 25.0% of co-stimulatory inhibitors and 1.0% to 2.0% with IL-17 or IL-23 inhibitors. Underlying disease, steroid dose greater than 7.5 to 10.0 mg, and comorbidities influence risk in individual patients. Opportunistic infections or reactivation of tuberculosis are rare.

> Lymphocyte depletion and blockade of T-cell activation and trafficking serve as therapeutic strategies for an enlarging number of immune-mediated diseases and malignancies. This review summarizes the infection risks associated to monoclonal antibodies that bind to the α chain of the interleukin-2 receptor, the cell surface glycoprotein CD52,

and members of α4- and β2-integrin families acting as cell-adhesion molecules. An outline of the mechanisms of action, approved indications and off-label uses, expected impact on the host immune response, and available clinical evidence is provided for each of these agents.

Anne Y. Liu

Targeting interleukins that drive innate inflammation has expanded treatments of autoinflammatory and autoimmune disorders. Interleukin (IL)-1 inhibition has proven useful for monogenic autoinflammatory syndromes, and IL-6 inhibition for autoimmune arthritides. Biological therapies impeding these pathways impair detection and containment of pathogens, particularly invasive bacteria, reflecting the importance of IL-1 and IL-6 in communicating danger throughout the immune system. Biologics targeting T helper type 2 inflammation are used to treat specific allergic, atopic, and eosinophilic diseases. They may impair protections against local herpesvirus reactivations while augmenting antiviral responses to respiratory viruses. Their risks with helminth exposures have yet to be defined.

Michael S. Abers and Michail S. Lionakis

The clearance of both tumors and microbes depends on highly coordinated immune responses that are sufficiently potent to kill malignant or microbial cells while avoiding immunopathology from an overly exuberant inflammatory response. A molecular understanding of the immune pathways that regulate these responses paved the way for the development of checkpoint inhibitors (CPIs) as a therapeutic strategy to boost endogenous antitumor immunity. CPIs have demonstrated survival benefits across a wide spectrum of cancers. While infectious complications of CPIs are uncommon, immune-related adverse events occur frequently and often require immunosuppressive therapies that increase the risk of infection.

Andrew Kin and Charles A. Schiffer

Tyrosine kinase inhibitors represent the standard of care for several diseases and drug targets in hematologic malignancies. Infectious complications vary by disease status and prior therapy, but overall incidence of infections generally is low. In chronic diseases, such as chronic myeloid leukemia and chronic lymphocytic leukemia, patients can remain on tyrosine kinase inhibitor therapy for many years, with few infectious complications from therapy. Bruton tyrosine kinase inhibitors overall are well tolerated in lymphoproliferative disorders, with long-term follow-up of many years in patients with chronic lymphocytic leukemia. Although opportunistic infections have been reported, they are uncommon and routine prophylaxis is not recommended.

have high risk of HBV reactivation (>10%), so antiviral prophylactic therapies are required. This review provides the different classes of biologics associated with HBV reactivation, stratifies the various reactivation risk levels by HBV status and biologic agent, and discusses management strategies.

JC Polyomavirus Infection Potentiated by Biologics

Ashrit Multani and Dora Y. Ho

The risk of JC polyomavirus encephalopathy varies among biologic classes and among agents within the same class. Of currently used biologics, the highest risk is seen with natalizumab followed by rituximab. Multiple other agents have also been implicated. Drug-specific causality is difficult to establish because many patients receive multiple immunomodulatory medications concomitantly or sequentially, and have other immunocompromising factors related to their underlying disease. As use of biologic therapies continues to expand, further research is needed into pathogenesis, treatment, and prevention of JC polyomavirus encephalopathy such that risk for its development is better understood and mitigated, if not eliminated altogether.

Fungal Infections Potentiated by Biologics

Matthew R. Davis, George R. Thompson III, and Thomas F. Patterson

Biologic therapies including monoclonal antibodies, tyrosine kinase inhibitors, and other agents represent a notable expansion in the pharmacotherapy armamentarium in treatment of a variety of diseases. Many of these therapies possess direct or indirect immunosuppressive and immunomodulatory effects, which have been associated with bacterial, viral, and fungal opportunistic infections. Careful screening of baseline risk factors before initiation, targeted preventive measures, and vigilant monitoring while on active biologic therapy mitigate these risks as use of biologics becomes more commonplace. This review compiles reported evidence of fungal infections associated with these agents with a focus on the tumor necrosis factor-α inhibitor class.

Mycobacterial Infections Potentiated by Biologics

Cassandra Calabrese and Kevin L. Winthrop

Biologic therapies have revolutionized the treatment of immune-mediated inflammatory diseases but are associated with an increased risk of serious and opportunistic infections, including tuberculosis and nontuberculous mycobacterial disease. Despite this increased risk, the overall risk-benefit ratio remains favorable with appropriate screening and risk assessment. Further population-based studies are needed to establish the risk of tuberculosis and nontuberculous mycobacterial disease with the new biologics. This article highlights the incidence and drug-specific risk of tuberculous and nontuberculous mycobacterial infection in the setting of biologics, screening and prevention, and treatment of latent tuberculosis in this setting.

Vaccinations and Biologics 425

Betty Hsiao, Aisha Khan, and Insoo Kang

The emergence of biologics has revolutionized the way physicians treat many autoimmune inflammatory conditions. Although biologics have become a vital component of the treatment approach to many inflammatory diseases, these agents may potentially disrupt the natural immune response against pathogens, thereby increasing the risk for infections. Some infections may be preventable or have a lessened risk through appropriate vaccinations; thus, vaccination history should be taken carefully in preparation for biologics and updated annually to maximize benefits while minimizing adverse effects. The objective of this review is to summarize recent articles, including guidelines, published that address vaccinations among patients on biologics.

INFECTIOUS DISEASE CLINICS OF NORTH AMERICA

Preface

Infections Related to Biologics

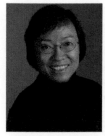 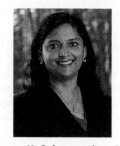

Dora Y. Ho, MD, PhD   Aruna K. Subramanian, MD
Editors

Biologics as a class of therapeutics are revolutionizing medicine by providing successful new treatment options for cancers, autoimmune diseases, neurodegenerative conditions, and many other devastating diseases. These drugs are large molecules that are manufactured using recombinant DNA technology in living systems, such as bacterial, fungal, animal, or plant cells. The field has expanded rapidly since 1982, when the first recombinant form of human insulin was approved by the Food and Drug Administration (FDA).[1] Today the vast majority of the world's top-selling medications are biologics. However, there were initial public fears of recombinant DNA technology, and there have been setbacks, such as when centoxin, a monoclonal antibody against the lipid A moiety of endotoxin thought to have great promise in gram-negative sepsis, was not approved by the FDA in 1992.[2] Thankfully, many hurdles were successfully overcome, and numerous biologic agents are now available to patients for previously untreatable conditions. There are currently over 1000 biologics in development, and the global biologics market is forecast to exceed $285 billion by 2023.[3]

Along with the promise of great benefit from the immunomodulatory effects of these biologics comes the risk of unintended consequences, including infection. Over the years it has become clear that each of these classes of agents has unique infectious risks that often correspond to their direct or indirect targets in the immune system.[4] The challenge for care providers is how to screen prior to administering the agents, what prophylaxis and preventative measures may be required, and how to predict for which infections to maintain a high index of suspicion.

When deciding on prophylaxis or treatment with antibiotics, there are multiple considerations to keep in mind. Not only do clinicians need to avoid promoting antimicrobial resistance with overuse of antibiotics, but also there are data showing that the use of antibiotics can render the biologic agents less effective through their effects on the gut microbiome.[5] Therefore, a thoughtful approach to understanding the

Infect Dis Clin N Am 34 (2020) xiii–xvi
https://doi.org/10.1016/j.idc.2020.04.001
0891-5520/20/© 2020 Published by Elsevier Inc.

infection risks of individual agents and providing prevention strategies is essential. Given the explosion of new agents on the market, it is becoming increasingly difficult for clinicians to keep up with such data. In this issue of *Infectious Diseases Clinics of North America*, the authors seek to provide timely guidance for clinicians caring for patients who are on biologics, by discussing the different classes of biologics and their infection risks in the first eight articles, then providing a survey of important infections potentiated by biologics with strategies to mitigate their risks in the following six articles.

This issue first addresses biologic drugs targeting B cells, which are widely used in treating B-cell proliferative malignancies and diseases where autoantibody production is responsible for pathologic condition. Their specific infection risks can be difficult to tease out given the frequent coadministration of other immunosuppressive agents, but there are unique risks that are critical for care providers to understand, with hepatitis B reactivation being a prominent example. Interestingly, the risks are not limited to the direct effects of hypogammaglobulinemia alone, so a nuanced look at these agents is required.

The next two articles address agents targeting T-cell activation, the majority of which are used in rheumatoid arthritis and psoriasis, and agents that directly inhibit T-cells function or target T-cell migration and chemotaxis, some of which are used to treat multiple sclerosis. The rates of serious infection are low with many of these drugs, with the exception of those like alemtuzumab. This agent can cause profound $CD4^+$ cell depletion and confers higher risks of infections, such as *Pneumocystis jirovecii* pneumonia.

Biologics that target the interleukin-1 (IL-1) and IL-6 pathways diminish inflammatory responses to pathogens and increase the risk of bacterial and opportunistic infections, while those that target the T-helper 2 cell pathway do not carry these same risks. Immune checkpoint inhibitors are being successfully used to treat a variety of solid tumors, improving outcomes in these conditions that were previously fatal. Unfortunate consequences of these agents include a 40% risk of immune-related adverse events, which often require the use of corticosteroids or other immunosuppressive agents. The infectious complications related to checkpoint inhibitors therefore include those related to the use of this enhanced immunosuppression as well.

Tyrosine kinase inhibitors (TKI) have demonstrated great success for patients with many hematologic diseases. Patients often are at risk of infections due to their underlying malignancy and prior chemotherapy, but understanding the additive risk of TKI is important. The TKIs used for solid tumors, including epidermal growth factor receptor inhibitors, are discussed separately, as are agents used to target the JAK-STAT signaling and complement pathways to abrogate inflammation.

The next six articles discuss important viral, fungal, and mycobacterial infections potentiated by biologics. There are existing guidelines on prophylaxis for herpesviruses, such as herpes simplex virus, varicella-zoster virus, and cytomegalovirus, in solid organ transplant and hematopoietic cell transplant recipients. However, strategies for prevention of reactivation of these viruses in patients on biologic agents are not available. Understanding which biologic agents potentiate the reactivation of herpesviruses is critical to targeting appropriate prevention strategies. Progressive multifocal leukoencephalopathy caused by JC polyomavirus can be a devastating opportunistic infection. Exploring the pathogenesis of JC polyomavirus and which biologics increase the risk of this condition is covered by the authors in this issue. Furthermore, a very important infectious risk for certain biologics is hepatitis B virus reactivation. This is preventable with the correct prophylactic approach; thus the authors' guidance in this area is very helpful.

Fungal infections can cause high morbidity and mortality and are especially important to consider with immunosuppression. The risk of certain fungal infections can be geographically limited, so correlating the epidemiology of infection to the biologic agents that increase the risks is key to correct diagnosis and treatment. Tumor necrosis factor-alpha inhibitors can especially predispose patients to both fungal and mycobacterial infections. The diagnosis of mycobacterial infections requires a high index of suspicion. In the 13th article, the authors discuss when screening for *Mycobacterium tuberculosis* is indicated and in which situations to consider nontuberculous mycobacterial infections.

One of the most important weapons in our armamentarium against infection is vaccination. The final article in this issue discusses the optimal use of vaccines in patients on biologics. Timing of immunization is important as vaccines should generally be given prior to starting immunosuppressive agents to optimize their efficacy and to reduce adverse effects when live vaccines are concerned. Understanding whom to target with vaccinations to maximize benefit while minimizing risk is the focus.

We are thankful to Consulting Editor, Dr Helen Boucher and Developmental Editor Donald Mumford, for inviting us to compile this issue on infections in biologics. We are especially thankful to all the authors, who are truly experts in their field, for their outstanding contributions to this issue of *Infectious Disease Clinics of North America.* The topics they have covered in great depth are of immense importance to practicing clinicians. The number of biologics and the indications for their use are growing exponentially. They provide great hope and promise for many of our patients. We truly believe the information and strategies covered in this issue will help clinicians mitigate the risk of infection associated with the use of these new agents and improve patient outcomes.

Dora Y. Ho, MD, PhD
Division of Infectious Diseases and
Geographic Medicine
Department of Medicine
Stanford University School of Medicine
300 Pasteur Drive, Lane Building L-135
Stanford, CA 94305, USA

Aruna K. Subramanian, MD
Division of Infectious Diseases and
Geographic Medicine
Department of Medicine
Stanford University School of Medicine
300 Pasteur Drive, Lane Building L-146
Stanford, CA 94305, USA

E-mail addresses:
jsbach@stanford.edu (D.Y. Ho)
asubram2@stanford.edu (A.K. Subramanian)

REFERENCES

1. Kinch MS. An overview of FDA-approved biologics medicines. Drug Discov Today 2015;20(4):393–8.

2. Warren HS, Danner RL, Munford RS. Anti-endotoxin monoclonal antibodies. N Engl J Med 1992;326(17):1153–7.
3. Available at: https://www.marketwatch.com/press-release/global-biologics-market-outlook-by-size-share-future-growth-and-forecast-from-2018-2023-2019-07-30. Accessed February 5, 2020.
4. Bongartz T, Sutton AJ, Sweeting MJ, et al. Anti-TNF antibody therapy in rheumatoid arthritis and the risk of serious infections and malignancies. JAMA 2006;295(19):2275–85.
5. Gopalakrishnan V, Spencer CN, Nezi L, et al. Gut microbiome modulates response to anti-PD-1 immunotherapy in melanoma patients. Science 2018;359(6371):97–103.

Infections Related to Biologics: Agents Targeting B Cells

Maria J. Leandro, MD, PhD

KEYWORDS

- B cells • Plasma cells • Serum immunoglobulins • B-cell targeting drugs
- Anti-CD20 • Anti-CD38 • Belimumab

KEY POINTS

- Biologic drugs targeting B cells are often relatively safe, but their use has been associated with serious infections, including opportunistic infections.
- Risk of infectious complications is often confounded by immunosuppressive factors associated with the disease itself being treated and previous and concomitant therapies.
- Detailed reports on effects on normal B cells, plasma cells, and serum immunoglobulin levels when B-cell targeted agents are used in lymphoproliferative diseases are often limited.
- Appropriate pretreatment screening, vaccination, and other prophylactic measures are important to decrease the risk of serious infectious complications.

INTRODUCTION

Biologic drugs targeting B cells have revolutionized the treatment of B-cell lymphoproliferative diseases and of various autoantibody-associated autoimmune diseases since the late 1990s. B cells are part of the adaptive immune system, and the immunoglobulins produced by the terminally differentiated plasma cells are an essential component of humoral immunity. B cells play different roles, some dependent on the presence of B cells per se and their direct interaction with antigens, with other immune cells and their production of cytokines and chemokines, others dependent on their differentiation into antibody-producing plasma cells.

Most biologics targeting B cells were developed for the treatment of B-cell lymphoproliferative diseases with the aim of killing malignant B cells, or malignant plasma cells, and/or of potentially making them more susceptible to other chemotherapeutic agents. These drugs are mostly monoclonal antibodies (mAbs) directed to molecules expressed on the lymphocyte cell surface. Many of these therapeutic agents rely on the patients' immune system to induce cytotoxicity by recruiting Fc

Centre for Rheumatology and Bloomsbury Rheumatology Unit, Division of Medicine, University College London, Rayne Building, 5 University Street, London WC1E 6JF, UK
E-mail address: maria.leandro@ucl.ac.uk

Infect Dis Clin N Am 34 (2020) 161–178
https://doi.org/10.1016/j.idc.2020.02.013 id.theclinics.com
0891-5520/20/© 2020 Elsevier Inc. All rights reserved.

gammaRc-bearing effector immune cells (natural killer [NK] cells, macrophages, neutrophils) for antibody-dependent cellular cytotoxicity (ADCC) or antibody-dependent cellular phagocytosis (ADCP) or by activating complement and inducing formation of the membrane attack complex (complement direct cytotoxicity, CDC). They can also induce transmembrane signaling and direct cell death (DCD) or interfere with cell-cycle and have cytostatic effects that can make malignant cells more susceptible to the effect of other chemotherapy agents. Some agents may interfere with the interaction between cancer cells and the microenvironment and tumor survival signals. When targeting cell surface molecules that typically internalize upon binding their ligand, the mAbs are sometimes conjugated to toxins that are then released inside the target cells and induce cell death.

Most of these agents are not specific for malignant B cells and also target normal B cells, and it is their effects on normal B cells per se, on plasma cells and/or on serum immunoglobulin levels, that have led to their use in autoimmune diseases but are also responsible for the associated risk of infections. In addition, some biologic agents are B cell–specific; others target molecules that are expressed by subsets of B cells and/or by plasma cells but also other cells of the immune system (T cells, NK cells, monocytes). Understandably, most reports on the use of these agents in B-cell malignancies are poor in detailed description of their effects on normal B cells, normal plasma cells, or total or antimicrobial-specific serum immunoglobulin levels.

In cancer trials, these agents are often used in combination with other chemotherapy agents as well as steroids, in patients previously treated with other cancer drugs, and in lymphoproliferative diseases that by themselves are associated with immunosuppression and increased risk of infections. Therefore, it is not always easy to discern the increased risk of infection that is specifically associated with each biologic agent. The same applies, although to a lesser extent, when looking at its use in patients with autoimmune diseases. In addition, many of these agents are associated with neutropenia, including both early- and late-onset neutropenia, which can contribute to the risk of infections.

When an infection occurs, the logical course of action is to discontinue the use of the drug involved, but, particularly in the cancer setting, this is not always feasible. In addition, several of these drugs not only exert their effect at the time that they are being administered and until complete clearance has occurred but also often have long-term effects in the immune system by causing prolonged B-cell depletion, by leading to a change in B-cell repertoire even after B-cell repopulation, by causing low total serum immunoglobulin levels, which may persist despite B-cell repopulation and/or by having direct, or indirect, prolonged effects on other immune cells, particularly T cells.

In clinical practice, it is the overall risk of infection that is important. Contributors will necessarily include the biologic drug that the patient is receiving or has received, the total amount of drug and exact administration schedule used, the disease process itself, previous and concomitant immunosuppressive therapies, the patient's age and concomitant diseases that may by themselves increase the risk of infections in general or of particular infections, and also the region where the patient lives and any endemic risk of particular infections. In this context, having detailed information on the direct and indirect effects of the various biologic drugs targeting B cells used is beneficial.

Although several of these B-cell targeting agents are relatively safe, knowledge of the infectious complications that have been associated with their use in the different contexts is important to inform the patient of the risks involved in starting these drugs as well as maintaining vigilance. It is important to remember that, in the case of rare infections, a true association may be difficult to prove in view of the small number of observed events. In addition, randomized controlled trials are powered to measure efficacy and not safety, and large open-label trials and cohort data are often difficult to interpret because of the large number of confounders. A multidisciplinary approach involving different specialties (cancer, autoimmune disease, and infectious disease specialists), including clinical immunologists in individual cases, can be useful.

This review focuses on the mechanisms of action of these biologic agents and their effects on normal B cells, plasma cells, and serum immunoglobulin levels, the infectious disease risks associated with their use and advisable prophylactic measures, including vaccination. Comprehensive reviews on the subject, including recent ones from the European Society of Clinical Microbiology and Infectious Diseases Study Group for Infections in Compromised Hosts, have previously been published.[1–3]

SPECIFIC AGENTS TARGETING B CELLS OR PLASMA CELLS

Tables 1 and 2 include the different B-cell targeting agents included in this review.

Biologic Drugs Targeting CD20

CD20 is a transmembrane phosphoprotein that plays a role in B-cell activation and proliferation. CD20 is a lineage-restricted molecule expressed in most normal B cells and by tumor cells in a large number of B-cell lymphoproliferative diseases. CD20 is first expressed by B-cell precursors at the pre-B-cell stage and is lost on terminal differentiation into plasma cells.[4]

There are 4 currently available anti-CD20 mAbs licensed for the treatment of different B-cell malignancies and/or autoantibody-associated autoimmune diseases: rituximab, ofatumumab, obinutuzumab, and ocrelizumab (see **Table 1**).[5–8] These antibodies deplete B cells by ADCP, ADCC, CDC and DCD, and the different agents differ in their relative potency to initiate different cytotoxic mechanisms. Differences relate to the exact epitope that they recognize on CD20, which influences their complement activating activity, internalization rate, and capacity to induce DCD, Fc modifications that increase binding to Fc gamma receptor on immune effector cells and their chimeric, humanized, or fully human structure.[9]

Anti-CD20 drugs induce a rapid and profound B-cell depletion in the peripheral blood. The extent of B-cell depletion in solid lymphoid tissues is less well known and variable.[4] Not all B cells that bind rituximab are depleted, and it is not known if cells coated with rituximab but not lysed have reduced function in vivo. Because CD20 is not expressed by hematopoietic stem cells and the earlier B-cell precursors (pro-B cells), B-cell repopulation of the peripheral blood usually starts once the drug has been cleared and seems to depend on the extent of the initial depletion and on the regenerative capacity of the individual's bone marrow.[10] B cell repopulation of the peripheral blood occurs usually 6 to 9 months after 1 standard cycle of treatment. Normal B-cell counts have been observed within 12 months after treatment, but in some patients, it can take longer for peripheral B cells to start repopulating and/or for B-cell counts to return to normal or to baseline levels.[4,11] B-cell repopulation occurs mainly with naïve B cells and the frequency of memory B cells, particularly switched memory B cells remain below baseline levels for prolonged periods of time in many patients studied.[11]

Normal plasma cells are not directly depleted by anti-CD20 drugs because they do not express CD20, but formation of new plasma cells is presumed to be reduced or prevented during the period of B-cell depletion. Following 1 standard course of treatment with anti-CD20 drugs, total serum immunoglobulin levels usually remain within the normal range (if normal at baseline) with immunoglobulin M (IgM) being the

Table 1
Description of biologic drugs that target B cells currently in clinical use

Agent Name	Agent Description	Target Cellular Expression	Mechanism of Action	Associated B-Cell Impaired Immunity	Year of Approval	Approved Indication
Rituximab	Type I anti-CD20 IgG1 mAb (chimeric)	B cells (including B-cell precursors from pre-B-cell stage, naïve and memory subsets); not expressed on plasma cells	B-cell depletion (normal and tumor B cells) by ADCC, ADCP, CDC, DCD	B-cell depletion, presumed prevention of formation of new plasma cells, hypogammaglobulinemia (particularly with repeated cycles)	1997 (FDA)/1998 (EMA)	NHL, CLL, RA, GPA, MPA, PV
Ofatumumab[a]	Type I anti-CD20 IgG1 mAb (fully human)	As for rituximab	As for rituximab	As for rituximab	2009 (FDA)/2010 (EMA, withdrawn May 2019 from outside United States)	CLL
Obinutuzumab	Type II anti-CD20 IgG1 mAb (humanized; glycoengineered)	As for rituximab	As for rituximab	As for rituximab	2013 (FDA)/2014 (EMA)	CLL, follicular lymphoma
Ocrelizumab	Type I anti-CD20 IgG1 mAb (humanized)	As for rituximab	As for rituximab	As for rituximab	2017 (FDA)/2018 (EMA)	MS

Drug	Type	Target cells	Mechanism	Effects on normal cells/immunoglobulin	Approval	Indication
Daratumumab	Anti-CD38 human IgG1 mAb	CD38 expressing cells including tumor and normal plasma cells, B-cell subsets, T-cell subsets, NK cells	Depletion of MM tumor cells (ADCC, CDC, DCD)	Depletion of a proportion of plasma cells and B cells; further decrease in total serum immunoglobulin levels	2015 (FDA)/2016 (EMA)	MM
Brentuximab vedotin	Anti-CD30 IgG1 mAb (chimeric) conjugated with antimicrotubule agent MMAE	CD30 expressing tumor cells, activated B (particular subset), T, and NK cells and monocytes	Depletion of CD30 expressing tumor cells (ADCC, CDC, DCD)	No detailed reports on effects on normal B cells, plasma cells, or serum immunoglobulin levels found in literature	2011 (FDA)/2012 (EMA)	Hodgkin lymphoma, anaplastic large cell lymphoma, cutaneous T-cell lymphoma
Blinatumomab	Bispecific CD19-directed CD3+ T-cell engager	B cells and plasma cells	Depletion of circulating CD19+ cells by T cells	No detailed reports on effects on normal circulating B cells, plasma cells, or serum immunoglobulins found in literature	2014 (FDA)/2015 (EMA)	B-precursor acute lymphoblastic leukemia
Inotuzumab ozogamicin	Anti-CD22 IgG4 mAb conjugated with a calicheamicin agent	B cells	Depletion of tumor and normal B cells (DCD)	No detailed reports on effects on normal circulating B cells, plasma cells, or serum immunoglobulins found in literature	2017 (FDA, EMA)	B-precursor acute lymphoblastic leukemia

(continued on next page)

Table 1
(continued)

Agent Name	Agent Description	Target Cellular Expression	Mechanism of Action	Associated B-Cell Impaired Immunity	Year of Approval	Approved Indication
Alemtuzumab	Anti-CD52 IgG1 humanized mAb	Mature B and T lymphocytes, lower expression in NK cells, monocytes, and macrophages PCs?	Depletion of CD52 expressing lymphocytes (ADCC, ADCP, CDC, DCD)	Profound lymphopenia, including B- and prolonged T-cell lymphopenia	2001 (FDA)/2001 EMA (withdrawn 2011, renewed 2013)	MS
Belimumab	Antisoluble BAFF (BLyS) IgG1 human mAb	Soluble BAFF	Binds soluble BAFF preventing it from binding to receptors on B cells (signaling involved in B-cell survival, activation, and maturation)	Decrease in circulating B-cell counts, in particular, naïve B-cell subsets (transitional and mature) Some decrease in serum total immunoglobulin levels, particularly IgM	2011 (FDA and EMA)	Systemic lupus erythematosus

Abbreviations: EMA, European Medicines Agency; FDA, Food and Drug Administration; GPA, granulomatosis with polyangiitis; MPA, microscopic polyangiitis; NHL, non-Hodgkin's lymphoma; PV, pemphigus vulgaris; RA, rheumatoid arthritis.
[a] The marketing authorization for Arzerra (ofatumumab) has been withdrawn at the request of the marketing authorization holder from outside the United States.

Table 2
Risk of neutropenia, risk of hypogammaglobulinemia, and specific infections risk associated with biologic drugs that target B cells currently in clinical use

Agent Name	Risk of Neutropenia	Risk of Low Immunoglobulins	Associated Opportunistic Infections Reported	Vaccination Recommended	Prophylaxis
Rituximab	Yes, including late neutropenia	Yes, particularly with repeated cycles of treatment or maintenance treatment; serum immunoglobulin levels should be monitored	PCP, CMV, herpes virus, PML, hepatitis C virus, hepatitis B virus reactivation, enterovirus	Pretreatment influenza and antipneumococcal vaccine; annual influenza vaccine	PCP prophylaxis in GPA/MPA and PV
Ofatumumab	As for rituximab	As for rituximab	As for rituximab	Same as rituximab	
Obinutuzumab	As for rituximab	As for rituximab	As for rituximab	Same as rituximab	
Ocrelizumab	As for rituximab	As for rituximab	As for rituximab	Same as rituximab	
Daratumumab	Yes	Transient worsening of low IgM and low IgA	Herpes zoster reactivation, CMV reactivation, CMV enterocolitis, cryptococcosis, hepatitis B reactivation, PCP	Same as rituximab	Herpes zoster reactivat on prophylaxis, PCP prophylaxis, HBV reactivation prophylaxis according to local guidelines
Brentuximab vedotin	Yes		PML, herpes zoster, CMV, PCP, hepatitis B reactivation	Same as rituximab	Herpes zoster reactivation prophylaxis, PCP prophylaxis
Blinatumomab	Yes		CMV, enterovirus, PCP, PML	Same as rituximab	
Inotuzumab ozogamicin	Yes		Limited data for specific infections	Same as rituximab	

(continued on next page)

Table 2
(continued)

Agent Name	Risk of Neutropenia	Risk of Low Immunoglobulins	Associated Opportunistic Infections Reported	Vaccination Recommended	Prophylaxis
Alemtuzumab	Yes (autoimmune neutropenia)		Herpes virus, listeriosis, TB reactivation, PML, PCP, hepatitis B reactivation, CMV (risk depends on dose)	Same as rituximab. herpes zoster vaccine pretreatment if appropriate	Herpes zoster reactivation prophylaxis, PCP prophylaxis, TB screening, CMV reactivation prophylaxis according to local guidelines (risk depends on dose)
Belimumab		Decreases in immunoglobulin levels with hypogammaglobulinemia reported	Herpes zoster reactivation, CMV reactivation, PML, Acinetobacter	Same as rituximab	

Abbreviation: CR, case reports.

more susceptible class and IgA being the least susceptible class. However, prolonged periods of treatment and/or repeated cycles of treatment increase the risk of prolonged hypogammaglobulinemia, which can be persistent even if the drug is discontinued and peripheral B-cell repopulation occurs. IgM is the immunoglobulin class most commonly affected by treatment with anti-CD20 mAbs, but low IgM by itself has not been consistently associated with an increased risk of infections. Persistently low IgG can be well tolerated but clearly carries a risk of severe or repeated infections as seen in other secondary hypogammaglobulinemias.[12-14] Response to vaccination in patients with low IgG can help assess the associated risk of infections. Therefore, serum immunoglobulin levels should be monitored in patients treated with anti-CD20 agents. Assessment of response to vaccination, antibiotic prophylaxis, and/or immunoglobulin replacement therapy should be considered as appropriate.[14] Risk of hypogammaglobulinemia is higher in pediatric patients when compared with adults.[15] Studies of rituximab in autoimmune diseases comparing changes in autoantibodies and antimicrobial antibodies showed more pronounced decreases in autoantibodies, presumably because their production is proportionally more dependent on formation of new plasma cells.[16]

Low levels of CD20 expression can be detected in a small percentage of peripheral blood T cells, but there are no data suggesting that rituximab's effect on these cells results in any further immunosuppression.[11]

All anti-CD20 mAbs have been associated with neutropenia, both early onset within the first 4 to 6 weeks after treatment and late onset more commonly seen around 4 to 6 months after the last anti-CD20 infusion. Drug-induced neutropenia can be well tolerated and resolve spontaneously but can also be symptomatic and associated with infections. Blood neutrophil counts should be measured before each course of rituximab, regularly up to 6 months after the last rituximab infusion and at any time the patient presents with signs or symptoms of infection.

Anti-CD20 agents are considered relatively safe, but serious infections, including opportunistic infections, have been reported even when these agents are used in monotherapy. Randomized controlled trials commonly do not show an increased risk of overall infections or of serious infections when compared with placebo in some of the diseases. In autoimmune diseases, if patients also have significant lymphopenia with very low CD4 or CD8 T-cell counts, treatment with anti-CD20 agents is relatively contraindicated.[5,8] Prophylaxis for pneumocystis pneumonia (PCP) is recommended in patients with ANCA-associated vasculitis and pemphigus vulgaris who require anti-CD20 agents.[5]

Serious infections reported with anti-CD20 drugs include herpes zoster primary infections and reactivation, hepatitis B virus reactivation, hepatitis C, cytomegalovirus (CMV) reactivation, enterovirus infections, PCP, and progressive multifocal leukoencephalopathy (PML).[1,2,5-8]

Patients with persistent hypogammaglobulinemia secondary to treatment with anti-CD20 agents may be more at risk of sinopulmonary infections by encapsulated microorganisms, such as pneumococcus, with a risk of bronchiectasis over time. Patients may also be at increased risk of sepsis by encapsulated microorganisms. Patients with humoral immunodeficiencies are susceptible to serious enterovirus infections, and cases of enterovirus encephalitis cases have been described in patients treated with rituximab and with obinutuzumab in association with hypogammaglobulinemia.[17]

Hepatitis B reactivation has been reported in patients treated with rituximab and other anti-CD20 agents, including fulminant hepatitis with fatal outcome.[5-8,11,18] Cases have been reported in patients who were hepatitis B surface antigen (HBsAg) -positive but also in patients who were hepatitis B core antibody–positive but

HBsAg-negative with or without positive anti-hepatitis B surface antibody. Most of these patients had lymphoproliferative diseases and were also exposed to chemotherapy. All patients being considered for treatment with anti-CD20 agents should have hepatitis B virus screening before initiation of therapy. If either HBsAg or hepatitis B core antibody is positive, advice from a liver expert before treatment is recommended. For patients HbsAg-negative, local guidelines differ, ranging from careful monitoring to prophylaxis with either lamivudine or other antiviral agents. Local guidelines will necessarily reflect different local hepatitis B virus (HBV) epidemiology, different baseline risks associated with disease being treated, and/or other concomitant therapies. Monitoring and/or prevention of reactivation antiviral treatment should be continued up to 6 to 12 months after completion of anti-CD20 therapy.

Very rare cases of PML have been reported following use of rituximab and other anti-CD20 agents. In lymphoproliferative diseases, in most of these cases, rituximab was used together with chemotherapy or as part of a hematopoietic stem cell transplant.

Vaccination with live vaccines is contraindicated during treatment with anti-CD20 and at least while the patient is peripherally B cell–depleted. Physicians should review the patient's vaccination status, and any vaccinations needed should be completed at least 4 weeks before the first administration of rituximab. Pretreatment vaccination with influenza vaccine and pneumococcal vaccine (at least if not previously done) is recommended. Annual influenza vaccine should be advised for patients previously treated or continuing treatment with anti-CD20 agents because the cellular immune response is preserved.[19] Humoral response rates to nonlive vaccines in patients previously treated with anti-CD20 agents are likely to be reduced particularly in patients with lymphoproliferative diseases and/or on concomitant therapies and particularly if vaccines are administered not long after anti-CD20 treatment and still at a time of B-cell depletion. Humoral responses to capsular pneumococcal polysaccharide vaccine and neoantigens are often reduced even 6 months after treatment. Mean pretreatment antibody titers against a panel of antigens (Streptococcus pneumoniae, influenza, mumps, rubella, varicella, tetanus toxoid) can be maintained following 1 course of treatment with rituximab.

Biologic Drugs Targeting CD38

CD38 is a transmembrane protein that regulates cell activation, proliferation, and adhesion. It has multiple functions participating in receptor-mediated cell adhesion and signaling and has enzymatic activity (it is an ADP ribosyl cyclase).[20] CD38 is widely expressed in many hematopoietic cells and in some nonhematopoietic cells. It is present in very early erythroid and myeloid precursors, precursor and mature B cells, normal plasma cells, thymocytes, T cells, and NK cells. It is highly expressed in malignant plasma cells in patients with multiple myeloma (MM), but relatively high levels of expression are also seen in normal plasma cells, early B and T cells, activated T cells, germinal center B cells, and NK cells.

Daratumumab is an anti-CD38 mAb. It kills CD38-expressing tumor cells by cytotoxic mechanisms, including ADCC, CDC, and apoptosis.[21] It also inhibits in vivo growth of CD38-expressing tumor cells and changes CD38 enzymatic activity in vitro. Daratumumab is licensed for the treatment of patients with MM.[22]

There is little published detailed information on depletion of normal B-cell lineage cells with daratumumab used in the treatment of MM patients. Circulating B cells expressing CD38 are depleted from the peripheral blood by treatment with daratumumab. Populations affected are, in particular, transitional naïve B cells, which express higher levels of CD38 and CD24, and also presumably mature naïve B cells and postgerminal center B cells because these were not found in the peripheral blood on MM patients under treatment with daratumumab.[23,24] To the author's knowledge, there are no published data with detailed information on depletion of B-cell precursors in the bone marrow or of germinal B cells in secondary lymphoid tissues, subpopulations that are known to express relatively high levels of CD38.

Normal plasma cells, because they express high levels of CD38, should be susceptible to daratumumab-mediated lysis. Daratumumab use in monotherapy decreased the frequency of normal plasma cells in bone marrow samples of MM patients both at 3 months and on reassessment upon disease progression, but a proportion of normal plasma cells survived daratumumab treatment.[25]

MM patients often have hypogammaglobulinemia before any treatment with daratumumab. Further decreases in total serum immunoglobulin levels following treatment with daratumumab have been described with data suggesting that normal IgG-secreting plasma cells are less sensitive to daratumumab compared with non-IgG-secreting plasma cells.[25]

Increases in T-cell clonality have been described following treatment with daratumumab possibly as a result of depletion of certain subsets of T cells.[24] NK cells express high levels of CD38 and are susceptible to daratumumab-mediated cell lysis. Decreases in absolute peripheral NK cell and in activated NK cell counts have been observed.[26,27] Red blood cells express low levels of CD38, and the presence of bound antibody can result in a positive indirect Coombs test that may persist for up to 6 months after last daratumumab infusion.[22]

Risk of infection in MM patients is high, and it is not always easy to separate the effect of the disease itself from the effect associated with individual treatments.[28,29] Serious infections reported in patients with MM treated with daratumumab include herpes zoster infections, CMV reactivation and CMV enterocolitis,[30,31] disseminated cryptococcosis,[32] hepatitis B virus reactivation, and PCP.[3] Viral reactivations are particularly frequent, and NK depletion may be a contributing factor. Prophylaxis for herpes zoster virus reactivation and PCP prophylaxis should be considered. Prophylaxis for hepatitis B virus reactivation should be considered according to the local guidelines. Monitoring should be continued for at least 6 months following the end of daratumumab therapy.

Vaccination status should be assessed before treatment. In a study looking at response to pneumococcal vaccination (conjugate vaccine followed 8 weeks later by unconjugated vaccine) and *Haemophilus influenzae* vaccination a median of 2 months after starting daratumumab, no significant differences were found when MM patients on daratumumab were compared with patients not on the drug.[4] In a subgroup of patients who received influenza vaccine, efficacy was low but similar to previously reported for MM patients not on daratumumab.[25]

Daratumumab can be associated with neutropenia and lymphopenia, and this may contribute to the risk of infections.

Biologic Drugs Targeting CD30

CD30 is a transmembrane glycoprotein member of the tumor necrosis factor receptor superfamily. It is characteristically expressed in certain hematologic malignancies, including Hodgkin lymphoma, anaplastic large cell lymphoma, and certain cutaneous T-cell lymphomas. Activated lymphocytes (T, B, and NK cells) and monocytes also express CD30. It regulates lymphocyte proliferation and cell death and has a critical role in the pathophysiology of Hodgkin disease and other CD30[+] lymphomas.[33]

Brentuximab vedotin is an anti-CD30 mAb covalently linked to an antimicrotubule agent monomethyl auristatin E (MMAE; ie, an antibody-drug conjugate). Brentuximab delivers MMAE directly to the CD30-expressing tumor cells. Binding of the antibody drug conjugate to CD30 initiates internalization of the complex, and MMAE is then released in lysosomes by proteolytic cleavage. MMAE binds to tubulin and disrupts the microtubule network, inducing cell-cycle arrest and ultimately apoptotic cell death.[33,34]

CD30 expression on B cells seems to be limited to activated large proliferating B cells located in lymph nodes in extrafollicular regions and at the edge of germinal centers.[35] To the author's knowledge, there are no published detailed reports describing specific effects on normal B cells, plasma cells, or serum immunoglobulin levels on patients treated with brentuximab vedotin.

Serious infections reported in patients treated with brentuximab vedotin include HBV reactivation, CMV reactivation, PCP, and PML.[3,34,36,37] Herpes virus reactivation and PCP prophylaxis should be considered as well as pretreatment vaccinations when appropriate.[3,34] Neutropenia occurs in patients treated with brentuximab vedotin and can contribute to the risk of infection.[34]

Biologic Drugs Targeting Both CD19 and CD3

Blinatumomab is a bispecific anti-CD19/anti-CD3 mAb. It leads to depletion of CD19-expressing circulating cells by T cells. It has a very short half-life compared with other mAbs and is given by continuous intravenous infusion. It is licensed for B-cell precursor acute lymphoblastic leukemia. Serious infections, including opportunistic infections, have been reported.[2,38] Neutropenia is associated with treatment with blinatumomab.[38]

Biologic Drugs Targeting CD22

Inotuzumab is an antibody-drug conjugate of an IgG4 anti-CD22 mAb covalently linked to N-acetyl-gamma-calicheamicin dimethylhydrazide, a cytotoxic product (ie, an antibody-drug conjugate). Binding of inotuzumab to CD22 on the B-cell surface is followed by internalization of the antibody-drug conjugate, intracellular release of the cytotoxic molecule, which induces DNA breaks with subsequent cell-cycle arrest and apoptotic cell death.[3,39] It is licensed for B-cell precursor acute lymphoblastic leukemia. Neutropenia has been reported in patients treated with inotuzumab.[39]

Biologic Drugs Targeting CD52

CD52 is a glycoprotein expressed at high levels in mature T and B cells and at lower levels on NK cells, monocytes, and macrophages. It is attached to the membrane by a glycosylphosphatidylinositol anchor. It is not expressed on bone marrow stem cells. Expression of CD52 has been described in 20% or more of normal plasma cells in bone marrow samples.[40]

Alemtuzumab is an IgG1 humanized mAb directed to CD52. It is currently licensed for treatment of multiple sclerosis (MS).[41] It was previously licensed for chronic lymphocytic leukemia (CLL), where it was used at much larger doses. It has been used off-label in other conditions. Alemtuzumab depletes CD52 expressing lymphocytes by ADCC and CDC. Profound depletion of T and B cells occurs while NK cells and monocytes decrease only marginally and transiently.[41–43] The profound depletion particularly of T cells is typically prolonged, leading to a prolonged decrease in cell-mediated immunity. Please refer to Mario Fernández-Ruiz and José María Aguado's article, "Direct T-Cell Inhibition and Agents Targeting T-Cell Migration and Chemotaxis", in this issue for further information regarding the effects of Alemtuzumab on T cells.

Alemtuzumab's effects on B cells are dose dependent and more profound at the doses previously used for the treatment of CLL. In MS, alemtuzumab depletes circulating B cells following each course of treatment with lowest levels detected 1 month after treatment. B-cell repopulation then follows with normal B-cell numbers usually attained within 6 months (frequently by 3 months). B-cell repopulation is similar to what is seen after hematopoietic cell transplant or rituximab with predominantly transitional and naïve B-cell populations. Recovery of memory B-cell populations is slower, so there are prolonged alterations of the B-cell pool in patients treated with alemtuzumab.

Nevertheless, it is the profound and more prolonged T-cell lymphopenia that more determines the risk of infection with the decreased cell-mediated immunity.[43] T-cell repopulation occurs more slowly than B-cell repopulation, and circulating T-cell numbers are usually still low by 12 months after treatment. Prolonged depletion, particularly of naïve T-cell clones and changes in T-cell repertoire upon repopulation, has been reported with treatment with alemtuzumab.[42]

Serious infections reported in patients treated with alemtuzumab include varicella zoster (both primary and reactivation), CMV (more frequent in the first 2 months after treatment), tuberculosis (TB) including reactivation, listeriosis including meningitis (usually within 1 month of treatment), PCP, and PML. Epstein-Barr virus–associated lymphoproliferative diseases have been reported. In CLL patients, invasive candidiasis, aspergillosis, and cryptococcal meningitis have been reported.[1,2,41]

Any vaccination needed should be administered at least 6 weeks before treatment with alemtuzumab. Herpes virus reactivation prophylaxis is recommended in all patients starting on the first day of each treatment course and continued for at least 2 months after the last dose, or when CD4 count is greater than 200 cells/mm³. Patients with no history of chickenpox or without previous vaccination against varicella zoster virus should be tested for antibodies to varicella-zoster virus. Vaccination should be considered if patients are antibody negative. PCP prophylaxis is recommended in patients with CLL receiving alemtuzumab treatment. CMV reactivation prophylaxis has also been used previously in CLL patients with recommendation to consider evaluation of CMV immune status before starting treatment with alemtuzumab.[44] All patients must be screened for active and latent TB before treatment. Patients should be advised to avoid uncooked or undercooked meats, soft cheeses, and unpasteurized dairy products at least 2 weeks before treatment and for a minimum of 1 month after because of the risk of listeriosis.

Because of the prolonged immunosuppression, patients should be monitored for at least 2 years after their last course of alemtuzumab. This monitoring includes screening for autoimmune conditions mentioned in later discussion. Annual human papillomavirus screening is recommended in female patients.

Alemtuzumab has been associated with the development of autoantibodies and autoimmune-mediated diseases and include autoimmune thyroid disease (most common, up to 36.8% of patients in clinical trials in MS), immune thrombocytopenic purpura, glomerulonephritis, and autoimmune hepatitis. It is important to take this into account when assessing a patient with possible infection. Autoimmune neutropenia has been infrequently reported in alemtuzumab trials. These autoimmune conditions can develop years after treatment.

Biologic Drugs Targeting B-Cell Activating Factor Belonging to the Tumor Necrosis Factor Family

B-cell activating factor belonging to the tumor necrosis factor family (BAFF) (also known as B-lymphocyte stimulator, BLyS) is a member of the tumor necrosis family that acts as a B-cell maturation, activation, and survival factor and also plays an important role in differentiation of B cells into immunoglobulin-producing plasma cells.

Belimumab is a human mAb against soluble BAFF. It blocks the binding of BAFF to its receptors on B cells. By decreasing the availability of soluble BAFF for signaling, it inhibits the survival of B cells and decreases differentiation of B cells into plasma cells. It is licensed for the treatment of systemic lupus erythematosus.[45]

Continuous belimumab treatment reduces peripheral B-cell counts, predominantly of naïve transitional and mature B-cell subsets.[46–48] Belimumab treatment has been associated with decrease of total serum immunoglobulin levels, more significantly of IgM and less so of IgA and IgG (for IgM decreases between 30% and 34%, for IgA between 16% and 29%, for IgG between 14% and 16% at 1 year) with some patients developing low IgM and rarely low IgG.[46,49,50] Following the initial decrease, levels for IgG and IgA tended to remain stable with some further decrease in IgM to a median of 46.6% over a total of 4 years.[51] Modest further decreases have been described on continuation of treatment over 7 years, including a decrease of 28% for IgG with 1.6% to 2.6% of the patients having levels less than 400 mg/dL.[52,53] No association between decreases in total immunoglobulin levels and risk of infections was found.

No significant effects on circulating T cells were described.[47,48]

Randomized controlled trials in systemic lupus erythematosus (SLE) have not shown an increased risk of infections in patients treated with belimumab compared with placebo.[46,49,50] Cases of serious infections in patients with SLE treated with belimumab include herpes zoster,[54] sepsis, and pneumonia caused by Acinetobacter[49,54]; disseminated CMV infection and CMV pneumonia[50,51]; coccidioidomycosis[51]; and PML.[55,56]

Live vaccines are contraindicated while on treatment with belimumab. Because of its mechanism of action, belimumab may interfere with response to vaccines. However, in an open-label trial, no significant differences were seen in the serologic response to the unconjugated pneumococcal vaccine between patients vaccinated before starting belimumab and those vaccinated after 6 months of treatment.[57] Treatment with belimumab also did not impair the capacity to respond to the conjugated pneumococcal vaccine.[58] The patient's vaccination status should be assessed before initiating treatment. In the phase 3 trials, belimumab treatment over 1 year was not associated with significant decreases in preexisting antitetanus toxoid, antipneumococcal, or anti-influenza virus antibody levels.[48,54]

SUMMARY

Several B-cell targeting biologic drugs are currently licensed for or used off-label in the treatment of different lymphoproliferative diseases of B-cell lineage cells and several autoantibody-associated autoimmune diseases. Some of these drugs are specific for B cells or plasma cells; others also target either T cells or other immune cells. The exact effects of these drugs on B cells, plasma cells, and/or serum immunoglobulin levels and their effect on response to vaccines are not always known in detail, particularly in the context of lymphoproliferative diseases. Although these biologic drugs can be relatively safe, they are associated with serious infections, including opportunistic infections. The risk of infection in the individual patient often reflects the effects of the drug being used but also of the disease itself and any previous or concomitant immunosuppressive therapies. It is important to be aware that some of these drugs may have long-lasting effects on the immune system, including changes in B-cell repertoire and secondary hypogammaglobulinemia. Patient education, pretreatment screening and vaccinations, prophylaxis measures, and/or monitoring for specific infections need to be considered when treating patients with these agents.

Multidisciplinary care, including a cancer or autoimmune disease specialist, an infectious disease specialist, and a clinical immunologist, may be of benefit in certain cases.

REFERENCES

1. Salvana EMT, Salata RA. Infectious complications associated with monoclonal antibodies and related small molecules. Clin Microbiol Rev 2009;22(2):274–90.
2. Mikulska M, Lanini S, Gudiol C, et al. ESCMID Study Group for Infections in Compromised Hosts (ESGICH) Consensus Document on the safety of targeted and biological therapies: an infectious diseases perspective (Agents targeting lymphoid cells surface antigens [1]: CD19, CD20 and CD52). Clin Microbiol Infect 2018;24:S71–82.
3. Drgona L, Gudiol C, Lanini S, et al. ESCMID Study Group for Infections in Compromised Hosts (ESGICH) Consensus Document on the safety of targeted and biological therapies: an infectious diseases perspective (Agents targeting lymphoid or myeloid cells surface antigens [II]: CD22, CD30, CD33, CD38, CD40, SLAMF-7 and CCR4. Clin Microbiol Infect 2018;24:S83–94.
4. Leandro MJ. B-cell subpopulations in humans and their differential susceptibility to depletion with anti-CD20 monoclonal antibodies. Arthritis Res Ther 2013; 15(Suppl 1):53.
5. Summary of product characteristics for rituximab, MabThera, as available in the EMC site on the 3rd of September 2019 – last updated July 2019.
6. Summary of product characteristics for ofatumumab, Arzerra, as available in the EMC site on the 3rd of September 2019 – last updated February 2015; Medicinal product no longer authorized.
7. Summary of product characteristics for obinutuzumab, Gazyvaro, as available in the EMC site on the 3rd of September 2019 – last updated April 2019.
8. Summary of product characteristics for ocrelizumab, Ocrevus, as available in the EMC site on the 3rd of September 2019 – last updated June 2019.
9. Marshall MJE, Stopforth RJ, Cragg MS. Therapeutic antibodies: what have we learnt from targeting CD20 and where are we going. Front Immunol 2017;8:1245.
10. Leandro MJ, Cooper N, Cambridge G, et al. Bone marrow B-lineage cells in patients with rheumatoid arthritis following rituximab therapy. Rheumatology (Oxford) 2007;46(1):29–36.
11. Leandro MJ, Cambridge G, Ehrenstein MR, et al. Reconstitution of peripheral blood B cells after depletion with rituximab in patients with rheumatoid arthritis. Arthritis Rheum 2006;54(2):613–20.
12. Shah S, Jaggi K, Greenberg K, et al. Immunoglobulin levels and infection risk with rituximab induction for anti-neutrophil cytoplasmic antibody-associated vasculitis. Clin Kidney J 2017;10:470–4.
13. Boleto G, Avouac J, Wipff J, et al. Predictors of hypogammaglobulinemia during rituximab maintenance therapy in rheumatoid arthritis: a 12-year longitudinal multi-center study. Semin Arthritis Rheum 2018;48:149–54.
14. Kado R, Sanders G, McCune WJ. Diagnostic and therapeutic considerations in patients with hypogammaglobulinemia after rituximab therapy. Curr Opin Rheumatol 2017;29:228–33.
15. Khojah AM, Miller ML, Klein-Gitelman MS, et al. Rituximab-associated hypogammagloblinemia in pediatric patients with autoimmune diseases. Pediatr Rheumatol 2019;17:61.

16. Cambridge G, Leandro MJ, Teodorescu M, et al. B cell depletion therapy in systemic lupus erythematosus, effect on autoantibody and antimicrobial profiles. Arthritis Rheum 2006;54:3612–22.

17. Eyckmans T, Wollants E, Janssens A, et al. Coxsackievirus A16 encephalitis during obinutuzumab therapy, Belgium, 2013. Emerg Infect Dis 2014;20(5):913–5.

18. Kusumoto S, ARcaini L, Hong X, et al. Risk of HBV reactivation in patients with B-cell lymphomas receiving obinutuzumab or rituximab chemotherapy. Blood 2019;133(2):137–46.

19. Arad U, Tzadok S, Amir S, et al. The cellular immune response to influenza vaccination is preserved in rheumatoid arthritis patients treated with rituximab. Vaccine 2011;29:1643–8.

20. Deaglio S, Vaisitti T, Billington R, et al. CD38/CD19: a lipid raft-dependent signalling complex in human B cells. Blood 2007;109(12):5390–8.

21. De Weers M, Tai Y-T, van der Veer MS, et al. Daratumumab, a novel therapeutic human CD38 monoclonal antibody, induces killing of multiple myeloma and other hematological tumors. J Immunol 2011;186:1840–8.

22. Spc for daratumumab, Darzalex, as available in the EMC site on the 3rd of September – last updated 03 July 2019.

23. Sims GP, Ettinger R, Shirota Y, et al. Identification and characterization of circulating human transitional B cells. Blood 2005;105(11):4390–8.

24. Krejcik J, Casneuf T, Nijhof IS, et al. Daratumumab depletes CD38+ immune regulatory cells, promotes T-cell expansion, and skews T-cell repertoire in multiple myeloma. Blood 2016;128(3):384–94.

25. Frerichs KA, Bosman PWC, van Velzen JF, et al. Effect of daratumumab on normal plasma cells, polyclonal immunoglobulin levels, and vaccination responses in extensively pre-treated multiple myeloma patients. Haematologica 2019. [Epub ahead of print].

26. Casneuf T, Xu XS, Adams HC III, et al. Effects of daratumumab on natural killer cells and impact on clinical outcomes in relapsed or refractory multiple myeloma. Blood Adv 2017;1(23):2105–14.

27. Nahi H, Chrobok M, Gran C, et al. Infectious complications and NK cell depletion following daratumumab treatment of multiple myeloma. PLoS One 2019;14(2): e0211927.

28. Moreau P, Attal M, Hulin C, et al. Bortezomib, thalidomide and dexamethasone with or without daratumumab before and after autologous stem-cell transplantation for newly diagnosed multiple myeloma (CASSIOPEIA): a randomised, open-label, phase 3 study. Lancet 2019;394(10192):29–38.

29. Blimark C, Holmberg E, Mellqvist UH, et al. Multiple myeloma and infections: a population-based study in 9235 multiple myeloma patients. Haematologica 2015;100(1):107–13.

30. Frerichs KA, Bosman PWC, Nijhof IS, et al. Cytomegalovirus reactivation in a patient with extensively pretreated multiple myeloma during daratumumab treatment. Clin Lymphoma Myeloma Leuk 2019;19(1):e9–11.

31. Lavi N, Okasha D, Sabo E, et al. Severe cytomegalovirus enterocolitis following daratumumab exposure in three patients with multiple myeloma. Eur J Haematol 2018. [Epub ahead of print].

32. Sato S, Kambe E, Tamai Y. Disseminated cryptococcosis in a patient with multiple myeloma treated with daratumumab, lenalidomide, and dexamethasone. Intern Med 2019;58:843–7.

33. Van der Weyden CA, Pileri SA, Feldman AL, et al. Understanding CD30 biology and therapeutic targeting: a historical perspective providing insight into future directions. Blood Cancer J 2017;7:e603.

34. Spc for brentuximab vedotin, Adcetris, as available in the EMC site on the 10th October – last updated February 2019.

35. Cattoretti G, Buttner M, Shaknovich R, et al. Nuclear and cytoplasmic AID in extrafollicular and germinal center B cells. Blood 2006;107:3967–75.

36. Carson KR, Newsome SD, Kin EJ, et al. Progressive multifocal leukoencephalopathy associated with brentuximab vedotin therapy. Cancer 2014;120:2464–71.

37. Jalan P, Mahajan A, Pandav V, et al. Brentuximab associated progressive multifocal leukoencephalopathy. Clin Neurol Neurosurg 2012;114:1335–7.

38. Spc for blinatumomab, Blincyto, as available in the EMC site on the 10th October – last updated October 2019.

39. Spc for inotuzumab ozogamicin, Besponsa, as available in the EMC site on the 10th of October 2019 – last updated August 2019.

40. Kumar S, Kimlinger TK, Lust Ja, et al. Expression of CD52 on plasma cells in plasma cell proliferative disorders. Blood 2003;102(3):1075–7.

41. Spc for alemtuzumab, Lemtrada, as available in the EMC site on the 1st October 2019 – last updated April 2019.

42. Osterborg A, Werner A, Halapi E, et al. Clonal CD8+ and CD52– T cells are induced in responding B cell lymphoma patients treated with Campath-1H (anti-CD52). Eur J Haematol 1997;58:5–13.

43. Thompson SA, Jones JL, Cox AL, et al. B-cell reconstitution and BAFF after alemtuzumab (Campath-1H) treatment of multiple sclerosis. J Clin Immunol 2010; 30(1):99–105.

44. O'Brien S, Ravandi F, Riehl T, et al. Valganciclovir prevents cytomegalovirus reactivation in patients receiving alemtuzumab-based therapy. Blood 2008;111(4): 1816–9.

45. Spc for belimumab, Benlysta, as available in the EMC site on the 3rd September 2019 – last updated July 2019.

46. Wallace DJ, Stohl W, Furie RA, et al. A phase II, randomized, double-blind, placebo-controlled, dose-ranging study of belimumab in patients with active systemic lupus erythematosus. Arthritis Rheum 2009;61(9):1168–78.

47. Jacobi AM, Huang W, Wand T, et al. Effect of long-term belimumab treatment on B cells in systemic lupus erythematosus. Extension of a phase II, double-blind, placebo-controlled, dose-ranging study. Arthritis Rheum 2010;62(1):201–10.

48. Stohl W, Hiepe F, Latinis KM, et al. Belimumab reduces autoantibodies, normalizes low complement levels, and reduces select B cell populations in patients with systemic lupus erythematosus. Arthritis Rheum 2012;64(7):2328–37.

49. Navarra SV, Guzman RM, Gallacher AE, et al. Efficacy and safety of belimumab in patients with active systemic lupus erythematosus : a randomised placebo-controlled, phase 3 trial. Lancet 2011;377:721–31.

50. Furie R, Petri M, Zamani O, et al. A phase III, randomized, placebo-controlled study of belimumab, a monoclonal antibody that inhibits B lymphocyte stimulator, in patients with systemic lupus erythematosus. Arthritis Rheum 2011;63(12): 3918–30.

51. Merrill JT, Ginzler EM, Wallace DJ, et al. Long-term safety profile of belimumab plus standard therapy in patients with systemic lupus erythematosus. Arthritis Rheum 2012;64(10):3364–73.

52. Ginzler EM, Wallace DJ, Merrill JT, et al. Disease control and safety of belimumab plus standard therapy over 7 years in patients with systemic lupus erythematosus. J Rheumatol 2014;41:300–9.
53. Furie RA, Wallace DJ, Aranow C, et al. Long-term safety and efficacy of belimumab in patients with systemic lupus erythematosus. Arthritis Rheumatol 2018; 70(6):868–77.
54. Chatham WW, Wallace DJ, Stohl W, et al. Effect of belimumab on vaccine antigen antibodies to influenza, pneumococcal, and tetanus vaccines in patients with systemic lupus erythematosus in the BLISS-76 trial. J Rheumatol 2012;39:163–1640.
55. Fredericks CA, Kvam KA, Bear J, et al. A case of progressive multifocal leukoencephalopathy in a lupus patient treated with belimumab. Lupus 2014;23:711–3.
56. Leblanc-Trudeau C, Masetto A, Bocti C. Progressive multifocal leukoencephalopathy associated with belimumab in a patient with systemic lupus erythematosus. J Rheumatol 2015;42:551–2.
57. Chatham W, Chadha A, Fettiplace J, et al. A randomized, open-label study to investigate the effect of belimumab on pneumococcal vaccination in patients with active, autoantibody-positive systemic lupus erythematosus. Lupus 2017; 26:1483–90.
58. Nagel J, Saxne T, GEborek P, et al. Treatment with belimumab in systemic lupus erythematosus does not impair antibody response to 13-valent pneumococcal conjugate vaccine. Lupus 2017;26:1072–81.

Risk of Serious Infection Associated with Agents that Target T-Cell Activation and Interleukin-17 and Interleukin-23 Cytokines

Stanford Shoor, MD

KEYWORDS

- Serious infection • Co-stimulatory molecule inhibitors • IL-17 and IL-23 inhibitors

KEY POINTS

- Abatacept and belatacept are monoclonal antibodies blocking co-stimulatory molecules of T-cell activation and are used in the treatment of rheumatoid arthritis and to prevent renal transplant rejection.
- Secukinumab, ixekizumab, and brodalumab are inhibitors of the cytokine interleukin (IL)-17 and are used in the treatment of psoriasis, psoriatic arthritis and ankylosing spondylitis. Secukinumab and ixekizumab are also approved for psoriatic arthritis and ankylosing spondylitis.
- Ustekinumab, tildrakizumab, guselkumab, and risankizumab inhibit IL-23 and are approved for use in psoriasis.
- Serious infections occur in a mean of 4.2% of patients on abatacept; 25% on belatacept, 1.2% on secukinumab, ixekizumab or brodalumab, 1.7% on ustikinumab and <1% to 1 % on IL-23 inhibitors.
- Host factors, such as underlying disease, steroid dose, and comorbidities must be considered in determining risk in individual patients.
- There are only sporadic case reports of opportunistic infection or tuberculosis reactivation on these drugs.

INTRODUCTION

Tumor necrosis factor (TNF) inhibitors, the first biological immunomodulators, bind TNF glycoprotein, the receptor of which is present in numerous immune and tissue-specific cells (**Table 1**). When stimulated by the TNF ligand, this causes generalized production of additional cytokines, recruitment of immune cells, and tissue

Stanford University, 1000 Welch Road Suite 203, Palo Alto, CA 94304, USA
E-mail address: sshoor@stanford.edu

Infect Dis Clin N Am 34 (2020) 179–189
https://doi.org/10.1016/j.idc.2020.02.001
0891-5520/20/© 2020 Elsevier Inc. All rights reserved.

Table 1
Co-Stimulatory & IL-17 & 23 inhibitors

Drug	Structure	Mechanism	Indications	Risk of Vs.				
				SI (%)	PBO	OI	TB	Notes
Abatacept (Orencia)	CTLA Fusion protein	$CD_{28,80/86}$ Co-stim-inhibitor	RA	4.2%[b,d]	Equal	N = 6[a]	0.14%	HSV/VZV 5.5%
Belatacept (Nulojix)	CTLA Fusion protein	$CD_{28,80/86}$ Co-stim-inhibitor	Renal transplant	25%[e]	NR	1–10%[c]	0.8%	EBV PTLD
Secukinumab (Cosentyx)	IL-17 Mab	1L-17i	Psoriasis Psor Arth AnkSpondy	1.2%	Equal	—	NR	0.8% to 6% localized candida
Ixekizumab (Taltz)	IL-17 Mab	1L-17i	Psoriasis, Psor Arth, AnkSpondy	1.3%		NR	NR	2.5% localized candida
Brodalumab (Siliq)	IL-17 Mab	IL-17 receptor	Psoriasis	1.2%	Equal	NR	NR	4% localized candida
Ustikinumab (Stelara)	1L-12/23Mab	IL-12/23i	Psoriasis Psor Arth	1.7%	Equal	NR	NR	—
Guselkinmab (Tremfya)	IL-23 Mab	IL-23i	Psoriasis	<1–1%	Equal	NR	NR	—
Tildrakizumab (Ilumya)	IL-23 Mab	IL-23i	Psoriasis	<1–1%	Equal	NR	NR	—
Risankizumab (Skyrizi)	IL-23 Mab	IL-23i	Psoriasis	<1–1%	Equal	NR	NR	—

Abbreviations: i, inhibitor; IL, interleukin; Mab, monoclonal antibody; NR, not reported; OI, opportunistic infection; PBO, placebo or comparator; PNA, pneumonia; PTLD, posttransplant lymphoproliferative disorder; Sof tis, soft tissue or articular; TB, tuberculosis; UTI, urinary tract infection or pyelonephritis; RA, rheumatoid arthritis; Psor Arth, psoriatic arthritis; AnkSpondy, ankylosing spondylitis. Overall rate of infection < TNF-I in 2 studies.

a Reported in only 3 studies: (2) aspergillus, (1) each systemic candidiasis, blastomycocis, histoplasmosis, atypical mycobacteria.

b Pneumonia, UTI, pyelonephritis, soft tissue or articular.

c Fungal.

d < TNFi.

e Equal versus cyclosporine.

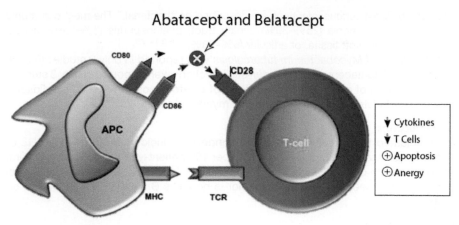

Fig. 1. Abatacept binds CD80 and CD86 and blocks costimulation. MHC, major histocompatibility complex; TCR, T-cell receptor.

inflammation. Inhibitors of T-cell activation and interleukin (IL)-17 and IL-23 inhibitors were developed to more selectively inhibit autoimmunity and reduce infection risk.[1]

In assessing risk of infection in an individual patient, one must consider host factors that may enhance it. Most but not all studies controlled for these covariates. These factors include the following:

- *The underlying disease* for which the patient is being treated. Patients with psoriatic and rheumatoid arthritis are at greater risk of infection simply as a result of their disease.[2,3]
- *Comorbidity.* The 12-month incidence of hospitalized infection in one study was as low as 3.7 to as high as 50.7 depending on the decile of an infection risk score.[4,5]
- *Treatment with corticosteroids.* Patients treated with biologics are often on corticosteroids, most commonly prednisone. Corticosteroids suppress immune activity and downstream inflammation via several mechanisms, and are known to result in increased risk of infection. Patients with rheumatoid arthritis on 7.5 to 10 mg of prednisone have a rate of serious bacterial infection as high as 13% and a relative risk of 1.93 for Herpes Zoster (HZ).[6–12]

INHIBITORS OF THE INTERACTION BETWEEN ANTIGEN PRESENTING OR DENDRITIC CELLS AND CD4 T LYMPHOCYTES

Abatacept and belatacept are monoclonal antibodies blocking co-stimulatory molecules of T-cell activation and are used in the treatment of rheumatoid arthritis and prevention of organ rejection in kidney transplants. These drugs are fusion proteins designed to interfere with the binding of $CD_{80/86}$ molecules on APCs/DC (antigen *presenting cells/dendritic cells*) with their CD_{28} receptors on the surface of CD_4 T cells, thus reducing T-cell activation[13] (**Fig. 1**).

Abatacept (Orencia)

The rate of serious infections with abatacept ranges from 0.25% to 13% (mean = 4.2%). When compared with placebo or other biologics (TNF inhibitors, rituximab, infliximab, tocilizumab) the relative risk averages 1.3 but is never statistically significant and in fact is reported to be 15% lower than TNF inhibitors and 1.5 times lower than tocilizumab. Most serious infections are described as "bacterial." The most commonly reported are pneumonia (25%–30%) urinary tract, pyelonephritis (3%–25%), sepsis (10%–15%), skin, soft tissue, or articular (6%–28%).[4–6,9,14–25]

Reactivation of *Mycobacterium tuberculosis* was reported in only 2 studies (0.06% and 0.23%) of abatacept.[16,26] Opportunistic infections were reported in only 3 studies. Two were cases of aspergillosis and 1 each of blastomycosis, systemic candidiasis, disseminated histoplasmosis, and atypical mycobacterium.[16,27,28]

Viral infections

When adjusted for multiple potential confounders, the incidence rate of either HZ or herpes simplex virus (HSV) infection is 5.49 per 100 patient-years for abatacept users, not significantly different from the other biologics.[12] Epstein-Barr virus (EBV) viral loads have not been found to increase nor is hepatitis B virus (HBV) reactivated on abatacept.[29,30]

Belatacept (Nulojix)

Belatacept is identical to abatacept except it has 2 specific amino acid substitutions that allow it to bind with greater avidity to CD 80 and 86, thus increasing its potency. It was designed specifically to prevent rejection of renal transplants.[31]

Serious infections occur in 10% to 38% (mean 25%) of patients on belatacept. In clinical trials comparing calcineurin inhibitors with belatacept, one study showed the incidence of serious infections was 10.6 per 100 patient-years in the belatacept in comparison with 13.3 in the calcineurin group. Two others found the opposite, one 10.9% belatacept versus 9.3% calcineurin, the other 38.2% of belatacept patients experiencing serious infection versus 23% of those on calcineurin inhibitors, a significant difference in univariate analysis that disappeared in multivariate analysis.[32–36]

In 3 studies that specified infections, urinary tract infections or pyelonephritis accounted for 31% to 50% of bacterial infections, the remainder being sepsis and pneumonia. Viral infections were described in 14% to 71% of belatacept patients, the most common being cytomegalovirus and BK virus.[34]

However, EBV-related posttransplant lymphoproliferative disorder has been found to be higher in patients on belatacept (1.5%) versus cyclosporine (0%), leading to the recommendation that the drug is contraindicated in patients who are EBV-negative.[37]

Opportunistic infections occurred in 1% to 10% of belatacept patients. Three studies reported serious fungal infections, 6 of 578 in a renal transplant study; 1 of 40 with cardiac transplant patients and 2 of 11 in a lung transplant study. In the renal transplant study (Durbach) the authors reported no significant difference between belatacept and cyclosporine patients. *Pneumocystis jirovecii* (PJP) has not been described in patients on PJP prophylaxis.[34–36,38,39]

Tuberculosis was noted in 4 (0.8%) of 578 patients on belatacept, 3 of which were from one site in an endemic area.[34]

INTERLEUKIN-17 AND INTERLEUKIN-23 INHIBITORS

In addition to TNF, 2 other cytokines have been found to be crucial in the development of psoriasis: IL-17 and IL-23. IL-17 is produced by activation of T_H17 lymphocytes, whereas IL-23 is secreted primarily by dermal DDs or APCs. Both of these cytokines have receptors on skin cells that upregulate the expression of psoriasis-related genes. This upregulation leads to excessive skin cell turnover: the hallmark of the disease. IL-17 and IL-23 inhibitors were developed to more specifically target these pathways, in the hope of reducing infectious complications and perhaps improving response.[40]

Interleukin-17 Inhibitors: Secukinumab (Cosentyx), Brodalumab (Siliq), and Ixekizumab (Taltz)

Secukinumab (Cosentyx)

Secukinumab is a monoclonal antibody designed to bind to the cytokine IL-17A and thus inhibit its activity in the pathogenesis of psoriasis, psoriatic arthritis, and ankylosing spondylitis: all indications for use of the drug.[41,42] Serious infections are seen in 1.0% to 1.4% of patients in clinical trials of secukinumab. Discontinuation due to serious adverse events in psoriatic arthritis was equivalent between secukinumab (1.3%) and placebo (2.1%)[43–47]

Because patients with hereditary deficiency in IL-17 have an increased risk for candida infections, IL-17 inhibiting antibodies carry with them the theoretic risk of candidiasis. However, Candida infections were reported in only 0.8% to 6.0% of secukinumab patients, all were superficial, mucocutaneous, and equivalent in placebo and secukinumab arms.[48]

No cases of active tuberculosis (TB) have been reported in a review of clinical trial data.[43,45,46]

A multicenter prospective study of patients with psoriasis with concurrent HBV or hepatitis C virus (HCV) infection treated with secukinumab found that 24% of patients with HBV who did *not* receive antiviral prophylaxis had disease reactivation but none of those receiving prophylaxis did. One of 14 (7%) of patients with HCV showed enhanced viral replication[49]

Brodalumab (Siliq)

Brodalumab differs from the other IL-17 inhibitors in that it is a monoclonal antibody directed against the receptor of IL-17A rather than directly against IL-17A. It is approved for the use of psoriasis.

Serious infections have been reported in 1.0 to 1.3 per 100 patient-years at 52 weeks but do not appear greater than comparators or placebo. Mucocutaneous candida infections are more common in brodalumab (3.5%–4%) versus placebo, ustekinumab, or etanercept, but none were systemic.[50–55] Although IL-17 cells play a role in host defense against *M tuberculosis*, *Listeria monocytogenes*, *Salmonella typhimurium*, *Staphylococcus aureus*, *Klebsiella pneumoniae*, and PJP, opportunistic infections were *not* reported in clinical trials of the IL-17 inhibitors.[50–55]

Ixekizumab (Taltz)

Ixekizumab is a IL-17A inhibitor that is approved for moderate-to-severe plaque psoriasis, psoriatic arthritis and ankylosing spondylitis. Serious infection occurs in 1% to 1.3% of patients on the drug versus 0% on placebo at 96 weeks. The incidence peaked at 24 to 36 weeks and remained stable over time. Superficial candida occurred in 2.6% versus 0.4% on placebo. Two cases of candida esophagitis were reported.[56–59]

Interleukin-23 Inhibitors: Ustekinumab (Stelara), Tildrakizumab (Ilumya), Guselkumab (Tremfya), and Risankizumab (Skyrizi)

These drugs inhibit IL-23, a cytokine that is upstream from T_H17 lymphocyte activation, and suppress lymphocyte production of IL-17, IL-12, and IL-22. They are all approved for the treatment of moderate to severe plaque like psoriasis; ustekinumab is also approved for psoriatic arthritis.

Ustekinumab (Stelara)

This was the first of the IL-23 inhibitors approved for the treatment of psoriasis and psoriatic arthritis. It is a monoclonal antibody that recognizes both the P40 and P19 protein subunits of IL-23. Because the P40 subunit is also present on IL-12, the drug suppresses both IL-23 and IL-12.

Serious infections have been recorded in 0.4% to 1.7% of patients, but did not appear to increase over time or be dose related. This was equivalent to placebo and less than in etanercept, adalimumab, and infliximab.[60–67]

Tildrakizumab (Ilumya)

Serious infections range from less than 1% to 1% with tildrakizumab. Although there have been isolated case reports of bacterial arthritis and epiglottis, selective IL-23 inhibitors are associated with a lower risk of Salmonella, Candida, and Mycobacterial infections in animals when compared with ustekinumab.[68–70]

Guselkumab (Tremfya)

Review of salient clinical trials of guselkumab for moderate-to-severe plaque psoriasis in which the drug was compared with placebo, ustekinumab, or adalimumab did *not* demonstrate an increased risk of serious infection. Three clinical trials with a total of 1123 subjects reported a total of 10 (0.8%) cases of serious infections (unspecified = 3, soft tissue = 4, bacterial arthritis = 1, bronchitis = 1).[71–78] Although there have been no reports of reactivation of TB, it is important to remember that patients with a history of active TB were excluded from participation in clinical trials of guselkumab. Unlike IL-17 inhibitors, IL-23 inhibitors have not been shown to increase the probability of mucocutaneous candida infections.[71–78]

Risankizumab (Skyrizi)

Risankizumab (RZB) is a selective anti–IL-23 antibody recently approved in the United States (4/19) for the treatment of psoriasis and is under investigation for psoriatic arthritis and inflammatory bowel disease.

The rate of serious infections has been reported as 1.0 to 1.6 per 100 patient-years in the RZB subjects versus 1.1 in placebo, 2.1 in adalimumab, and 5.3 in ustekinumab. No paired statistics were reported, and the rates remained stable over time. The most common serious infections were cellulitis (0.2/100 patient-years), pneumonia (0.2/100 patient-years), and sepsis (0.3/100 patient-years). There were no cases of active TB in any group. Mucocutaneous candidiasis was noted in 3.4%.

No systemic opportunistic infections were described.[79–81]

DISCLOSURE

The author received funding from Stanford University and Hospitals and Pfizer for a study in Patient Centered Care in Rheumatoid Arthritis.

REFERENCES

1. Olesen CM, Coskun M, Peyrin-Biroulet L, et al. Mechanisms behind efficacy of tumor necrosis factors inhibitors in inflammatory bowel disease. Pharmacol Ther 2016;159:110–9.

2. Doran MF, Crowson CS, Pond GR, et al. Frequency of infection in patients with rheumatoid arthritis compared with controls: a population-based study. Arthritis Rheum 2002;46:2287–93.

3. Mikuls TR, Saag KG, Criswell LA, et al. Mortality risk associated with rheumatoid arthritis in a prospective cohort of older women: results from the Iowa Women's Health Study. Ann Rheum Dis 2002;61(11):994–9.

4. Yun H, Xie F, Delzell E, et al. Comparative risk of hospitalized infection associated with biologic agents in rheumatoid arthritis patients enrolled in medicare. Arthritis Rheumatol 2016;68(1):56–66.

5. Mori S, Yoshitama T, Hidaka T, et al. Comparative risk of hospitalized infection between biological agents in rheumatoid arthritis patients: a multicenter retrospective cohort study in Japan. PLoS One 2018;12(6):e0179179.

6. George MD, Baker JF, Winthrop K, et al. Risk of biologics and glucocorticoids in patients with rheumatoid arthritis undergoing arthroplasty. a cohort Study. Ann Intern Med 2019;170:825–36.

7. Wolfe F, Caplan L, Michaud K. Treatment for rheumatoid arthritis and the risk of hospitalization for pneumonia: associations with prednisone, disease-modifying antirheumatic drugs, and anti-tumor necrosis factor therapy. Arthritis Rheum 2006;54:628–34.

8. Greenberg JD, Reed G, Kremer JM, et al. Association of methotrexate and tumor necrosis factor antagonists with risk of infectious outcomes including opportunistic infections in the CORRONA registry. Ann Rheum Dis 2010;69:380–6.

9. Curtis JR, Yang S, Patkar NM, et al. Risk of hospitalized bacterial infections associated with biologic treatment among US Veterans with rheumatoid arthritis. Arthritis Care Res 2014;66(7):990–7.

10. Lacaille D, Guh DP, Abrahamitic M, et al. Use of nonbiologic disease-modifying antirheumatic drugs and risk of infection in patients with rheumatoid arthritis. Arthritis Rheum 2008;59(8):1074–81.

11. Stuck AE, Minder CE, Frey FJ. Risk of infectious complications in patients taking glucocorticosteroids. Rev Infect Dis 1989;11:954–63.

12. Curtis JR, Xie F, Yun H, et al. Real-word comparative risk of herpes virus infections in tofacitinib and biologic treated patients with rheumatoid arthritis. Ann Rheum Dis 2016;75:1843–7.

13. Kremer J, Westhovens R, Leon M, et al. Treatment of rheumatoid arthritis by selective inhibition of T-cell activation with fusion protein CTLA4Ig. N Engl J Med 2003;349(20):1907–15.

14. Mariette X, Gottenberg JE, Ravaud P, et al. Registries in rheumatoid arthritis and autoimmune diseases: data from the French registries. Rheumatology 2011;50: 222–9.

15. Tank ND, Karelia BN, Bhavisha N, et al. Biological response modifiers in rheumatoid arthritis: systematic review and meta-analysis of Safety. J Pharmacol Pharmacother 2017;8(3):92–105.

16. Simon TA, Askling J, Lacaille D, et al. Infections requiring hospitalization in the abatacept clinical development program: an epidemiological assessment. Arthritis Res Ther 2010;12:1–11.

17. Salliot C, Dougados M, Gossec L. Risk of serious infections during rituximab, abatacept and anakinra treatments for rheumatoid arthritis: meta-analysis of randomised placebo-controlled trials. Ann Rheum Dis 2009;68:25–32.

18. Pawar A, Rishi I, Desai J, et al. Risk of serious infections in tocilizumab versus other biologic drugs in patients with rheumatoid arthritis: a multi-database cohort study. Ann Rheum Dis 2019;78:456–64.

19. Schiff M, Pritchard C, Huffstutter JE, et al. The 6-month safety and efficacy of abatacept in patients with rheumatoid arthritis who underwent a washout after anti-tumour necrosis factor therapy or were directly switched to abatacept: the ARRIVE trial. Ann Rheum Dis 2009;68:1708–14.

20. Lederballe Grøn K, Arkema EV, Glintborg B, et al. Risk of serious infections in patients with rheumatoid arthritis treated in routine care with abatacept, rituximab and tocilizumab in Denmark and Sweden. Ann Rheum Dis 2019;78:320–7.

21. Singh JA, Cameron C, Noorbaloochi S, et al. Risk of serious infection in biological treatment of patients with rheumatoid arthritis: a systematic review and meta-analysis. Lancet 2015;386(9990):258–65.

22. Vieira MC, Zwillich SH, Jansen JP, et al. Tofacitinib versus biologic treatment in patient with active rheumatoid arthritis who have had an inadequate response to tumor necrosis factor inhibitors: results from a network meta-analysis. Clin Ther 2016;38(12):2628–41.

23. Singh JA, Wells GA, Christensen R, et al. Adverse effects of biologics: a network meta-analysis and Cochrane overview. Cochrane Database Syst Rev 2011;(2):CD008794.

24. Singh JA, Wells GA, Christensen R, et al. Adverse effects of biologics: a network meta-analysis and Cochrane overview. Cochrane Database of Systematic Reviews 2011, Issue 2. The Cochrane Collaboration. London: John Wiley & Sons Ltd; 2011. p.1-57.

25. Montastruc F, Renoux C, Hudson M, et al. Abatacept initiation in rheumatoid arthritis and the risk of serious infection: a population-based study. Semin Arthritis Rheum 2019;48(6):1053–8.

26. Souto A, Maneiro JR, Salgado E, et al. Risk of tuberculosis in patients with chronic immune-mediated inflammatory diseases treated with biologics and tofacitinib: a systematic review and meta-analysis of randomized controlled trials and long-term extension studies. Rheumatology 2014;53:1872–85.

27. Jain N, Doyon JB, Lazarus JE, et al. A case of disseminated histoplasmosis in a patient with rheumatoid arthritis on abatacept. J Gen Intern Med 2018;33(5): 769–72.

28. Schiff M. Abatacept treatment for rheumatoid arthritis. Rheumatology 2011;50(3): 437–49.

29. Nathalie- Balandraud N, Texier G, Massy E, et al. Long-term treatment with abatacept or tocilizumab does not increase Epstein-Barr virus load in patients with rheumatoid arthritis - A three years retrospective study. PLoS One 2017; 12(2):1–13.

30. Padovan M, Filippini M, Tincani A, et al. Safety of abatacept in rheumatoid arthritis with serologic evidence of past or present hepatitis B virus infection. Arthritis Care Res 2016;68(6):738–43.

31. Larsen CP, Pearson TC, Adams AB, et al. Rational development of LEA29Y (belatacept), a high-affinity variant of CTLA4-Ig with potent immunosuppressive properties. Am J Transplant 2005;5:443–53.

32. Ippoliti G, D'Armini AM, Lucioni M, et al. Introduction to the use of belatacept: a fusion protein for the prevention of posttransplant rejection. Biologics 2012;6: 355–62.

33. Vincenti F, Rostaing L, Grinyo J, et al. Belatacept and long-term outcomes in kidney transplantation. N Engl J Med 2016;374(26):2600–1.

34. Durrbach A, Pestanab JM, Pearsonc T, et al. A phase III study of belatacept versus cyclosporine in kidney transplant from extended criteria donors (BENEFIT-EXT Study). Am J Transplant 2010;10:547–57.

35. Neuwirt H, Leitner-Lechner I, Kerschbaum J, et al. Efficacy and safety of belatacept treatment in renal allograft recipients at high cardiovascular risk – a single center experience. J Clin Med 2019;8(1164):1–12.

36. Grinyó JM, Rial M, Alberu J, et al. Safety and efficacy outcomes 3 years after switching to belatacept from a calcineurin inhibitor in kidney transplant recipients: results from a phase 2 randomized trial. Am J Kidney Dis 2017;69(5):587–94.
37. Larsen CP, Grinyó J, Medina-Pestana J, et al. Belatacept-based regimens versus a cyclosporine A-based regimen in kidney transplant recipients: 2-year results from the BENEFIT and BENEFIT-EXT studies. Transplantation 2010;90(12): 1528–35.
38. Launay, M, Guitard, J, Dorent, et al. Belateacept-based immunosuppression: a calcineurin inhibitor-spraing, regimen in heart transplant patients. To be presented at the ASTS Winter Symposium. American Society of Transplant Surgeons. Miami, Florida, January 9-12, 2020.
39. Iasella CJ, Winstead RJ, Moore CA, et al. Maintenance belatacept-based immunosuppression in lung transplantation recipients who failed calcineurin inhibitors. Transplantation 2018;102(1):171–7.
40. Mease PJ. Inhibition of interleukin-17, interleukin-23 and the TH17 cell pathway in the treatment of psoriatic arthritis and psoriasis. Curr Opin Rheumatol 2015;27(2): 127–33.
41. Hueber W, Patel DD, Dryja T, et al. Effects of AIN457, a fully human antibody to interleukin-17A, on psoriasis, rheumatoid arthritis, and Uveitis. Sci Transl Med 2010;2(52):52–72.
42. Jin W, Dong C. IL-17 cytokines in immunity and inflammation. Emerg Microbes Infect 2013;2(1):1–5.
43. Deodhar A, Mease PJ, McInnes IB, et al. Long-term safety of secukinumab in patients with moderate-to-severe plaque psoriasis, psoriatic arthritis, and ankylosing spondylitis: integrated pooled clinical trial and post-marketing surveillance data. Arthritis Res Ther 2019;21:1–11.
44. Zhang L, Yang H, Chen O, et al. Adverse drug events observed with 150mg versus 300mg secukinumab for the treatment of moderate to severe plaque psoriasis A systematic review and meta-analysis. Medicine 2019;98(2):1–8.
45. Reich K, Armstrong AW, Langley RG, et al. Andrew Blauvelt Guselkumab versus secukinumab for the treatment of moderate-to-severe psoriasis (ECLIPSE): results from a phase 3, randomised controlled trial. Lancet 2019;394:831–9.
46. Mease P, van der Heijide D, Landewe R, et al. Secukinumab improves active psoriatic arthritis symptoms and inhibits radiographic progression: primary results from the randomised, double-blind, phase III FUTURE 5 study. Ann Rheum Dis 2018;77:890–7.
47. Mrowietz U, Bachelez H, Burden DA, et al. Secukinumab for moderate-to-sever palmoplantar pustular psoriasis: Result of the 2 PRECISE study. J Am Acod Dermatol 2019;80(5):1344–52.
48. Puel A, Cypowyj S, Bustamante J, et al. Chronic mucocutaneous candidiasis in humans with inborn errors of interleukin-17 immunity. Science 2011; 332(6025):65–8.
49. Chiu HY, Hui RC, Huang YH, et al. Safety profile of secukinumab in treatment of patients with psoriasis and concurrent hepatitis B or C: a multicentric prospective cohort study. Acta Derm Venereol 2018;98:829–34.
50. Galluzzo M, D'adamio S, Bianchi L, et al. Brodalumb for the treatment of psoriasis. Expert Rev Clin Immunol 2016;12(12):1255–71.
51. Puig L. Brodalumab: the first anti-IL-17 receptor agent for psoriasis. Drugs Today (Barc) 2017;53(5):283–95.
52. Papp KA, Leonardi C, Menter A, et al. Brodalumab, an antiinterleukin-17-receptor antibody for psoriasis. N Engl J Med 2012;366(13):1181–9.

53. Papp KA, Reich K, Paul C, et al. A prospective phase III, randomized, double-blind, placebo-controlled study of brodalumab in patients with moderate-to-severe plaque psoriasis. Br J Dermatol 2016;175(2):273–86.

54. Lebwohl M, Strober B, Menter A, et al. Phase 3 studies comparing brodalumab with ustekinumab in psoriasis. N Engl J Med 2015;373(14):1318–28.

55. Attia A, Abousouk AI, Hussien A. Safety and efficacy of brodalumb for moderate -to- severe plaque psoriasis. Clin Drug Investig 2017;37:439–51.

56. Zachariae C, Gordon K, Kimball B. Efficacy and safety of ixekizumab over 4 years of open-label treatment in a phase 2 study in chronic plaque psoriasis. J Am Acad Dermatol 2018;79(2):294–301.

57. van der Heijde D, Cheng-Chung Wei J, Dougados M, et al. Ixekizumab, an interleukin-17A antagonist in the treatment of ankylosing spondylitis or radiographic axial spondyloarthritis in patients previously untreated with biological disease-modifying anti-rheumatic drugs (COAST-V): 16 week results of a phase 3 randomised, double-blind, active-controlled and placebo-controlled trial. Lancet 2018;392(10163):2441–51.

58. Mease P, Roussou E, Burmester GR. Safety of ixekizumab in patients with psoriatic arthritis: results from a pooled analysis of three clinical trials. Arthritis Care Res 2019;71(3):367–78.

59. Okubo Y, Mabuchi 1 T, Iwatsuki K. Long-term efficacy and safety of ixekizumab in Japanesepatients with erythrodermic or generalized pustular psoriasis: subgroup analyses of an open-label, phase 3 study (UNCOVER-J). J Eur Acad Dermatol Venereol 2019;33:325–32.

60. Gómez-García F, Epstein D, Isla-Tejera B, et al. Short-term efficacy and safety of new biologic agents targeting IL -23/Th17 pathway for moderate to severe plaque psoriasis: a systematic review and network meta -analysis. Br J Dermatol 2017; 176(3):594–603.

61. Lebwohl M, Leonardi C, Griffiths CE, et al. Long-term safety experience of ustekinumab in patients with moderate-to-severe psoriasis (Part I or II): results from analyses of general safety parameters from pooled phase 2 and 3 clinical trials. J Am Acad Dermatol 2012;66(5):731–41.

62. Gordon KB, Papp KA, Langley RG, et al. Long-term safety experience of ustekinumab in patients with moderate to severe psoriasis (Part II of II): results from analyses of infections and malignancy from pooled phase II and III clinical trials. J Am Acad Dermatol 2012;66(5):742–51.

63. Kimball AB, Papp KA, Wasfi Y, et al, PHOENIX 1 Investigators. Long-term efficacy of ustekinumab in patients with moderate-to-severe psoriasis treated for up to 5 years in the PHOENIX 1 study. J Eur Acad Dermatol Venereol 2013;27(12): 1535–45.

64. Langley RG, Lebwohl M, Krueger GG, et al. PHOENIX 2 Investigators. Long-term efficacy and safety of ustekinumab, with and without dosing adjustment, in patients with moderate-to-severe psoriasis: results from the PHOENIX 2 study through 5 years of follow-up. Br J Dermatol 2015;172(5):1371–83.

65. Papp K, Gottlieb AB, Naldi L, et al. Safety surveillance for ustekinumab and other psoriasis treatments fthe psoriasis longitudinal assessment and registry (PSOLAR). J Drugs Dermatol 2015;14(7):706–14.

66. Mocko P, Kawalec P, Pilc A. Safety profile of biologic drugs in the therapy of Crohn disease: a systematic review and network metaanalysis. Pharmacol Rep 2016;68(6):1237–43.

67. Jauregui-Amezaga A, Somers M, De Schepper H, et al. Next generation of biologics for the treatment of Crohn's disease: an evidence based- review on ustekinumab. Clin Exp Gastroenterol 2017;10:293–301.
68. Pithadia DJ, Reynolds KA, Lee FB, et al. Tildrakizumab in the treatment of psoriasis: Latest evidence and place in therapy. Ther Adv Chronic Dis 2019;10:1–9.
69. Santostefano M, Herzyk D, Montgomery D, et al. Nonclinical safety of tildrakizumab, a humanized anti–IL-23p19 monoclonal antibody, in nonhuman primates. Regul Toxicol Pharmacol 2019;108:1–8.
70. Reich K, Papp KA, Blauvelt A, et al. Tildrakizumab versus placebo or etanercept for chronic plaque psoriasis (reSURFACE 1 and reSURFACE 2): results from two randomised controlled, phase 3 trials. Lancet 2017;390:276–88.
71. Nogueira M, Torres T. Guselkumab for the treatment of psoriasis–evidence to date. Drugs Context 2019;8:212594.
72. Yang E, Smith MP, Ly K, et al. Evaluating guselkimab: an anti-IL-23 antibody for the treatment of plaque psoriasis. Drug Des Devel Ther 2019;13:1993–2000.
73. Nemoto O, Hirose K, Shibata S, et al. Safety and efficacy of guselkumab in Japanese patients with moderate-to-severe plaque psoriasis: a randomized, placebo-controlled, ascending-dosestudy. Br J Dermatol 2018;178(3):689–96.
74. Blauvelt A, Papp KA, Griffiths CE, et al. Efficacy and safety of guselkumab, an anti-interleukin-23 monoclonal antibody, compared with adalimumab for the continuous treatment of patients with moderate to severe psoriasis: results from the phase III, double-blinded, placebo- and active comparator–controlled VOYAGE 1 trial. J Am Acad Dermatol 2017;76(3):405–17.
75. Reich K, Armstrong AW, Foley P, et al. Efficacy and safety of guselkumab, an anti-interleukin-23monoclonal antibody, compared with adalimumab for the treatment of patients with moderate to severe psoriasis with randomized withdrawal and retreatment: results from the phase III,double-blind, placebo- and active comparator-controlled VOYAGE 2 trial. J Am Acad Dermatol 2017;76(3):418–31.
76. Langley RG, Tsai T-F, Flavin S, et al. Efficacy and safety of guselkumab in patients with psoriasis who have an inadequate response to ustekinumab: results of the randomized, double-blind, phase III NAVIGATE trial. Br J Dermatol 2018; 178(1):114–23.
77. Sano S, Kubo H, Morishima H, et al. Guselkumab, a human interleukin-23 monoclonal antibody in Japanese patients with generalized pustular psoriasis and erythrodermic psoriasis: efficacy and safety analyses of a 52-week, phase 3, multicenter, open-label study. J Dermatol 2018;45(5):529–39.
78. Conti HR, Gaffen SL. IL-17-mediated immunity to the opportunistic fungal pathogen candida albicans. J Immunol 2015;195(3):780–8.
79. Leonardi C, Bachelez H, Wu J, et al. Long-term safety of risankizumab in patients with moderate to severe psoriasis: analysis of pooled clinical trial data. J Am Acad Dermatol 2019;81(4):AB234.
80. Strober B, Blauvelt A, Menter A, et al. Risankizumab treatment is associated with low and consistent infection rates over time in patients with moderate to severe psoriasis: analysis of pooled clinical trial data. J Am Acad Dermatol 2019; 81(4):AB234.
81. Reich K, Gooderham M, Thaçi D, et al. Risankizumab compared with adalimumab in patients with moderate-to-severe plaque psoriasis (IMMvent): a randomised, double-blind, active-comparator-controlled phase 3 trial. Lancet 2019; 394(10198):576–86.

Direct T-cell Inhibition and Agents Targeting T-cell Migration and Chemotaxis

Mario Fernández-Ruiz, MD, PhD[a,b],*, José María Aguado, MD, PhD[a,b,c]

KEYWORDS

- Basiliximab • Daclizumab • Alemtuzumab • Natalizumab • Vedolizumab
- Efalizumab • Infection

KEY POINTS

- Basiliximab and daclizumab are monoclonal antibodies (mAbs) targeting CD25 (α chain of the interleukin-2 receptor) that induce no lymphodepletion. Used as induction therapy in solid organ transplant recipients, anti-CD25 agents are not associated with an apparent impact on the susceptibility to overall or opportunistic infection.

- Alemtuzumab is an anti-CD52 mAb that exerts a profound and sustained T-cell depletion. In patients with B-cell chronic lymphocytic leukemia and other hematological malignancies, alemtuzumab increases the rate of overall infection and predisposes to opportunistic events such as *Pneumocystis jirovecii* pneumonia.

- Mucocutaneous herpes is the most relevant infection observed with alemtuzumab at the substantially lower doses administered for multiple sclerosis (MS), requiring acyclovir prophylaxis.

- Natalizumab is an anti-α4-integrin subunit mAb approved for MS that may cause progressive multifocal leukoencephalopathy (PML). This risk increases with JC virus seropositivity, duration of therapy, and previous immunosuppression. Because of its gut-selective mode of action, this complication has not been reported with vedolizumab (anti-α4β7-integrin mAb).

- Efalizumab is an anti-CD11a (α-subunit of the LFA-1 integrin) mAb that was approved for the treatment of psoriasis. The occurrence of various PML cases led to its withdrawal from the US market in 2009.

Funding sources: This research was partially supported by Plan Nacional de I + D + I 2013 to 2016 and Instituto de Salud Carlos III, Subdirección General de Redes y Centros de Investigación Cooperativa, Spanish Ministry of Science and Innovation, Spanish Network for Research in Infectious Diseases (REIPI RD16/0016/0002) –co-financed by the European Development Regional Fund (EDRF) *"A way to achieve Europe"*. M. Fernández-Ruiz holds a research contract "Miguel Servet" (CP 18/00073) from the Spanish Ministry of Science and Innovation, Instituto de Salud Carlos III.

[a] Unit of Infectious Diseases, Hospital Universitario "12 de Octubre", Instituto de Investigación Sanitaria Hospital "12 de Octubre" (imas12), Madrid, Spain; [b] Spanish Network for Research in Infectious Diseases (REIPI RD16/0016/0002), Instituto de Salud Carlos III, Madrid, Spain; [c] School of Medicine, Universidad Complutense, Madrid, Spain
* Corresponding author. Unit of Infectious Diseases, Hospital Universitario "12 de Octubre", Centro de Actividades Ambulatorias, 2ª planta, bloque D. Avda.de Córdoba, s/n, Madrid 28041, Spain.
E-mail address: mario_fdezruiz@yahoo.es

INTRODUCTION

The advent over the past decades of the so-called biological (or targeted) therapies has revolutionized the management of malignancies and immune-mediated disorders such as multiple sclerosis (MS), inflammatory bowel disease (IBD), or psoriasis. This expanding armamentarium is not exempt from risks to the host, namely an increased susceptibility to infection. The theoretic effect of a given monoclonal antibody (mAb) and the expected safety profile may be anticipated by considering its specific site of action on the immune system.[1] The present review is focused on mAbs that induce direct T-cell inhibition (by targeting the interleukin-2 receptor [IL-2R] or the cell-surface glycoprotein CD52) or block T-cell trafficking and extravasation from the vascular compartment to inflamed tissues (by targeting cell-adhesion molecules such as integrins). An overview of the associated risks of infectious complications is provided in **Table 1**.

INTERLEUKIN-2 RECEPTOR INHIBITORS: BASILIXIMAB AND DACLIZUMAB

Basiliximab (Simulect, Novartis) is a mouse-human chimeric immunoglobulin G (IgG1) mAb targeting the 55-kDa α chain of the heterotrimeric IL-2R.[2] Daclizumab (Zenapax, Roche) is a humanized IgG1 mAb that targets an epitope largely shared by basiliximab on the extracellular domain of the CD25 molecule.[3] In the 1970s IL-2 emerged as a pleiotropic cytokine playing an instrumental role in T-cell differentiation and homeostasis.[4] It was later recognized as a T-cell growth factor essential for the generation of effector, memory, and regulatory subsets.[5] Heterotrimerization of the α chain in the IL-2R complex initiates the sequential recruitment of the β and γ_c subunits and confers high-affinity properties to the IL-2–binding site.[6] CD25 blockade prevents the transition of IL-2R to the high-affinity state and, subsequently, interrupts clonal expansion of activated T cells and cytokine release. In addition to the corresponding structure (chimeric vs humanized) and dosing regimens, both agents differ in their half-life, which is estimated as approximately 7 days for basiliximab and up to 3 weeks for daclizumab.

Basiliximab was approved in 1998 by the Food and Drug Administration (FDA) and the European Medicines Agency (EMA) to prevent acute graft rejection in adult and pediatric patients undergoing kidney transplantation (KT). The FDA had granted a similar approval to daclizumab in 1997, followed by the EMA 2 years later. Off-label uses of both agents include the prevention of rejection in other types of solid organ transplantation (SOT) and the treatment of steroid-refractory acute graft-versus-host disease (GVHD).[7] The production of daclizumab, however, was discontinued by the manufacturer in October 2008 for commercial reasons.[8] More recently, long-term daclizumab therapy was approved for relapsing forms of MS as a monthly subcutaneous (SC) injection (Zinbryta, Biogen, and Abbvie).[9] The emergence of severe autoimmune adverse events—such as meningoencephalitis, hepatitis, and drug reaction with eosinophilia and systemic symptoms—led to the definitive withdrawal of daclizumab in 2018.[10]

The inhibition of IL-2/IL-2R binding and the subsequent downstream signaling pathway prevents T-cell activation and proliferation without inducing cell lysis. Thus, basiliximab and daclizumab do not exert a lymphocyte-depleting effect, in contrast to other agents also used as induction therapy such as polyclonal antithymocyte globulin (ATG) preparations. Moreover, CD25 is selectively expressed on CD4+ and CD8+ T-cells on T-cell receptor activation and on regulatory T cells (T_{reg}).[4,11] It is plausible that this rather specific action, which preserves the functionality of other effector mechanisms, justify the minor impact on the susceptibility to posttransplant infection

Table 1
Summary of infection risks associated with agents targeting interleukin-2 receptor, CD52, and cell-adhesion molecules

Agent	Risk of PCP	Risk of HSV/VZV	Risk of LTBI Reactivation	Risk of PML	Specific Comments
Basiliximab, daclizumab	No	No	No	No	No apparent increase in infection risk when used as induction therapy in SOT recipients. Slightly higher infection rate with daclizumab than placebo in MS trials (clinical development program stopped due to autoimmune events)
Alemtuzumab	Yes	Yes	Yes	Yes[a]	Substantially lower infection risk when used for MS compared with B-CLL and other hematological malignancies
Natalizumab	No	No (consider prophylaxis in selected cases)[b]	No (consider screening in selected cases)[c]	Yes	PML risk minimization strategy based on clinical vigilance, monitoring for anti-JCV antibody index, and repeated MRI scans
Vedolizumab	No	No	No[d]	No[e]	Lower infection risk due to gut-specific mode of action
Efalizumab	No	No	No	Yes	Withdrawn from the market in 2009

Abbreviations: B-CLL, B-cell chronic lymphocytic leukemia; HSV, herpes simplex virus; JCV, John Cunningham polyomavirus; LTBI, latent tuberculosis infection; PCP, *Pneumocystis jirovecii* pneumonia; PML, progressive multifocal leukoencephalopathy; SOT, solid organ transplantation; VZV, varicella zoster virus.

[a] Low to unknown risk; **please see the article by Ashrit Multani and Dora Y. Ho,** "Viral Infections Potentiated by Biologics (and Prevention) - JC Polyomavirus," in this issue for further details.

[b] Patients with previous immunosuppressive therapy or frequent oral or genital herpes simplex recurrences.

[c] Patients with previous immunosuppressive therapy or coming from high-incidence countries.

[d] Despite low theoretic risk, screening for LTBI was required in pivotal trials and recommended per prescription label.

[e] No cases of vedolizumab-associated PML reported to date.

associated with anti-CD25 mAbs given as induction therapy, particularly in comparison with ATG.

Kalil and colleagues[12] performed a large meta-analysis on 70 randomized clinical trials (RCTs) with 10,106 SOT recipients (mainly kidney and liver). Induction therapy with lymphocyte-depleting agents (rabbit and, to a lesser extent, horse ATG) was used in approximately half of the studies (n = 3377), and anti-CD25 mAbs in the remaining trials (n = 6729), with basiliximab and daclizumab equally represented. The risk of opportunistic infection was significantly lower for anti-CD25 mAbs compared with controls (odds ratio [OR]: 0.80; 95% confidence interval [CI]: 0.68–0.94; P-value = .009). Differences were mainly driven by the occurrence of viral infection and cytomegalovirus (CMV) disease. Adjustment by the type of maintenance immunosuppression did not change these results. Because of the lack of head-to-head trials, an adjusted indirect comparison concluded that anti-CD25 induction was associated with a 59% reduction in the infection risk compared with ATG, with the difference consistent across the different types of infection except fungal infection. The somewhat unexpected protective effect of anti-CD25 mAbs when compared with no induction was attributed to the requirement of lower maintenance immunosuppression levels.[12]

A more recent meta-analysis restricted to 8 RCTs (n = 1153) that directly compared induction with basiliximab or ATG in KT recipients did not find significant differences in 1-year rates of overall infection (OR: 0.90; 95% CI: 0.48–1.68; P-value = .73). On the other hand, the incidence of posttransplant de novo malignancy was lower with basiliximab (OR: 0.26; 95% CI: 0.08–0.78; P-value = .02), supporting the notion that IL-2 blockade exerts a less profound impact on the T-cell–mediated immunity than lymphocyte-depleting preparations.[13] Although the cumulative doses of daclizumab (1 mg/Kg on the day of transplantation and then every 2 weeks for a total of 5 doses) are higher than those of basiliximab (20 mg on days 0 and 4 with no adjustment for body weight), the comparison of both mAbs in a meta-analysis that comprised 6 RCTs (n = 509) did not reveal significant differences in terms of overall or CMV infection.[14]

An RCT comparing induction therapy with basiliximab and alemtuzumab—an anti-CD52 mAb that induces sustained T-cell depletion, as discussed later—among 852 KT recipients did not find significant differences in the incidence of serious or opportunistic infections, although human BK polyomavirus (BKPyV) viremia was more common in the alemtuzumab arm.[15] These results are in apparent contradiction to those reported from a previous RCT, in which the rate of overall infection was higher with alemtuzumab than basiliximab (35% vs 22%; P-value = .02).[16] Nevertheless, differences in maintenance immunosuppression make difficult a direct comparison between both studies. Inconsistencies in the reporting of posttransplant infection across RCTs comparing alemtuzumab and anti-CD25 mAbs or ATG have been also noted.[17] Regarding other SOT groups, alemtuzumab was associated with a higher risk of death from infectious causes and posttransplant lymphoproliferative disorder than basiliximab after lung transplantation.[18] The risk of disseminated fungal infection has also been reported to be significantly increased with alemtuzumab induction as compared with basiliximab in a mixed SOT population.[19]

Anti-CD25 induction has not been associated with an apparent increase in the susceptibility to specific opportunistic pathogens in the KT population, such as BKPyV,[20] P jirovecii pneumonia (PCP),[21] or adenoviruses.[22] Because of the absence of lympho-depleting effects, there is no evidence to assume that these agents would individually affect the posttransplant kinetics of CMV-specific CD4+ and CD8+ T cells.[23–25] Clinical experience derived from large multicenter registries seems to support the safety of anti-CD25 mAbs in terms of CMV infection or disease.[26–28] Accordingly, current guidelines do not contain specific recommendations for the administration of antiviral prophylaxis against CMV on the sole basis of the use of anti-CD25 induction therapy in SOT recipients.[29–31]

Although the clinical development program of daclizumab for MS has been discontinued,[10] data from pivotal RCTs for this indication constitute a reminder that long-term CD25 blockade is still associated to a minor but significant increase in the absolute risk of infection.[32] Such an impact would be outweighed by the contributing role of maintenance immunosuppression with short courses of anti-CD25 therapy used as induction in the SOT setting. Patients with relapsing MS randomized to receive monthly SC daclizumab (150 or 300 mg) for 52 to 144 weeks experienced a slightly higher rate of infections compared with the control group (placebo or interferon [IFN] β-1a), mostly in the form of urinary tract infection, upper respiratory tract infection, and pharyngitis.[33–35] The 3-year analysis of an open-label extension study reported a cumulative incidence of 5% for orolabial herpes simplex virus (HSV) infection and only 2 cases (0.5%) of opportunistic infection (vulvovaginal candidiasis and pulmonary tuberculosis in a patient from an endemic area who had received daclizumab for 2.5 years).[36] As commented earlier, the occurrence of severe autoimmune phenomena involving the central nervous system (CNS) was revealed as the major safety concern.[37]

ANTI-CD52 AGENTS: ALEMTUZUMAB

Alemtuzumab is a humanized IgG1 mAb targeted against CD52, a 21- to 28-kDa glycosylphosphatidylinositol-anchored cell surface glycoprotein highly expressed on thymocytes, monocytes, mature peripheral blood B and T cells, and natural killer cells (but not on plasma cells or CD34+ hematopoietic stem cells). Moreover, CD52 is also present at high density on lymphoid and, to a lesser extent, myeloid leukemic blasts.[38,39] This mAb was first approved by the FDA and EMA in 2001 (under the names of Campath and MabCampath, respectively [Genzyme Corporation]) for patients with B-cell chronic lymphocytic leukemia (B-CLL) that had been treated with alkylating agents and fludarabine.[40] In addition, alemtuzumab has been used for other CD52-positive lymphoproliferative disorders (such as T-cell prolymphocytic leukemia and cutaneous T-cell lymphomas), as induction therapy in patients undergoing SOT and as part of reduced-intensity conditioning regimens to prevent GVHD after allogeneic hematopoietic stem cell transplantation.[41] The therapeutic potential of anti-CD52 mAbs in CNS demyelinating diseases had been investigated for decades. In 2013 alemtuzumab (marketed under the name of Lemtrada) received EMA approval for adult patients with active relapsing-remitting MS, whereas the FDA approval for relapsing forms came 1 year later. It should be noted that dosing and administration schedules largely differ according to the indication. In patients with B-CLL, alemtuzumab is initiated at a dose of 3 mg daily with progressive escalation to a maintenance regimen of 30 mg three times per week for a maximum of 12 weeks (leading to cumulative doses greater than 1000 mg). In contrast, the licensed regimen for MS is 12 mg daily for 5 consecutive days, with a second 3-day course given 12 months later (retreatment with up to 2 additional courses has been recently approved by the EMA). Therefore, the cumulative dose throughout 1 year is approximately one-tenth of that used in hematological malignancies.[42]

On binding to cell surface CD52, alemtuzumab induces leukemic cell lysis through complement-dependent cytotoxicity and antibody-dependent cell-mediated cytotoxicity. Caspase-independent apoptosis has also been demonstrated in B-CLL cell lines.[43] This mode of action leads to profound and sustained lymphodepletion, which manifests by 2 to 4 weeks from the first dose. Median CD4$^+$ and CD8$^+$ T-cell counts remained less than 25% from baseline levels beyond 9 months among patients with B-CLL who received alemtuzumab as first-line therapy.[44] This T-cell-depleting effect is even more dramatic for heavily treated patients with refractory or relapsed leukemia receiving purine analogues or bendamustine. Even at the lower doses used in MS, each treatment course rapidly depletes peripheral blood T and B cells, with the lowest values typically found after 1 month.[42] Recovery to the normal range can take 8 months for B cells and up to 3 years for CD4$^+$ and CD8$^+$ T cells, although lymphocyte counts rarely return to baseline values.[45] In addition, anti-CD52 therapy leads to a distinctive pattern of cellular repopulation, with a relative increase in T_{reg} and memory subsets and reduced proinflammatory Th1 and Th17 responses within the overall T-cell population.[32] Because hematopoietic stem cells lack CD52, alemtuzumab does not interfere with early hematopoietic development.

The infection risk associated with alemtuzumab varies according to the indication and dosing regimen.[46] Given the larger cumulative doses administered and the contribution of additional factors, patients with B-CLL and other lymphoproliferative disorders face the greatest risk. A meta-analysis of 5 RCTs (n = 845) on B-CLL concluded that the use of alemtuzumab increased the risk of overall (risk ratio [RR]: 1.32; 95% CI: 1.01–1.74; P-value = .04) and CMV infection (RR: 10.52; 95% CI: 1.42–77.68; P-value = .02) compared with antileukemia therapy alone.[47] On the other hand, PCP represents a well-established complication that results from the CD4$^+$ T-cell lymphodepletion induced by CD52 blockade, the concomitant use of corticosteroids and conventional chemotherapy (such as fludarabine, alkylating agents, or vincristine), and the detrimental impact of the underlying lymphoproliferative disorder on the cell-mediated immunity. In a pooled analysis of 7 RCTs (n = 417), PCP prophylaxis was recommended until 2 months after completion of alemtuzumab therapy. The cumulative incidence of PCP was 0.9% (4/417), and the only cases occurred in patients who were not receiving anti-Pneumocystis prophylaxis.[48] Other serious, although rare, infections associated with alemtuzumab in hematological malignancies (with chemotherapy regimens based on purine analogues playing a contributing role) include progressive multifocal leukoencephalopathy (PML),[49,50] invasive aspergillosis,[51] norovirus-related chronic diarrhea,[52] and severe hepatitis C reactivation.[53]

Although the rate of infectious complications in phase 3 RCTs leading to alemtuzumab approval for relapsing-remitting MS was higher than with the comparator (SC IFN β-1a), most of them were mild or moderate in severity. Urinary and upper respiratory tract infections, mucocutaneous herpes, and non-complicated herpes zoster (HZ) were the predominant events.[54,55] The notable cumulative incidence of HSV infection (which ranged from 13% to 16%) led to a protocol amendment requiring the use of acyclovir prophylaxis for participants allocated to alemtuzumab. No other prophylaxis was routinely administered. A pooled 6-year analysis across the alemtuzumab clinical development program for MS showed that the infection risk peaked after the first course to decline thereafter. In detail, HSV infections were most common during the first month following each treatment course and markedly decreased with acyclovir prophylaxis (from 4.9% to 0.5% and from 2.4% to 0.8% for the first and second courses, respectively).[56] This modest increase in the susceptibility to infection contributes to the overall positive benefit-risk profile of alemtuzumab for the treatment of MS. Nevertheless, serious opportunistic infections, such as nocardiosis,[57] CMV disease,[58] listeriosis with CNS involvement,[59,60] or invasive pulmonary aspergillosis,[61] have emerged during postmarketing use. Although uncommon, neutropenia may occur following alemtuzumab therapy.[62] A case of probable PML based on clinical symptoms and radiological features after a second course of alemtuzumab has been recently reported.[63] The risk of reactivation of latent tuberculosis infection (LTBI) is increased due to alemtuzumab-induced T-cell depletion, although only 2 cases of active tuberculosis were reported in pivotal phase 3 trials.[62,63]

As previously commented, some,[16,18] but not all,[15] studies suggest that induction therapy with alemtuzumab in SOT recipients may result in an increased incidence of infection as compared with anti-CD25 mAbs, ATG, or no induction. It should be noted that the dosing used in this patient population (usually a single 30 mg dose) is substantially lower than that recommended for other indications. A meta-analysis based on 6 RCTs (n = 446) that investigated the role of alemtuzumab induction for KT found no significant effect on the risk of overall (RR: 1.00; 95% CI: 0.74–1.35; P-value = 0 .989) or CMV infection (RR: 0.70; 95% CI: 0.38–1.30; P-value = 0.263).[64] A single-center retrospective study with a large cohort of mixed SOT recipients that received alemtuzumab (n = 726) reported in fact that the risk of posttransplant infection was slightly lower when compared with the basiliximab group, although this difference was mainly driven by a lower rate of urinary tract infection (likely due to lower requirements of antirejection therapy). However, the incidence of disseminated fungal infection, mainly invasive candidiasis, was higher with alemtuzumab (OR: 4.76; 95% CI: 1.58–14.28; P-value = .003).[19] Similar findings have been reported for small bowel transplant recipients.[65] Thus, although induction with alemtuzumab seems to have no effect on the overall incidence of posttransplant infection, the severity of episodes would be increased.

Various risk-minimization strategies should be implemented in patients treated with alemtuzumab (**Table 2**). Anti-*Pneumocystis* prophylaxis with trimethoprim/sulfamethoxazole should be given in hematological patients and SOT recipients from the initiation of therapy to at least 6 months after its completion.[66] Alternative agents include aerosolized pentamidine, dapsone, and atovaquone. The use of valganciclovir prophylaxis against CMV is recommended among CMV-seropositive SOT for 3 to 6 months.[29–31] Antiviral prophylaxis against HSV with acyclovir should be given to patients with MS from the first day of each alemtuzumab cycle and be maintained for at least 2 months or until the CD4+ T-cell count recovers to greater than or equal to 200 cells/μL.[67] A similar recommendation would apply to CMV-seronegative SOT recipients (because valganciclovir offers appropriate protection against HSV and varicella zoster virus). Monitoring of CD4+ T-cell counts could be also useful to guide the duration of anti-CMV and anti-*Pneumocystis* prophylaxes.[29] Baseline screening for LTBI (followed by appropriate therapy if needed) is mandatory, as well as for hepatitis B and C virus. Annual human papillomavirus screening should be offered to female patients. Age-appropriate inactivated vaccines should be administered, with particular emphasis on seasonal influenza vaccination. Finally, patients should avoid the ingestion of undercooked meats, soft cheeses, and unpasteurized dairy products from 2 weeks before the initiation of alemtuzumab to at least 1 month after discontinuation of therapy to minimize the risk of invasive listeriosis.[46,67]

ANTIINTEGRIN AGENTS: NATALIZUMAB, VEDOLIZUMAB, AND EFALIZUMAB

T-cell trafficking involves several processes (priming, homing, recirculation, or retention) that may serve as potential therapeutic targets in immune-mediated conditions such as MS or IBD. Integrins are key mediators of cell-to-matrix and cell-to-cell adhesive interactions that are expressed as transmembrane heterodimers in almost every cell type. Integrins are formed by dimerization of one α- and one β-subunit. So far, 18 α-integrin and 8 β-integrin subunits have been identified, which combine to form at least 25 different αβ heterodimers.[68] Therefore, mAbs may target the integrin molecule

Table 2
Risk minimization strategies recommended for patients receiving alemtuzumab therapy

Infection	Recommended Prophylaxis or Preventive Measure	Timing
PCP	Trimethoprim/sulfamethoxazole (single-strength [80/400 mg] tablet daily or double-strength [160/800 mg] tablet daily or three times weekly) *Alternatives:* aerosolized pentamidine (300 mg monthly), dapsone (100 mg daily), atovaquone (1500 mg daily)	From the initiation of therapy to at least 6 mo after completion (or, alternatively, until CD4$^+$T-cell count $\geq$200 cells/μL)
HSV and VZV infection[a]	HSV-seropositive patients: acyclovir (200 mg twice daily)[b] *Alternatives:* valacyclovir (500 mg twice daily), famciclovir (500 mg twice daily)	MS patients: from the first day of each treatment cycle for at least 2 mo (or, alternatively, until CD4$^+$T-cell count $\geq$200 cells/μL) Hematological patients: from the initiation of therapy to at least 1 mo after completion[c]
CMV infection/disease	CMV-seropositive SOT recipients: antiviral prophylaxis with valganciclovir (900 mg daily [with dosage adjustment according to renal function]) CMV-seropositive hematological patients: antiviral prophylaxis or preemptive therapy guided by CMV-DNA detection	CMV-seropositive SOT recipients: 3–6 mo from transplantation
HBV reactivation	Serologic screening for chronic or resolved infection (HBsAg, anti-HBs IgG, anti-HBc IgG $\pm$ HBV-DNA) and referral to liver specialists if positive[d]	Baseline (before initiating therapy)
HCV reactivation	Serologic screening for chronic (anti-HCV IgG, HCV antigen) and referral to liver specialists if positive	Baseline (before initiating therapy)

HPV-related cancers	Annual HPV screening in female patients	
Active tuberculosis	Screening for LTBI as per local practice (TST and/or IGRA) and appropriate therapy if needed	Baseline (before initiating therapy)
Invasive listeriosis	*Listeria*-free diet (avoidance of undercooked meats, soft cheeses, and unpasteurized dairy products)	From 2 wk before the initiation of therapy to at least 1 mo after completion
Toxoplasmosis	*Toxoplasma* seronegative patients only: avoidance of raw or undercooked meat and contact with cat feces	From 2 wk before the initiation of therapy to at least 1 mo after completion

Abbreviations: CMV, cytomegalovirus; HBV, hepatitis B virus; HCV, hepatitis C virus; HPV, human papillomavirus; IGRA, interferon-γ release assay; TST, tuberculin skin test; VZV, varicella zoster virus.

[a] SOT recipients under anti-CMV prophylaxis with valganciclovir do not need additional antiviral prophylaxis against HSV or VZV.[104]

[b] Acyclovir doses used in pivotal MS trials. Higher doses (400 mg every 8–12 hours) are usually recommended for hematological patients.[105]

[c] Optimal duration of antiviral prophylaxis is not well established for hematological patients.

[d] Antiviral prophylaxis (entecavir or tenofovir) should be administered from the initiation of therapy to at least 6 to 12 months after completion to HBsAg-positive patients (or HBsAg-negative/anti-HBc-positive patients with detectable HBV-DNA). Antiviral prophylaxis (entecavir, tenofovir, or lamivudine) or alternatively close monitoring for HBV-DNA with preemptive treatment should be administered to HBsAg-negative/anti-HBc-positive patients to prevent reactivation of occult HBV infection.[106]

either at a monomer or a heterodimer level, resulting in the therapeutic blockade of a set of integrins or only one specific member, respectively. This variable specificity will dictate the expected safety profile and associated infectious complications.[69]

Natalizumab

Natalizumab (Tysabri, Elan Pharmaceuticals, and Biogen Idec) is a humanized IgG4 mAb targeting the α4-integrin subunit that constituted the first antiintegrin agent approved for clinical use. The α4 chain dimerizes with either the β1 subunit or the β7 subunit to form 2 different integrins, α4β1 (also known as very late antigen [VLA]-4]) and α4β7, respectively. VLA-4 is expressed on virtually all leukocytes (except mature granulocytes) and mediates binding to endothelial cell layers, including the blood-brain barrier (BBB), via vascular cell adhesion molecule (VCAM)-1. The VLA-4/VCAM-1 interaction is required for immune cell trafficking into the CNS. By blocking the α4β1 integrin (VLA-4), natalizumab abrogates T-cell migration across the BBB leading to reduced CNS inflammation.[70] This agent gained FDA regulatory approval to treat relapsing-remitting MS in November 2004. Four years later, natalizumab was also approved for moderate-to-severe Crohn disease (CD).[71]

Natalizumab seemed to be well tolerated across phase 3 RCTs leading to approval for MS[72,73] and CD.[74] However, the first cases of PML in natalizumab-treated patients recruited in pivotal trials were early reported.[75–77] This circumstance led to a voluntary suspension of marketing in February 2005. Natalizumab was reintroduced in the US market in 2006 with a black-box warning for PML and under a restricted distribution program (Tysabri Outreach: Unified Commitment to Health).[32] The EMA has approved natalizumab as monotherapy only for patients with highly active or rapidly evolving forms of relapsing-remitting MS despite an adequate course with at least one disease-modifying agent.

The natalizumab-induced impairment of homeostatic CNS immune surveillance results in the reactivation of the John Cunningham polyomavirus (JCV), a nonenveloped double-stranded DNA virus that infects oligodendrocytes, with subsequent white matter demyelination and development of clinical PML. The JCV seroprevalence in the general population increases with age and reaches ~60% to 70% beyond the sixth decade,[78] with a yearly seroconversion rate of about 7%.[79] Based on more than 150,000 patients treated with natalizumab worldwide, the overall incidence of PML has been estimated in 4.22 cases per 1000 patients.[32] Three clinical risk factors have been identified: treatment duration (with the greatest increase in risk occurring after 2 years of therapy), exposure to JCV (as assessed by a positive status for anti-JCV IgG antibodies), and previous or even remote history of immunosuppressive therapy (including relatively mild agents such as methotrexate). The incidence among JCV-seropositive patients was estimated at 3.87 cases per 1000 natalizumab-treated patients, as compared with 0 cases per 1000 in seronegative individuals. By combining these variables into a risk stratification algorithm, different categories may be established, with expected PML incidences ranging from less than 0.09 cases per 1000 patients in the lowest-risk subgroup to 11.1 cases per 1000 patients in the highest-risk category.[80] The quantification of anti-JCV IgG titers by enzyme-linked immunosorbent assay (ELISA) has been proved to provide further refinement in risk prediction. The anti-JCV antibody index is the normalized ratio between the signal (in optical densities) obtained from the patient's serum and that from a cutoff calibrator prepared with pooled sera collected from JCV-seropositive healthy volunteers. Patients not previously treated with immunosuppressive agents with an index value less than or equal to 0.9 carried a risk of 0.1 PML cases per 1000 during the first 24 months of therapy, which gradually increased up to 0.4 per 1000 with 49 to

72 months of exposure. In contrast, the expected incidence during the first 24 months among patients with an index greater than 1.5 was of 1.0 cases per 1,000, reaching 10.12 per 1000 between months 49 to 72.[81] An FDA-cleared second-generation ELISA test (STRATIFY JCV, Focus Diagnostics) is now commercially available.[82] For more information, please refer to Ashrit Multani and Dora Y. Ho's article, "Viral Infections Potentiated by Biologics (and Prevention) - JC Polyomavirus," in this issue on JC virus.

Because the prognosis of natalizumab-associated PML critically depends on early recognition, risk minimization strategies rely on continuous clinical vigilance, monitoring of anti-JCV antibody index, and cerebral MRI.[32] Typical clinical and radiological characteristics are detailed in **Box 1**. All patients should be assessed for anti-JCV IgG antibodies before initiating natalizumab. An index cutoff value of greater than 1.5 constitutes a reasonable threshold to guide the clinical decision process. According to recent recommendations from an expert panel, JCV-seronegative patients, as well as those who are JCV-seropositive with an initial index less than or equal to 1.5, should be retested every 6 months beyond the first year. Patients with an index greater than 1.5 are to be already considered at high risk and no further testing is required. Cerebral MRI with diffusion-weighted imaging and fluid-attenuated inversion recovery should be performed at baseline and repeated at scheduled intervals according to the JCV serostatus and antibody index levels. JCV-seropositive patients who choose to remain on natalizumab therapy should have annual MRI scans during the first 18 months of therapy. Thereafter, the frequency of monitoring should be increased to a least 6-month intervals for patients with an index less than or equal to 1.5 and 3- to 4-month intervals for those with index greater than 1.5. Annual MRI scanning would suffice for JCV-seronegative patients. Any new lesions on subsequent MRI that were not evident on the previous most recent scan should trigger clinical consideration and further investigation is necessary (ie, JCV PCR testing on cerebrospinal fluid specimens).[83]

Box 1

Main clinical and radiological features of progressive multifocal leukoencephalopathy in patients treated with natalizumab

Clinical presentation
- Subacute (weeks) onset and progressive course
- Aphasia, behavioral and neuropsychological alterations, visual deficits, hemiparesis, and seizures

MRI features
- Large (>3 cm) lesions in a unifocal, multifocal, or widespread distribution
- Subcortical location rather than periventricular
- Frequent involvement of cortical gray matter (50% of cases), posterior fossa less commonly affected
- No mass effect even in large lesions
- T2-weighted sequences: diffuse hyperintensity (often with punctate microcystic appearance) within the lesions
- T1-weighted sequences: lightly hypointensity at onset, with signal intensity decreasing over time
- Paramagnetic contrast enhancement in less than 50% of cases at the time of presentation (often patchy or punctate appearance)
- Diffusion-weighted imaging: hyperintense appearance of acute lesions

Adapted from McGuigan C, Craner M, Guadagno J, Kapoor R, Mazibrada G, Molyneux P, et al. Stratification and monitoring of natalizumab-associated progressive multifocal leukoencephalopathy risk: recommendations from an expert group. J Neurol Neurosurg Psychiatry 2016;87:117-25; with permission.

A recent study from France found an annual reduction of 23.0% in the crude incidence of natalizumab-associated PML since 2013 (in contrast to the steady increase observed before that year), supporting the efficacy of this risk minimization strategy.[84] Treatment of natalizumab-associated PML includes immediate drug discontinuation and clearance from the bloodstream through plasma exchange or immunoadsorption.[69]

Vedolizumab

Vedolizumab (Entyvio, Takeda Pharmaceuticals) is a humanized IgG1 mAb that targets α4β7 integrin, a cell surface glycoprotein variably expressed on circulating B and T cells. A central event in the pathogenesis of IBD is the homing of T cells to the gut. Vedolizumab selectively blocks the interaction between α4β7 integrin and its natural partner, the mucosal addressin cell adhesion molecule 1, which is constitutively expressed on high endothelial venules of Peyer patches, mesenteric lymph nodes, and postcapillary venules of the intestinal lamina propria.[85] Vedolizumab-mediated α4β7 integrin blockade selectively inhibits the migration of memory T cells into inflamed gastrointestinal tissue and, unlike natalizumab, no effect is expected on the α4β1-dependent CNS homing via VCAM-1.[86] Vedolizumab was approved in 2014 by the FDA and EMA for the treatment of adult patients with moderate-to-severe active CD and ulcerative colitis (UC) who had an inadequate response to standard therapies or antitumor necrosis factor (TNF-α) agents.[87]

The gut-selective mode of action of vedolizumab should theoretically lead to a lower infection risk, although the cumulative experience is still more limited than with other biological agents approved for IBD. A recent meta-analysis pooled 3 pivotal RCTs (n = 1262) and evaluated the infection risk associated with antiintegrin agents (vedolizumab or natalizumab) given as maintenance therapy for up to 52 weeks in patients with UC or CD. None of these mAbs was associated with a statistically significant risk of overall infection, regardless of the underlying IBD (RR [for patients with CD]: 1.10, 95% CI: 0.97–1.25; RR [for patients with UC]: 1.02; 95% CI: 0.88–1.16).[88] The most commonly reported events were upper respiratory tract infection and influenza. Serious infections such as sepsis, *Clostridioides difficile*–associated diarrhea, CNS listeriosis, or tuberculosis occurred very rarely (≤0.6% of patients) in pivotal RCTs.[89–91] No differences were found between patients treated with antiintegrin agents or placebo in the rate of opportunistic infection (0.5% vs 0.0%) either. The incidence of opportunistic infection, albeit low, was numerically higher across all trials in the treatment arms of anti-TNF-α trials than that observed with antiintegrin agents.[88] An integrated summary of safety data from 6 RCTs identified that prior anti-TNF-α failure and concomitant narcotic analgesic use acted as risk factors for infection in patients with UC, whereas concomitant corticosteroid therapy also predicted infection among patients with CD.[92]

Real-world clinical data seem to confirm this relatively minor impact of vedolizumab on the susceptibility to infection. A multicenter propensity score–matched analysis reported a trend toward a lower risk of serious infections in patients with IBD receiving vedolizumab monotherapy than in those under anti-TNF-α agents (4.1% vs 10.1%), although the difference was attenuated when biological therapy was combined with corticosteroids and other immunosuppressive agents. No significant differences in the risk of serious infection was observed after adjusting for clinical covariates between patients treated with vedolizumab or adalimumab (an anti-TNF-α mAb) in an administrative claims-based analysis.[93] Because α4β7 integrin is a unique gut-homing marker, the use of vedolizumab has not been associated with side effects in the CNS. Considering the exposure time to vedolizumab across RCTs (3326 and

906 participants were exposed for ≤24 and > 24 months, respectively) and assuming a JCV seroprevalence of 50%, it has been estimated that at least 6 to 7 PML cases would have been expected in the clinical development program had the risk been similar to that of natalizumab. However, no cases of PML have been reported to date.[92] The theoretic risk of LTBI reactivation is not expected to be increased, and there were only 4 cases of pulmonary tuberculosis in patients from high-incidence countries (accounting for 0.1 cases per 100 patient-years) in the vedolizumab arms of pivotal RCTs.[89–91] Nevertheless, it should be noted that LTBI had to be excluded as per study protocol before patient inclusion. Given than corticosteroids and other immunosuppressive agents are frequently needed during the course of IBD, baseline screening for LTBI should be performed according to local practices. Finally, according to the to the prescription label the administration of vedolizumab should be postponed (or *temporarily discontinued*) in patients with active uncontrolled severe infection.

Efalizumab

Efalizumab (Raptiva, Genentech Inc.) is a humanized IgG1 mAb targeting the α-subunit (CD11a) of the lymphocyte function–associated antigen 1(LFA-1) integrin.[94] LFA-1 is a member of the β2-integrin family, which are heterodimers composed of a common β subunit (CD18) and a variable α chain (CD11a in the case of LFA-1). β2 integrins are expressed on leukocytes and mediate cell-adhesion and migration. In addition to other ligands, LFA-1 binds to the intercellular adhesion molecule 1, an Ig superfamily member present on the surface of endothelial cells, epidermal keratinocytes, and antigen-presenting cells. By inhibiting T-cell activation in the lymph nodes, trafficking from the circulation into dermal and epidermal tissues, and subsequent reactivation in these sites (all of them instrumental events in the pathogenesis of psoriasis), LFA-1 blockade lead to significant and sustained clinical improvement in psoriatic patients.[95] Efalizumab received approval in 2004 for the treatment of severe plaque psoriasis in adult patients who were unresponsive or intolerant to other options, such as methotrexate or cyclosporine.

Phase 1/2[96] and 3[97–99] RCTs did not note a meaningful risk of infectious complications, which occurred at rates similar to those in the placebo groups. Most common events among patients treated with efalizumab for 12 weeks included viral upper respiratory tract infection, streptococcal pharyngitis, impetigo, HSV infection, and cellulitis, and no evidence emerged of increased susceptibility to opportunistic pathogens or clinically relevant laboratory abnormalities.[97] This safety profile seemed to be confirmed for an extended 24-week regimen.[99] No cases of HZ were observed in a large population-based database of psoriatic patients receiving biological therapies, although the number of efalizumab-treated participants was low.[100]

In October 2008 the FDA issued a first warning of the occurrence of PML associated with efalizumab use. The diagnosis of PML was confirmed in 3 patients (leading to a fatal outcome in 2 of them despite various courses of plasma exchange) and 1 additional case was clinically suspected. All the patients had been treated with efalizumab monotherapy for more than 3 years.[101] Impaired transendothelial migration by peripheral T cells was demonstrated in vitro in 2 patients, as well as a steady increase in migratory capacity following plasma exchange. In addition, this therapy prompted proliferative reconstitution of primed central T cells, with the subsequent expansion of peripheral CD4+ and CD8+ T cells with an effector memory phenotype.[102] Because of these emerging safety concerns, the EMA's Committee on Medicinal Products for Human Use concluded that there was not enough evidence to identify a group of psoriatic patients for whom the potential benefits of efalizumab would outweigh the associated risk of PML. Therefore, European and Canadian regulatory agencies recommend the suspension of the marketing authorization in February and June 2009, respectively. The manufacturer had voluntarily withdrawn efalizumab from the United States market as of April 2009.[103]

DISCLOSURE

The authors have nothing to disclosure.

REFERENCES

1. Fernandez-Ruiz M, Meije Y, Manuel O, et al. ESCMID Study Group for Infections in Compromised Hosts (ESGICH) consensus document on the safety of targeted and biological therapies: an infectious diseases perspective (Introduction). Clin Microbiol Infect 2018;24(Suppl 2):S2–9.
2. Onrust SV, Wiseman LR. Basiliximab. Drugs 1999;57:207–13 [discussion: 14].
3. Wiseman LR, Faulds D. Daclizumab: a review of its use in the prevention of acute rejection in renal transplant recipients. Drugs 1999;58:1029–42.
4. Malek TR. The biology of interleukin-2. Annu Rev Immunol 2008;26:453–79.
5. Abbas AK, Trotta E, R Simeonov D, et al. Revisiting IL-2: biology and therapeutic prospects. Sci Immunol 2018;3 [pii:eaat1482].
6. Robb RJ, Greene WC, Rusk CM. Low and high affinity cellular receptors for interleukin 2. Implications for the level of Tac antigen. J Exp Med 1984;160: 1126–46.
7. Funke VA, de Medeiros CR, Setubal DC, et al. Therapy for severe refractory acute graft-versus-host disease with basiliximab, a selective interleukin-2 receptor antagonist. Bone Marrow Transplant 2006;37:961–5.
8. Chouhan KK, Zhang R. Antibody induction therapy in adult kidney transplantation: a controversy continues. World J Transplant 2012;2:19–26.
9. Milo R, Osherov M. Daclizumab and its use in multiple sclerosis treatment. Drugs Today (Barc) 2017;53:7–18.
10. Daclizumab withdrawn from the market worldwide. Drug Ther Bull 2018;56:38.
11. Boyman O, Sprent J. The role of interleukin-2 during homeostasis and activation of the immune system. Nat Rev Immunol 2012;12:180–90.
12. Kalil AC, Florescu MC, Grant W, et al. Risk of serious opportunistic infections after solid organ transplantation: interleukin-2 receptor antagonists versus polyclonal antibodies. A meta-analysis. Expert Rev Anti Infect Ther 2014;12:881–96.
13. Wang K, Xu X, Fan M. Induction therapy of basiliximab versus antithymocyte globulin in renal allograft: a systematic review and meta-analysis. Clin Exp Nephrol 2018;22:684–93.
14. Sun ZJ, Du X, Su LL, et al. Efficacy and safety of basiliximab versus daclizumab in kidney transplantation: a meta-analysis. Transplant Proc 2015;47:2439–45.
15. 3C Study Collaborative Group, Haynes R, Harden P, Judge P, et al. Alemtuzumab-based induction treatment versus basiliximab-based induction treatment in kidney transplantation (the 3C Study): a randomised trial. Lancet 2014;384: 1684–90.
16. Hanaway MJ, Woodle ES, Mulgaonkar S, et al. Alemtuzumab induction in renal transplantation. N Engl J Med 2011;364:1909–19.
17. Morgan RD, O'Callaghan JM, Knight SR, et al. Alemtuzumab induction therapy in kidney transplantation: a systematic review and meta-analysis. Transplantation 2012;93:1179–88.

18. Furuya Y, Jayarajan SN, Taghavi S, et al. The impact of alemtuzumab and basiliximab induction on patient survival and time to bronchiolitis obliterans syndrome in double lung transplantation recipients. Am J Transplant 2016;16: 2334–41.

19. Safdar N, Smith J, Knasinski V, et al. Infections after the use of alemtuzumab in solid organ transplant recipients: a comparative study. Diagn Microbiol Infect Dis 2010;66:7–15.

20. Radtke J, Dietze N, Fischer L, et al. Incidence of BK polyomavirus infection after kidney transplantation is independent of type of immunosuppressive therapy. Transpl Infect Dis 2016;18:850–5.

21. de Boer MG, Kroon FP, le Cessie S, et al. Risk factors for *Pneumocystis jirovecii* pneumonia in kidney transplant recipients and appraisal of strategies for selective use of chemoprophylaxis. Transpl Infect Dis 2011;13:559–69.

22. Florescu DF, Islam MK, Mercer DF, et al. Adenovirus infections in pediatric small bowel transplant recipients. Transplantation 2010;90:198–204.

23. Higdon LE, Trofe-Clark J, Liu S, et al. Cytomegalovirus-responsive CD8(+) T cells expand after solid organ transplantation in the absence of CMV disease. Am J Transplant 2017;17:2045–54.

24. Abate D, Saldan A, Fiscon M, et al. Evaluation of cytomegalovirus (CMV)-specific T cell immune reconstitution revealed that baseline antiviral immunity, prophylaxis, or preemptive therapy but not antithymocyte globulin treatment contribute to CMV-specific T cell reconstitution in kidney transplant recipients. J Infect Dis 2010;202:585–94.

25. Bestard O, Lucia M, Crespo E, et al. Pretransplant immediately early-1-specific T cell responses provide protection for CMV infection after kidney transplantation. Am J Transplant 2013;13:1793–805.

26. San Juan R, Aguado JM, Lumbreras C, et al. Impact of current transplantation management on the development of cytomegalovirus disease after renal transplantation. Clin Infect Dis 2008;47:875–82.

27. Manuel O, Kralidis G, Mueller NJ, et al. Impact of antiviral preventive strategies on the incidence and outcomes of cytomegalovirus disease in solid organ transplant recipients. Am J Transplant 2013;13:2402–10.

28. Fernández-Ruiz M, Arias M, Campistol JM, et al. Cytomegalovirus prevention strategies in seropositive kidney transplant recipients: an insight into current clinical practice. Transpl Int 2015;28:1042–54.

29. Torre-Cisneros J, Aguado JM, Caston JJ, et al. Management of cytomegalovirus infection in solid organ transplant recipients: SET/GESITRA-SEIMC/REIPI recommendations. Transplant Rev (Orlando) 2016;30:119–43.

30. Kotton CN, Kumar D, Caliendo AM, et al. The third international consensus guidelines on the management of cytomegalovirus in solid-organ transplantation. Transplantation 2018;102:900–31.

31. Razonable RR, Humar A. Cytomegalovirus in solid organ transplant recipients-guidelines of the American Society of Transplantation Infectious Diseases Community of Practice. Clin Transplant 2019;33(9):e13512.

32. McGinley MP, Moss BP, Cohen JA. Safety of monoclonal antibodies for the treatment of multiple sclerosis. Expert Opin Drug Saf 2017;16:89–100.

33. Gold R, Giovannoni G, Selmaj K, et al. Daclizumab high-yield process in relapsing-remitting multiple sclerosis (SELECT): a randomised, double-blind, placebo-controlled trial. Lancet 2013;381:2167–75.

34. Giovannoni G, Gold R, Selmaj K, et al. Daclizumab high-yield process in relapsing-remitting multiple sclerosis (SELECTION): a multicentre, randomised, double-blind extension trial. Lancet Neurol 2014;13:472–81.
35. Kappos L, Wiendl H, Selmaj K, et al. Daclizumab HYP versus Interferon Beta-1a in relapsing multiple sclerosis. N Engl J Med 2015;373:1418–28.
36. Gold R, Radue EW, Giovannoni G, et al. Safety and efficacy of daclizumab in relapsing-remitting multiple sclerosis: 3-year results from the SELECTED open-label extension study. BMC Neurol 2016;16:117.
37. Stork L, Bruck W, von Gottberg P, et al. Severe meningo-/encephalitis after daclizumab therapy for multiple sclerosis. Mult Scler 2019;25:1618–32.
38. Hale G. The CD52 antigen and development of the CAMPATH antibodies. Cytotherapy 2001;3:137–43.
39. Xia MQ, Hale G, Lifely MR, et al. Structure of the CAMPATH-1 antigen, a glycosylphosphatidylinositol-anchored glycoprotein which is an exceptionally good target for complement lysis. Biochem J 1993;293(Pt 3):633–40.
40. Tibes R, Keating MJ, Ferrajoli A, et al. Activity of alemtuzumab in patients with CD52-positive acute leukemia. Cancer 2006;106:2645–51.
41. Gribben JG, Hallek M. Rediscovering alemtuzumab: current and emerging therapeutic roles. Br J Haematol 2009;144:818–31.
42. Li Z, Richards S, Surks HK, et al. Clinical pharmacology of alemtuzumab, an anti-CD52 immunomodulator, in multiple sclerosis. Clin Exp Immunol 2018; 194:295–314.
43. Stanglmaier M, Reis S, Hallek M. Rituximab and alemtuzumab induce a nonclassic, caspase-independent apoptotic pathway in B-lymphoid cell lines and in chronic lymphocytic leukemia cells. Ann Hematol 2004;83:634–45.
44. Lundin J, Porwit-MacDonald A, Rossmann ED, et al. Cellular immune reconstitution after subcutaneous alemtuzumab (anti-CD52 monoclonal antibody, CAMPATH-1H) treatment as first-line therapy for B-cell chronic lymphocytic leukaemia. Leukemia 2004;18:484–90.
45. Hill-Cawthorne GA, Button T, Tuohy O, et al. Long term lymphocyte reconstitution after alemtuzumab treatment of multiple sclerosis. J Neurol Neurosurg Psychiatry 2012;83:298–304.
46. Mikulska M, Lanini S, Gudiol C, et al. ESCMID Study Group for Infections in Compromised Hosts (ESGICH) Consensus Document on the safety of targeted and biological therapies: an infectious diseases perspective (Agents targeting lymphoid cells surface antigens [I]: CD19, CD20 and CD52). Clin Microbiol Infect 2018;24(Suppl 2):S71–82.
47. Skoetz N, Bauer K, Elter T, et al. Alemtuzumab for patients with chronic lymphocytic leukaemia. CochraneDatabase Syst Rev 2012;(2):CD008078.
48. Cordonnier C, Cesaro S, Maschmeyer G, et al. Pneumocystis jirovecii pneumonia: still a concern in patients with haematological malignancies and stem cell transplant recipients. J Antimicrob Chemother 2016;71:2379–85.
49. Isidoro L, Pires P, Rito L, et al. Progressive multifocal leukoencephalopathy in a patient with chronic lymphocytic leukaemia treated with alemtuzumab. BMJCase Rep 2014;2014 [pii:bcr2013201781].
50. Noreña I, Fernández-Ruiz M, Aguado JM. Viral infections in the biologic therapy era. Expert Rev Anti Infect Ther 2018;16:781–91.
51. Anoop P, Stanford M, Saso R, et al. Ocular and cerebral aspergillosis in a non-neutropenic patient following alemtuzumab and methyl prednisolone treatment for chronic lymphocytic leukaemia. J Infect Chemother 2010;16:150–1.

52. Ronchetti AM, Henry B, Ambert-Balay K, et al. Norovirus-related chronic diarrhea in a patient treated with alemtuzumab for chronic lymphocytic leukemia. BMC Infect Dis 2014;14:239.
53. Anoop P, Wotherspoon A, Matutes F. Severe liver dysfunction from hepatitis C virus reactivation following alemtuzumab treatment for chronic lymphocytic leukaemia. Br J Haematol 2010;148:484–6.
54. Coles AJ, Twyman CL, Arnold DL, et al. Alemtuzumab for patients with relapsing multiple sclerosis after disease-modifying therapy: a randomised controlled phase 3 trial. Lancet 2012;380:1829–39.
55. Cohen JA, Coles AJ, Arnold DL, et al. Alemtuzumab versus interferon beta 1a as first-line treatment for patients with relapsing-remitting multiple sclerosis: a randomised controlled phase 3 trial. Lancet 2012;380:1819–28.
56. Wray S, Havrdova E, Snydman DR, et al. Infection risk with alemtuzumab decreases over time: pooled analysis of 6-year data from the CAMMS223, CARE-MS I, and CARE-MS II studies and the CAMMS03409 extension study. Mult Scler 2019;25:1605–17.
57. Penkert H, Delbridge C, Wantia N, et al. Fulminant central nervous system nocardiosis in a patient treated with alemtuzumab for relapsing-remitting multiple sclerosis. JAMA Neurol 2016;73:757–9.
58. Aguirre C, Meca-Lallana V, Sanchez P, et al. Cytomegalovirus primary infection in a patient with multiple sclerosis treated with alemtuzumab. Mult Scler Relat Disord 2019;35:270–1.
59. Holmoy T, von der Lippe H, Leegaard TM. *Listeria monocytogenes* infection associated with alemtuzumab - a case for better preventive strategies. BMC Neurol 2017;17:65.
60. Pappolla A, Midaglia L, Boix Rodriguez CP, et al. Simultaneous CMV and Listeria infection following alemtuzumab treatment for multiple sclerosis. Neurology 2019;92:296–8.
61. Russo CV, Sacca F, Paternoster M, et al. Post-mortem diagnosis of invasive pulmonary aspergillosis after alemtuzumab treatment for multiple sclerosis. Mult Scler 2020;26(1):123–6.
62. Maniscalco GT, Cerillo I, Servillo G, et al. Early neutropenia with thrombocytopenia following alemtuzumab treatment for multiple sclerosis: case report and review of literature. Clin Neurol Neurosurg 2018;175:134–6.
63. Gerevini S, Capra R, Bertoli D, et al. Immune profiling of a patient with alemtuzumab-associated progressive multifocal leukoencephalopathy. Mult Scler 2019;25:1196–201.
64. Zheng J, Song W. Alemtuzumab versus antithymocyte globulin induction therapies in kidney transplantation patients: a systematic review and meta-analysis of randomized controlled trials. Medicine (Baltimore) 2017;96:e7151.
65. Silva JT, San-Juan R, Fernandez-Caamano B, et al. Infectious complications following small bowel transplantation. Am J Transplant 2016;16:951–9.
66. Maertens J, Cesaro S, Maschmeyer G, et al. ECIL guidelines for preventing *Pneumocystis jirovecii* pneumonia in patients with haematological malignancies and stem cell transplant recipients. J Antimicrob Chemother 2016;71:2397–404.
67. Epstein DJ, Dunn J, Deresinski S. Infectious complications of multiple sclerosis therapies: implications for screening, prophylaxis, and management. OpenForum Infect Dis 2018;5:ofy174.
68. Caswell PT, Vadrevu S, Norman JC. Integrins: masters and slaves of endocytic transport. Nat Rev Mol Cell Biol 2009;10:843–53.

69. Redelman-Sidi G, Michielin O, Cervera C, et al. ESCMID Study Group for Infections in Compromised Hosts (ESGICH) Consensus Document on the safety of targeted and biological therapies: an infectious diseases perspective (Immune checkpoint inhibitors, cell adhesion inhibitors, sphingosine-1-phosphate receptor modulators and proteasome inhibitors). Clin Microbiol Infect 2018;24(Suppl 2):S95–107.

70. Yednock TA, Cannon C, Fritz LC, et al. Prevention of experimental autoimmune encephalomyelitis by antibodies against alpha 4 beta 1 integrin. Nature 1992; 356:63–6.

71. Natalizumab. AN 100226, anti-4alpha integrin monoclonal antibody. Drugs R D 2004;5:102–7.

72. Polman CH, O'Connor PW, Havrdova E, et al. A randomized, placebo-controlled trial of natalizumab for relapsing multiple sclerosis. N Engl J Med 2006;354: 899–910.

73. Rudick RA, Stuart WH, Calabresi PA, et al. Natalizumab plus interferon beta-1a for relapsing multiple sclerosis. N Engl J Med 2006;354:911–23.

74. Sandborn WJ, Colombel JF, Enns R, et al. Natalizumab induction and maintenance therapy for Crohn's disease. N Engl J Med 2005;353:1912–25.

75. Langer-Gould A, Atlas SW, Green AJ, et al. Progressive multifocal leukoencephalopathy in a patient treated with natalizumab. N Engl J Med 2005;353: 375–81.

76. Kleinschmidt-DeMasters BK, Tyler KL. Progressive multifocal leukoencephalopathy complicating treatment with natalizumab and interferon beta-1a for multiple sclerosis. N Engl J Med 2005;353:369–74.

77. Van Assche G, Van Ranst M, Sciot R, et al. Progressive multifocal leukoencephalopathy after natalizumab therapy for Crohn's disease. N Engl J Med 2005;353:362–8.

78. Bozic C, Richman S, Plavina T, et al. Anti-John Cunnigham virus antibody prevalence in multiple sclerosis patients: baseline results of STRATIFY-1. Ann Neurol 2011;70:742–50.

79. Aladro Y, Terrero R, Cerezo M, et al. Anti-JC virus seroprevalence in a Spanish multiple sclerosis cohort: JC virus seroprevalence in Spain. J Neurol Sci 2016; 365:16–21.

80. Bloomgren G, Richman S, Hotermans C, et al. Risk of natalizumab-associated progressive multifocal leukoencephalopathy. N Engl J Med 2012;366:1870–80.

81. Plavina T, Subramanyam M, Bloomgren G, et al. Anti-JC virus antibody levels in serum or plasma further define risk of natalizumab-associated progressive multifocal leukoencephalopathy. Ann Neurol 2014;76:802–12.

82. Lee P, Plavina T, Castro A, et al. A second-generation ELISA (STRATIFY JCV DxSelect) for detection of JC virus antibodies in human serum and plasma to support progressive multifocal leukoencephalopathy risk stratification. J Clin Virol 2013;57:141–6.

83. McGuigan C, Craner M, Guadagno J, et al. Stratification and monitoring of natalizumab-associated progressive multifocal leukoencephalopathy risk: recommendations from an expert group. J Neurol Neurosurg Psychiatry 2016;87: 117–25.

84. Vukusic S, Rollot F, Casey R, et al. Progressive multifocal leukoencephalopathy incidence and risk stratification among natalizumab users in France. JAMA Neurol 2019. [Epub ahead of print].

85. Nakache M, Berg EL, Streeter PR, et al. The mucosal vascular addressin is a tissue-specific endothelial cell adhesion molecule for circulating lymphocytes. Nature 1989;337:179–81.
86. Zundler S, Becker E, Weidinger C, et al. Anti-Adhesion therapies in inflammatory bowel disease-molecular and clinical aspects. Front Immunol 2017;8:891.
87. Scribano ML. Vedolizumab for inflammatory bowel disease: from randomized controlled trials to real-life evidence. World J Gastroenterol 2018;24:2457–67.
88. Shah ED, Farida JP, Siegel CA, et al. Risk for overall infection with Anti-TNF and Anti-integrin agents used in IBD: a systematic review and meta-analysis. Inflamm Bowel Dis 2017;23:570–7.
89. Sandborn WJ, Feagan BG, Rutgeerts P, et al. Vedolizumab as induction and maintenance therapy for Crohn's disease. N Engl J Med 2013;369:711–21.
90. Feagan BG, Rutgeerts P, Sands BE, et al. Vedolizumab as induction and maintenance therapy for ulcerative colitis. N Engl J Med 2013;369:699–710.
91. Sands BE, Feagan BG, Rutgeerts P, et al. Effects of vedolizumab induction therapy for patients with Crohn's disease in whom tumor necrosis factor antagonist treatment failed. Gastroenterology 2014;147:618–27.e3.
92. Colombel JF, Sands BE, Rutgeerts P, et al. The safety of vedolizumab for ulcerative colitis and Crohn's disease. Gut 2017;66:839–51.
93. Singh S, Facciorusso A, Dulai PS, et al. Comparative risk of serious infections with biologic and/or immunosuppressive therapy in patients with Inflammatory bowel diseases: a systematic review and meta-analysis. Clin Gastroenterol Hepatol 2019. https://doi.org/10.1016/j.cgh.2019.02.044.
94. Efalizumab.Anti-CD11a monoclonal antibody–Genentech/Xoma, HU 1124, hu1124, xanelim. Drugs R D 2002;3:40–3.
95. Krueger JG. The immunologic basis for the treatment of psoriasis with new biologic agents. J Am Acad Dermatol 2002;46:1–23 [quiz: -6].
96. Gottlieb AB, Krueger JG, Wittkowski K, et al. Psoriasis as a model for T-cell-mediated disease: immunobiologic and clinical effects of treatment with multiple doses of efalizumab, an anti-CD11a antibody. Arch Dermatol 2002;138:591–600.
97. Gordon KB, Papp KA, Hamilton TK, et al. Efalizumab for patients with moderate to severe plaque psoriasis: a randomized controlled trial. JAMA 2003;290:3073–80.
98. Lebwohl M, Tyring SK, Hamilton TK, et al. A novel targeted T-cell modulator, efalizumab, for plaque psoriasis. N Engl J Med 2003;349:2004–13.
99. Menter A, Gordon K, Carey W, et al. Efficacy and safety observed during 24 weeks of efalizumab therapy in patients with moderate to severe plaque psoriasis. Arch Dermatol 2005;141:31–8.
100. Dreiher J, Kresch FS, Comaneshter D, et al. Risk of Herpes zoster in patients with psoriasis treated with biologic drugs. J Eur Acad Dermatol Venereol 2012;26:1127–32.
101. Carson KR, Focosi D, Major EO, et al. Monoclonal antibody-associated progressive multifocal leucoencephalopathy in patients treated with rituximab, natalizumab, and efalizumab: a review from the Research on Adverse Drug Events and Reports (RADAR) Project. Lancet Oncol 2009;10:816–24.
102. Schwab N, Ulzheimer JC, Fox RJ, et al. Fatal PML associated with efalizumab therapy: insights into integrin alpha-L-beta-2 in JC virus control. Neurology 2012;78:458–67 [discussion: 65].
103. DeFrancesco L. RIP Raptiva? Nat Biotechnol 2009;27:303.

104. Lee DH, Zuckerman RA, AST Infectious Diseases Community of Practice. Herpes simplex virus infections in solid organ transplantation: guidelines from the American Society of Transplantation Infectious Diseases Community of Practice. Clin Transplant 2019;33:e13526.

105. Sandherr M, Hentrich M, von Lilienfeld-Toal M, et al. Antiviral prophylaxis in patients with solid tumours and haematological malignancies–update of the Guidelines of the Infectious Diseases Working Party (AGIHO) of the German Society for Hematology and Medical Oncology (DGHO). Ann Hematol 2015;94: 1441–50.

106. Sarmati L, Andreoni M, Antonelli G, et al. Recommendations for screening, monitoring, prevention, prophylaxis and therapy of hepatitis B virus reactivation in patients with haematologic malignancies and patients who underwent haematologic stem cell transplantation-a position paper. Clin Microbiol Infect 2017;23: 935–40.

Infectious Implications of Interleukin-1, Interleukin-6, and T Helper Type 2 Inhibition

Anne Y. Liu, MD[a,b],*

KEYWORDS

- Anakinra • Canakinumab • Rilonacept • Tocilizumab • Sarilumab • Siltuximab
- Dupilumab • Mepolizumab

KEY POINTS

- Biologics targeting the interleukin (IL)-1 pathway (eg, anakinra, canakinumab, and rilonacept) impair innate inflammatory signals. They increase the risk of bacterial infections, including pneumonia and sepsis, and may increase the risk of bacterial and fungal opportunistic infections.
- Biologics targeting the IL-6 pathway (eg, tocilizumab, sarilumab, and siltuximab) impair innate inflammatory responses to trauma and pathogens, including tissue repair and adaptive immunity. They increase the risk of bacterial infections, of opportunistic infections including tuberculosis and herpes zoster, and of gastrointestinal perforation. Infectious risks are especially augmented when used in combination with other immunomodulatory medications.
- Biologics targeting the T helper type 2 (Th2) pathway (eg, dupilumab, mepolizumab, reslizumab, benralizumab, and omalizumab) do not significantly increase bacterial, most viral, and opportunistic infections. Dupilumab may increase extracutaneous localized herpesvirus infections in atopic dermatitis patients.
- Pre-biologic screening recommendations and protocols might decrease the associated incidence of tuberculosis, viral hepatitides, helminth infections, and live vaccine-associated infections. These precautions make a clear assessment of their infectious risks impractical.

INTRODUCTION

Interleukin-blocking therapies have expanded the treatment options for patients with rare, monogenic conditions with minimal treatment options, as well as those with severe presentations of common diseases that are refractory to traditional therapies.

[a] Division of Infectious Diseases and Geographic Medicine, Department of Medicine, Stanford University School of Medicine, Stanford, CA 94305, USA; [b] Division of Allergy/Immunology/Rheumatology, Department of Pediatrics, Stanford University School of Medicine, Stanford, CA 94305, USA
* 269 Campus Drive, CCSR Building, Stanford, CA 94305.
E-mail address: anneliu@stanford.edu

Infect Dis Clin N Am 34 (2020) 211–234
https://doi.org/10.1016/j.idc.2020.02.003
0891-5520/20/© 2020 Elsevier Inc. All rights reserved.

These therapies can act on targets that are expressed and act widely, by acting on the interleukin, the receptor, or associated regulatory molecules (**Table 1**).

This article reviews US Food and Drug Administration (FDA)-approved biologic therapies that block:

- Interleukin (IL)-6 signaling: tocilizumab, sarilumab, and siltuximab
- IL-1 signaling: anakinra, canakinumab, and rilonacept
- T helper type 2 (Th2)-related signaling: dupilumab (IL-4/IL-13), mepolizumab (IL-5), reslizumab (IL-5), benralizumab (IL-5), and omalizumab (IgE). Although not an interleukin-directed therapy, omalizumab is included here because of its functional relatedness to Th2 signaling.

Therapies that target IL-17 and IL-12/IL-23 will be discussed separately.

Infectious complications may occur infrequently in the context of clinical trials in which certain infection-related risk factors were exclusion criteria [e.g., pre-existing immunocompromising conditions, human immunodeficiency virus (HIV), or viral hepatitides]. Many clinical trials discussed herein excluded patients with a history of tuberculosis (TB) and/or required screening for and treatment of latent TB infection. Geographically focused infections such as endemic fungi may not be appreciated in multicenter trials that aggregate subjects of disparate geography. With few exceptions, most clinical trials discussed here were conducted among populations with low prevalence of TB and helminth infections. Real-world risks of blocking these immunologic pathways may be revealed only with retrospective registry data, case reports, and other observational data.

For this review, randomized clinical trials (mostly Phase III), open-label extension studies, and pooled data from clinical trials were reviewed if they tracked infections as adverse events. Meta-analyses and registry data were reviewed that aggregated infection data, particularly serious infections. Small case series and selected case reports were included if they described rare or opportunistic infections (OIs) that developed in the setting of one of these biologic therapies.

INTERLEUKIN-6
Biology of IL-6

IL-6 production is normally triggered by tissue damage or inflammation, an innate response to infections and injuries.[1] Pathogen-associated molecular patterns (PAMPs) and damage-associated molecular patterns (DAMPs) released by tissue destruction stimulate IL-6 production by a wide variety of cell types, particularly endothelial cells, smooth muscle cells, and immune cells that include T cells, B cells, neutrophils, and monocytes.[2] IL-6 exerts a wide range of tissue effects, including induction of acute phase reactant production, fever, tissue repair, angiogenesis, and hematopoiesis. Notably, IL-6 augments neutrophil chemotaxis and bone marrow egress, without affecting neutrophil function and apoptosis.[3] IL-6 does not have a well-defined role in maintenance of tuberculous granulomas as TNFα does. IL-6 contributes to adaptive immunity by promoting T cell proliferation and differentiation (while suppressing regulatory T cells), as well as antibody production via activated B cells and plasmablast expansion.[2,4]

IL-6 signaling occurs through the cell-bound IL-6 receptor (IL-6R) and the soluble IL-6R (sIL-6R).[5] Cell-bound IL-6R signaling has anti-inflammatory and regenerative effects via activity in hepatocytes and various immune cells. sIL-6R signaling triggers proinflammatory processes through endothelial and smooth muscle cells. IL-6 production should be transient and terminate when environmental stress factors are

Table 1
IL-1, IL-6, and Th2-blocking therapies

Drug (Year of Approval)	Target/Class	US Food and Drug Administration-Approved Indications	Vaccine Considerations (Pretreatment)	Tuberculosis Screening Pretreatment Recommended?	Infectious Considerations
Tocilizumab (2011)	IL-6R mAb	• Moderate to severe RA without adequate response to DMARDs • Giant cell arteritis • Polyarticular juvenile idiopathic arthritis • Systemic juvenile idiopathic arthritis ≥2 y of age • Cytokine release syndrome during CAR T-cell therapy ≥2 y of age	Live vaccines contraindicated Inactivated vaccines recommended	Yes	• Boxed warning for serious infection with concomitant immunosuppression • Bacterial infections, especially pneumonia, increased • Gastrointestinal perforation increased • Increase in OIs and TB • Possible loss of HBsAb during treatment
Sarilumab (2017)	IL-6R mAb	• Moderate to severe RA without adequate response to DMARDs		Yes	• Boxed warning for serious infection with concomitant immunosuppression • Bacterial infections, especially pneumonia, increased • Gastrointestinal perforation increased
Siltuximab (2014)	IL-6 mAb	• Multicentric Castleman disease (HIV- and HHV-8 negative)		No recommendation	• No specific TB screening recommendation given, but reasonable to do • Bacterial infections, especially pneumonia, may be increased

(continued on next page)

Table 1
(continued)

Drug (Year of Approval)	Target/Class	US Food and Drug Administration-Approved Indications	Vaccine Considerations (Pretreatment)	Tuberculosis Screening Pretreatment Recommended?	Infectious Considerations
Anakinra (2001)	IL-1ra (antagonist) homolog	• NOMID • Moderate to severe active RA failed DMARDs ≥18 y of age	Live vaccines contraindicated Inactivated vaccines recommended	Yes	• Increased bacterial infections, especially pneumonia and cellulitis • Increased sepsis with concomitant steroids • Infrequent OIs
Canakinumab (2009)	IL-1β mAb	• CAPS ≥4 y of age • sJIA ≥2 y of age • Familial Mediterranean fever • Hyper IgD syndrome • TRAPS		Yes	• Increased bacterial infections, especially pneumonia, skin/soft tissue, intraabdominal abscess, colitis, sepsis • Infrequent OIs
Rilonacept (2008)	Decoy receptor for IL-1	• CAPS ≥12 y of age		No recommendation	• Serious infections reported, mostly bacterial
Dupilumab (2017)	IL-4Ra mAb	• Moderate to severe atopic dermatitis ≥12 y of age • Moderate to severe asthma (eosinophilic or steroid-dependent) ≥12 y of age • Poorly controlled chronic rhinosinusitis with nasal polyps in adults	Live vaccines contraindicated	No recommendation	• No overall increase in infections • Decreased cutaneous bacterial and viral infections • Decreased influenza • Increased localized HSV and VZV infections • Unknown risk of helminth infections

Mepolizumab (2015)	IL-5 mAb	• Severe eosinophilic asthma ≥6 y of age • Eosinophilic granulomatosis with polyangiitis in adults	Zoster vaccination recommended prior to initiation	No recommendation	• No significant increase in infections • Poorly defined risk of herpes zoster • Unknown risk of helminth infections
Reslizumab (2016)	IL-5 mAb	• Severe eosinophilic asthma in adults	None		• No significant increase in infections • Poorly defined risk of herpes zoster • Unknown risk of helminth infections
Benralizumab (2017)	IL-5Ra mAb	• Severe eosinophilic asthma ≥12 y of age	None		• No significant increase in infections • Unknown risk of helminth infections
Omalizumab (2003)	IgE mAb	• Moderate to severe allergic asthma ≥6 y of age • Chronic idiopathic urticaria ≥12 y of age	None	No recommendation	• No significant increase in infections • Reduces respiratory virus-associated exacerbations • May increase risk of helminth infections • Possible role in ABPA treatment

removed, and dysregulation of the IL-6 axis has been implicated in multiple chronic inflammatory diseases, including rheumatoid arthritis (RA), multicentric Castleman disease (MCD), giant cell arteritis, and juvenile idiopathic arthritis (JIA), among others.

Tocilizumab

Tocilizumab is a recombinant humanized immunoglobulin G1 (IgG1) antibody specific for the IL-6 receptor (IL-6R). It blocks IL-6 binding to both cell-bound IL-6R and sIL-6R.[6] The FDA approved tocilizumab in 2010 for use in adults with moderate to severe RA not responding adequately to 1 or more traditional disease modifying antirheumatic drugs (DMARD). Additional indications now include: giant cell arteritis, polyarticular juvenile JIA and systemic JIA in individuals 2 years of age or older, and severe or life-threatening cytokine release syndrome for chimeric antigen receptor (CAR) T-cell therapy in patients 2 years of age or older. Both tocilizumab and sarilumab carry a boxed warning for serious infection, particularly with concomitant immunosuppressants. Most tocilizumab trials excluded patients with active infections, history of TB including latent, history of hepatitis B and C, and HIV.

Data from clinical trials and open-label extension trials for RA have shown that tocilizumab increases infection risk in a dose-dependent manner, particularly with bacterial infections such as pneumonia and cellulitis, as well as with upper respiratory tract infections (URTIs) and nasopharyngitis.[7–18] In aggregated data from multiple clinical trials, incidence rates of serious infections for control, tocilizumab 4 mg/kg, and tocilizumab 8 mg/kg treated groups were 3.5, 3.5, and 4.9 cases per 100 patient-years.[19] OIs included TB despite prescreening, local and systemic candidiasis, fungal infections (no further information), nontuberculous mycobacterial infections, *Pneumocystis jiroveci* pneumonia (PJP), and cryptococcal pneumonia. Most OIs occurred at the higher 8 mg/kg dose. Higher rates of gastrointestinal perforations were noted on tocilizumab.

Subsequent cumulative analyses and meta-analyses have identified up to a twofold risk of serious infections compared with placebo.[20–23] The most common serious infection was pneumonia, occurring at an incidence similar to that of patients on TNFα inhibitors, followed by herpes zoster and other bacterial infections (staphylococcal and streptococcal skin, soft tissue, and joint infections, gram-negative infections, pyelonephritis, and sepsis). Herpes zoster incidence with tocilizumab was similar to that seen with abatacept, rituximab, and TNFα inhibitors.[24,25] Rare infections associated with tocilizumab have included PJP, coccidioidomycosis, aspergillosis, and *Alcaligenes* spp infection. Disseminated cryptococcosis occurred in a patient treated with tocilizumab, cyclosporine, and prednisolone.[26]

Risk factors for serious infections in RA patients treated with tocilizumab include advanced age (≥65 year old), prolonged disease duration (≥10 years), pre-existing lung conditions, and concomitant therapy with methotrexate, corticosteroids, and other DMARDs.[23,27,28] In a French RA registry, serious infections were associated with positive anticitrullinated protein antibody, higher initial RA severity, higher initial neutrophil counts (>5 K/μL), and concurrent leflunomide.[29] Tocilizumab-associated neutropenia (3%–6%) is not associated with serious infections, consistent with IL-6 involvement in neutrophil chemotaxis but not function.[30]

Fewer data exist on tocilizumab-associated infections for the non-RA indications, including JIA and CAR-T cell-associated cytokine release syndrome.[31] Trials for polyarticular JIA and systemic JIA reported few infections overall,[32–34] but a pediatric JIA registry detected more infections – predominantly viral – with tocilizumab (15.5/100 person-years) than with TNFα inhibitors, with 6.5% infections classified as severe or very severe.[35]

Assessment of TB risk from biologics may be limited in clinical trials.[36] Reported cases have been a mix of de novo and reactivated infections, developing months to years after starting tocilizumab. Reactivations occurred despite prior treatment of latent infection. Most were pulmonary or pleural disease, with rare disseminated infections.[20,21,28,37] TB risk with tocilizumab is probably lower than with TNFα inhibitors but still bears pretreatment screening and chemoprophylaxis. Routine screening during treatment is advisable given the risk of asymptomatic seroconversion.[38]

Hepatitis B reactivation has been reported during tocilizumab treatment, although definitions of reactivation vary.[39] In a group of patients with positive hepatitis B assays prior to tocilizumab who did not receive chemoprophylaxis, over 40% of patients with baseline positive surface antigens experienced reactivation (by viral DNA), while none of those with positive core antibodies and negative surface antigens reactivated.[40] These observations have been corroborated by others.[41] Of the patients with positive hepatitis B surface antibodies before tocilizumab, 19% became seronegative on tocilizumab, concerning for loss of antigen-specific humoral immunity. Chemoprophylaxis may have a role in preventing reactivation in patients with chronic hepatitis B.[40]

Sarilumab

Sarilumab is a fully human monoclonal antibody that binds IL-6R both in its membrane-bound and soluble forms to abrogate IL-6 signaling. The FDA approved sarilumab in 2017 for use in patients with moderate to severe active RA without adequate response to DMARDs. Like tocilizumab, it carries a boxed warning of serious infections, especially with concomitant immunosuppression, and TB screening is recommended before and during treatment. Most sarilumab studies included an exclusion screen for TB.

Infections with sarilumab are substantially increased in a dose-dependent manner when used in combination with other DMARDs (usually methotrexate), and have most commonly been bacterial infections such as pneumonia and cellulitis.[42–46] Incidence rates of serious infections with sarilumab monotherapy and in combination with DMARDs were 1.0 and 3.7 cases per 100 person-years, respectively.[47] Gastrointestinal perforations occurred only on combination therapy. For common infections, sarilumab risk may be similar to that of TNFα inhibition.[48] As in tocilizumab studies, sarilumab-associated neutropenia did not affect infection risk. Localized herpes zoster was the most common OI but was not increased compared with controls; other OIs and TB were rare.[42,49] Two cases of PJP were reported from a cohort in which approximately 50% were taking corticosteroids.[46] *Mycobacterium chelonae* was implicated in a case of sarilumab injection site infection.[50]

Siltuximab

Siltuximab is a mouse-human chimeric IgG1 type monoclonal antibody that binds IL-6, preventing its interaction with soluble and cell-bound IL-6R. The FDA approved siltuximab in 2014 for use in patients with MCD who are HIV-negative and human herpesvirus-8 (HHV-8)-negative. Because siltuximab did not bind viral IL-6 in vitro, patients who were HIV-seropositive or HHV-8 viremic were excluded based on their greater possibility of circulating HHV-8-generated IL-6.[51] IL-6 is produced in excess in MCD and may contribute to its clinical manifestations, including lymphadenopathy, lymphoproliferation, constitutional symptoms, and autoinflammation.[52]

Siltuximab appears to have an infection risk profile similar to that of tocilizumab and sarilumab. The limited literature on siltuximab in MCD suggests an increase in respiratory viral and typical bacterial infections including pneumonia, without OIs or viral reactivations (with a substantial proportion on acyclovir or valacyclovir prophylaxis).[51,53,54] Bacterial infections were also increased in myelodysplastic syndrome patients, but not in other malignancies studied.[54–56]

INTERLEUKIN-1
Biology of IL-1

IL-1 contributes to innate inflammatory signals through its 2 forms, IL-1α and IL-1β. IL-1α acts as an innate danger indicator when released by endothelial and epithelial cells upon cell necrosis, and plays a critical role in sterile inflammation.[57] IL-1β is produced by myeloid cells as pro-IL-1β and is activated upon cleavage by caspase-1.[58] Caspase-1 activation requires assembly of inflammasomes that contribute to innate responses to viruses and bacteria.[59,60] IL-1β is involved in fever induction, pain sensitization, bone and cartilage destruction, and production of acute-phase reactants. Both IL-1α and IL-1β bind IL-1 receptor type 1 (IL-1R1), leading to transcription of proinflammatory genes.

To counter-regulate self-sustaining IL-1 activity, several endogenous molecules diminish IL-1 activity. These include: IL-1Ra (antagonist) that binds IL-1R1 without permitting intracellular signaling and competitively blocks IL-1α and IL-1β binding; IL-1 receptor type 2 (IL-1R2), which lacks a cytoplasmic domain and thus acts as a trap for IL-1α/IL-1β; and soluble IL-1R2, which binds pro-IL-1β and prevents cleavage by caspase-1.[58,61]

Unchecked activation of caspase-1 and IL-1β results in systemic and multiorgan sterile inflammation. IL-1 mediated inflammation contributes to some autoimmune diseases (eg, RA) and is central in autoinflammatory disorders such as familial Mediterranean fever (FMF) and cryopyrin-associated periodic syndromes (CAPS). These autoinflammatory diseases are characterized by fevers, arthritis, serositis, rashes, and sterile abscesses, with neutrophilia and elevated inflammatory markers. CAPS are caused by *NLRP3* mutations that encode abnormal cryopyrin protein (an inflammasome component) and include familial cold autoinflammatory syndrome (FCAS), Muckle-Wells syndrome (MWS), and neonatal onset multi-inflammatory disease (NOMID).

Multiple animal models of *Mycobacterium tuberculosis* have demonstrated a possible protective role for IL-1 in controlling mycobacterial infections.[62–64] Its relative contribution compared with other cytokines (eg, TNFα), however, is not well understood.[63,65]

Anakinra

Anakinra is a recombinant nonglycosylated homolog of human IL-1Ra, the IL-1R1 antagonist, and blocks IL-1 signaling.[58] FDA-approved indications include NOMID at any age and moderate to severe active RA in patients ≥18 years of age who have failed DMARDs. Reported off-label uses have included other CAPS, FMF and other periodic fever syndromes, adult-onset Still disease (AOSD), JIA, gout, and recurrent pericarditis.[66] Anakinra is cleared rapidly compared with monoclonal antibodies, a feature that may be desirable in patients at high risk for infectious complications. Many anakinra trials excluded ongoing infections, viral hepatitis, and HIV.

Anakinra increased serious infections compared with placebo controls in RA patients regardless of comorbidities (5.4/100 PY vs 1.65/100 PY).[67(p200),68,69] The most common serious infections were pneumonia and cellulitis, and limited microbiologic data revealed typical bacteria (eg, *Streptococcus pneumoniae*) in pneumonias and *S aureus* in bone/joint infections, without TB or OIs (in populations of low TB incidence). Additional infections appeared in the open-label extension trial including intraabdominal bacterial infections, osteomyelitis, and pyelonephritis, as well as 3 OIs: atypical mycobacterial infection, histoplasmosis, and esophageal candidiasis.[69] Sepsis rates increased with continued anakinra exposure in patients on concomitant steroids. The addition of anakinra to etanercept for RA increased infection risk compared with etanercept monotherapy, including herpes zoster.[70] Anakinra trials in CAPS and other rare disorders have found a similar infection profile as the larger RA studies,[71,72] as have subsequent observational and registry data.[73–75] Viral OI risk appears to be low. TB reactivation on anakinra has been sparsely reported but can be extrapulmonary.[76,77] Screening for latent TB is recommended prior to anakinra treatment.

Canakinumab

Canakinumab is a fully human mAb that selectively blocks IL-1β and does not interact with other IL-1 family members. The FDA has approved its use in CAPS for patients 4 years of age and older, systemic JIA in patients 2 years of age and older, and adults and children with familial Mediterranean fever, hyper IgD syndrome/mevalonate kinase deficiency, and tumor necrosis factor receptor-associated periodic syndrome (TRAPS).

In small clinical trials for systemic JIA and rare autoinflammatory syndromes, canakinumab increased risk of infections including serious bacterial infections (pneumonia, skin/soft-tissue infections, intraabdominal abscess).[78–80] Similar infections were seen in open-label studies.[81,82] Large trials of canakinumab use in gout, diabetes mellitus (DM), and atherosclerosis have corroborated this infectious risk and profile,[83–85] with serious infections in 1.8% of canakinumab-treated gout patients compared to 0% in placebo controls.[83] Pseudomembranous colitis and fatal infections and sepsis were significantly increased in a large trial of patients with atherosclerosis.[85] OIs and TB were rare in clinical trials. One child with MWS on combination immunosuppression had multiple viral infections including Epstein-Barr virus, suspected parvovirus, mumps meningitis, and herpes zoster.[82]

TB risk on canakinumab appears to be low,[85–87] but TB screening is still recommended before treatment. Invasive fungal infections have only rarely been reported, including a patient with uncontrolled diabetes who developed orbital invasion from an *Aspergillus fumigatus* ethmoid sinus mycetoma.[88]

Rilonacept

Rilonacept is a dimeric fusion protein that acts as a decoy receptor for IL-1α and IL-1β, preventing signaling through endogenous IL-1R1.[89,90] Rilonacept joins the ligand-binding domains of the extracellular portion of the human IL-1R and the Fc region of human IgG1. Its FDA-approved indication is CAPS for patients 12 years of age and older, including FCAS and MWS. Much of its safety data comes from trials in other diseases.

Randomized trials of rilonacept did not detect an increased risk of infection when studied for CAPS, gout, systemic JIA, and systemic sclerosis.[34,91–95] However, the serious infections reported in clinical trials and in observational data have been similar in nature if not frequency to those noted with anakinra and canakinumab.[96–98]

T HELPER TYPE 2
Biology of Th2

Th2 type immunity mediates inflammation characteristic of both helminth infections and allergic disorders.[99,100] Innate inflammatory signals such as IL-33 and thymic stromal lymphopoietin (TSLP) promote differentiation of Th2 cells that produce IL-4, IL-5, and IL-13. IL-4 promotes B cell class switching and antigen-specific IgE production. IL-13 contributes to epithelial cell proliferation and goblet cell differentiation with mucus hypersecretion. IL-5 induces eosinophil maturation, differentiation, mobilization, activation, and survival.[101] Eosinophils contribute to tissue remodeling, airway hyperreactivity, and further Th2 inflammation. Antigen-specific IgE is free or constitutively bound to the high-affinity IgE receptor, and antigen binding triggers receptor cross-linking to produce many features of allergic inflammation.

Dupilumab

Dupilumab is a fully human mAb that binds to IL-4Rα, a receptor subunit common to both IL-4 and IL-13 receptors.[102] It thus produces a broad inhibition of Th2 inflammation. Dupilumab is currently FDA approved for moderate/severe atopic dermatitis (AD) inadequately controlled with topical steroids for patients 12 years of age and older, moderate/severe asthma of eosinophilic phenotype or corticosteroid dependence for patients 12 years of age and older, and for adults with inadequately controlled chronic rhinosinusitis with nasal polyps.

None of the dupilumab clinical trials reported an overall increased risk of serious infection, which is corroborated by pooled analyses and observational studies.[103–107] Differences in infection types have not appeared in asthma, sinusitis, and eosinophilic esophagitis trials.[105,106,108–111] In contrast, AD patients may experience a reduction in cutaneous bacterial and viral infections, but an increase in extracutaneous localized herpesvirus infections.

Adults with AD exhibited a dupilumab-associated reduction in serious infections (RR 0.38), including bacterial skin infections such as folliculitis and cellulitis (RR 0.44) but an increase in bacterial conjunctivitis.[103,112] However, a smaller AD study in adolescents comparing 2 doses of dupilumab found more skin infections with the higher dose.[113] AD patients have a tenfold risk of methicillin-resistant S aureus (MRSA) colonization; impaired keratinocyte antimicrobial peptide production may permit S aureus growth.[114,115] Dupilumab may reduce bacterial infections by restoring an impaired skin barrier, reducing S aureus colonization,[116] and/or altering the underlying immunologic milieu.

Viral infections appear to be increased overall in AD patients on dupilumab, with notably increased herpesvirus infections and a slight increase in nasopharyngitis and URTI, but a decrease in influenza.[103,117] Herpesvirus infections were predominantly mucosal herpes simplex virus (HSV) infections; herpes zoster and herpes zoster ophthalmicus also occurred in clinical trials.[104,112] HSV uveitis and varicella zoster virus (VZV) meningitis have been reported in AD patients.[118] Risks with viral hepatitides are unknown as this was a clinical trial exclusion, but chemoprophylaxis could be considered.[119]

However, dupilumab may have a protective effect against cutaneous viral infections, with a notably decreased incidence of eczema herpeticum.[103] Dupilumab initiation was also associated with rapid clearance of previously persistent, refractory molluscum contagiosum in a series of patients with severe AD.[120]

The mechanism for increased extracutaneous herpesvirus infections with dupilumab is unknown. Th2 immunity may not contribute significantly to the antiviral response, but other IL-4 producing cells such as natural killer T cells do have antiviral activity.[121,122]

An inflammatory conjunctivitis has emerged in patients with severe AD on dupilumab.[104,117,123,124] Most cases appear to be noninfectious, although HSV keratitis and uveitis and herpes zoster ophthalmicus should be entertained. Risk factors include higher AD severity and history of conjunctivitis.[123,124] Patients with dupilumab-associated conjunctivitis should be referred to an ophthalmologist.[125]

No endoparasitic infections developed in 7 AD trials, and ectoparasitic infections were rare; however, dupilumab trials were not conducted in populations with high prevalence of parasitosis.[103] Pending further study, dupilumab should be avoided or used with caution in patients at risk of helminth infections, and prescreening and treatment should be considered.

Currently live vaccines are contraindicated in patients receiving dupilumab, although the risks have not been studied. Dupilumab did not reduce specific antibody responses to tetanus (Tdap) and meningococcal (MPSV4) vaccines.[126]

Mepolizumab

Mepolizumab is a humanized mAb specific for human IL-5, which binds free IL-5 and prevents its binding to the IL-5 receptor. FDA-approved indications include severe eosinophilic asthma in patients 6 years of age and older and eosinophilic granulomatosis with polyangiitis (EGPA) in adults.

No increased risk of infection was detected in mepolizumab-treated patients in eosinophilic asthma, eosinophilic chronic obstructive pulmonary disease (COPD), and EGPA trials.[127–132] Infections reported in open-label and other observational studies most commonly included nasopharyngitis and URTIs, with several cases of HSV, herpes zoster, and *Candida* (not otherwise specified), and 1 case of pulmonary TB.[133–136] When studied for hypereosinophilic syndrome at a dose 7.5 times higher than that approved for asthma, mepolizumab-treated patients had more URTIs and bronchitis without increased serious infections.[137] The only OI was PJP in a patient who seroconverted HIV during the study.[138] TB prescreening was not required. Zoster vaccination is recommended in older patients prior to mepolizumab initiation.

Allergic bronchopulmonary aspergillosis (ABPA) is characterized by eosinophilic airway inflammation with bronchiectasis, *A fumigatus*-specific IgE, and elevated total IgE in asthmatic and cystic fibrosis patients.[139] Use of mepolizumab therapy in ABPA has been associated with clinical improvement and reduced corticosteroid requirements.[140–143]

The risk of parasitic infections is unknown. Given the role of eosinophils in clearing parasite infestations, caution should be taken in using mepolizumab in high-risk patients; screening and monitoring may be warranted.

Reslizumab

Like mepolizumab, reslizumab is a humanized mAb directed against IL-5. It is FDA approved as add-on therapy for adults with eosinophilic asthma. In asthma and eosinophilic esophagitis studies, reslizumab did not significantly increase risk of viral, bacterial, or fungal infections.[144–146] In fact, reslizumab-treated asthmatics demonstrated a trend toward fewer respiratory infections. Patients with helminth infections were excluded. No OIs or helminthic infections were noted.

Benralizumab

Benralizumab is an afucosylated, humanized IgG1 mAb directed against the IL-5Rα subunit and has a cytolytic effect on IL-5R-expressing cells. It induces a rapid depletion of eosinophils and basophils via antibody-dependent cell-mediated cyto-toxicity.[147] The FDA has approved benralizumab for add-on maintenance therapy for severe eosinophilic asthma ≥12 years of age.

In clinical trials of benralizumab for eosinophilic asthma and COPD, no increased risk in infections has been found, and no unusual infections or OIs occurred.[148–154] Benralizumab may decrease respiratory infections as well as increase pyrexia.[155,156] Disseminated herpes zoster 5 days after benralizumab initiation was reported in a patient with chronic eosinophilic pneumonia who was also on prednisolone and cyclophosphamide.[157]

There is no recommendation on zoster vaccination prior to benralizumab initiation. Benralizumab did not impair antibody responses to inactivated influenza immunization by hemagglutination inhibition and microneutralization assays.[158]

Omalizumab

Omalizumab is a humanized IgG1 mAb directed against free IgE and blocks IgE inter-action with the high- and low-affinity IgE receptors, FcεRI and CD23/FcεRII, respec-tively.[159] FcεRI is expressed on mast cells, basophils, eosinophils, plasmacytoid dendritic cells (pDCs), and Langerhans cells. CD23 is expressed on B cells and antigen-presenting cells. Omalizumab does not recognize receptor-bound IgE and thus cannot trigger receptor cross-linking and downstream signaling. It is FDA approved for moderate/severe persistent asthma with perennial sensitization for pa-tients 6 years of age and older, and chronic idiopathic urticaria for patients 12 years of age and older.

Since early omalizumab trials over 20 years ago,[160,161] there have been more than 150 clinical trials of this agent. Many key asthma trials were reviewed by Humbert and colleagues.[162] Overall, omalizumab has not been associated with increased infections in asthmatics; rather, a trend toward decreased rates of sinusitis and respiratory infec-tions has been observed.[163,164] Herpesvirus infections and OIs were rare to nil. Smaller trials in patients with chronic idiopathic urticaria detected more URTIs and sinusitis, compared with placebo.[165]

Omalizumab has exhibited protective activity against respiratory viruses.[166] Respi-ratory viruses are closely linked to asthma pathophysiology, with a major role in asthma exacerbations and a possible pathogenic contribution to the development of asthma.[167,168] Atopic patients experience a peak in asthma exacerbations in autumn, attributed in large part to viral infections. Omalizumab can eliminate seasonal increases in exacerbations and can decrease the duration of rhinovirus shed-ding.[166,169,170] This effect has been credited to a boosting of pDC production of anti-viral alpha interferons seen when omalizumab prevents IgE binding on pDCs.[166,171]

High IgE levels typical of ABPA would have excluded these patients from earlier omalizumab trials. Yet, omalizumab may be an effective treatment for reducing ABPA exacerbations and allowing corticosteroid tapering, despite IgE levels greater than 1000 IU/mL.[172–174]

IgE is increased in helminth infections and may play a role in infection clear-ance.[175–177] Although soil-transmitted helminths may infect approximately 2 billion people worldwide,[178] most of the trials discussed were conducted in populations with low burdens of parasitic infections. A single clinical trial addressed helminth risk in high-exposure patients.[179] Omalizumab treatment was associated with an in-crease in helminth infections (odds ratio [OR] 1.47) that did not reach statistical signif-icance. Most infections occurred with *Ascaris lumbricoides*, hookworm species, *Trichuris trichiura*, *Enterobius vermicularis*, and enteric protozoa. In animal models, anti-IgE antibodies have had mixed effects on parasite burden.[175] Case reports of

omalizumab-associated helminth infections are sparse.[180] No specific screening recommendations exist for parasitic infections before omalizumab. It is reasonable to
screen patients from endemic areas for parasitic infections prior to initiation and, if
ongoing exposures are expected, during treatment.

SUMMARY

This article has reviewed the known infectious risks of biologic therapies that act upon
IL-1, IL-6, and Th2 signaling. Appropriate caution should be taken when exposing patients who are on concomitant immunosuppression or at risk for latent tuberculosis
infection to IL-1 and IL-6 pathway inhibitors. Although the Th2-blocking agents exhibit
fairly benign infectious profiles, their risks in parasite-endemic areas have only been
minimally explored. Their potential to reduce specific bacterial and viral infections
may shed light on the counterbalancing mechanisms in Th2 inflammation.

DISCLOSURE

Dr A.Y. Liu has served on a medical advisory board for Sanofi Regeneron.

REFERENCES

1. Tanaka T, Kishimoto T. The biology and medical implications of interleukin-6.
   Cancer Immunol Res 2014;2(4):288–94.
2. Rose-John S, Winthrop K, Calabrese L. The role of IL-6 in host defence against
   infections: immunobiology and clinical implications. Nat Rev Rheumatol 2017;
   13(7):399–409.
3. Wright HL, Cross AL, Edwards SW, et al. Effects of IL-6 and IL-6 blockade on
   neutrophil function in vitro and in vivo. Rheumatology (Oxford) 2014;53(7):
   1321–31.
4. Kishimoto T. The biology of interleukin-6. Blood 1989;74(1):1–10.
5. Schett G. Physiological effects of modulating the interleukin-6 axis. Rheumatology (Oxford) 2018;57(Suppl_2):ii43–50.
6. Sato K, Tsuchiya M, Saldanha J, et al. Reshaping a human antibody to inhibit the
   interleukin 6-dependent tumor cell growth. Cancer Res 1993;53(4):851–6.
7. Smolen JS, Beaulieu A, Rubbert-Roth A, et al. Effect of interleukin-6 receptor inhibition with tocilizumab in patients with rheumatoid arthritis (OPTION study): a
   double-blind, placebo-controlled, randomised trial. Lancet 2008;371(9617):
   987–97.
8. Emery P, Keystone E, Tony HP, et al. IL-6 receptor inhibition with tocilizumab improves treatment outcomes in patients with rheumatoid arthritis refractory to
   anti-tumour necrosis factor biologicals: results from a 24-week multicentre randomised placebo-controlled trial. Ann Rheum Dis 2008;67(11):1516–23.
9. Genovese MC, McKay JD, Nasonov EL, et al. Interleukin-6 receptor inhibition
   with tocilizumab reduces disease activity in rheumatoid arthritis with inadequate
   response to disease-modifying antirheumatic drugs: the tocilizumab in combination with traditional disease-modifying antirheumatic drug therapy study.
   Arthritis Rheum 2008;58(10):2968–80.
10. Jones G, Sebba A, Gu J, et al. Comparison of tocilizumab monotherapy versus
    methotrexate monotherapy in patients with moderate to severe rheumatoid
    arthritis: the AMBITION study. Ann Rheum Dis 2010;69(1):88–96.
11. Kremer JM, Blanco R, Brzosko M, et al. Tocilizumab inhibits structural joint dam-
    age in rheumatoid arthritis patients with inadequate responses to methotrexate:

results from the double-blind treatment phase of a randomized placebo-controlled trial of tocilizumab safety and prevention of structural joint damage at one year. Arthritis Rheum 2011;63(3):609–21.

12. Jones G, Wallace T, McIntosh MJ, et al. Five-year efficacy and safety of tocilizumab monotherapy in patients with rheumatoid arthritis who were methotrexate- and biologic-naive or free of methotrexate for 6 months: the AMBITION study. J Rheumatol 2017;44(2):142–6.

13. Nishimoto N, Hashimoto J, Miyasaka N, et al. Study of active controlled monotherapy used for rheumatoid arthritis, an IL-6 inhibitor (SAMURAI): evidence of clinical and radiographic benefit from an x ray reader-blinded randomised controlled trial of tocilizumab. Ann Rheum Dis 2007;66(9):1162–7.

14. Nishimoto N, Miyasaka N, Yamamoto K, et al. Study of active controlled tocilizumab monotherapy for rheumatoid arthritis patients with an inadequate response to methotrexate (SATORI): significant reduction in disease activity and serum vascular endothelial growth factor by IL-6 receptor inhibition therapy. Mod Rheumatol 2009;19(1):12–9.

15. Nishimoto N, Miyasaka N, Yamamoto K, et al. Long-term safety and efficacy of tocilizumab, an anti-IL-6 receptor monoclonal antibody, in monotherapy, in patients with rheumatoid arthritis (the STREAM study): evidence of safety and efficacy in a 5-year extension study. Ann Rheum Dis 2009;68(10):1580–4.

16. Yazici Y, Curtis JR, Ince A, et al. Efficacy of tocilizumab in patients with moderate to severe active rheumatoid arthritis and a previous inadequate response to disease-modifying antirheumatic drugs: the ROSE study. Ann Rheum Dis 2012;71(2):198–205.

17. Burmester GR, Rubbert-Roth A, Cantagrel A, et al. A randomised, double-blind, parallel-group study of the safety and efficacy of subcutaneous tocilizumab versus intravenous tocilizumab in combination with traditional disease-modifying antirheumatic drugs in patients with moderate to severe rheumatoid arthritis (SUMMACTA study). Ann Rheum Dis 2014;73(1):69–74.

18. Maini RN, Taylor PC, Szechinski J, et al. Double-blind randomized controlled clinical trial of the interleukin-6 receptor antagonist, tocilizumab, in European patients with rheumatoid arthritis who had an incomplete response to methotrexate. Arthritis Rheum 2006;54(9):2817–29.

19. Schiff MH, Kremer JM, Jahreis A, et al. Integrated safety in tocilizumab clinical trials. Arthritis Res Ther 2011;13(5):R141.

20. Genovese MC, Rubbert-Roth A, Smolen JS, et al. Longterm safety and efficacy of tocilizumab in patients with rheumatoid arthritis: a cumulative analysis of up to 4.6 years of exposure. J Rheumatol 2013;40(6):768–80.

21. Nishimoto N, Ito K, Takagi N. Safety and efficacy profiles of tocilizumab monotherapy in Japanese patients with rheumatoid arthritis: meta-analysis of six initial trials and five long-term extensions. Mod Rheumatol 2010;20(3):222–32.

22. Navarro G, Taroumian S, Barroso N, et al. Tocilizumab in rheumatoid arthritis: a meta-analysis of efficacy and selected clinical conundrums. Semin Arthritis Rheum 2014;43(4):458–69.

23. Teitsma XM, Marijnissen AKA, Bijlsma JWJ, et al. Tocilizumab as monotherapy or combination therapy for treating active rheumatoid arthritis: a meta-analysis of efficacy and safety reported in randomized controlled trials. Arthritis Res Ther 2016;18(1):211.

24. Tran CT, Ducancelle A, Masson C, et al. Herpes zoster: risk and prevention during immunomodulating therapy. Joint Bone Spine 2017;84(1):21–7.

25. Yun H, Xie F, Delzell E, et al. Risks of herpes zoster in patients with rheumatoid arthritis according to biologic disease-modifying therapy. Arthritis Care Res 2015;67(5):731–6.
26. Nishioka H, Takegawa H, Kamei H. Disseminated cryptococcosis in a patient taking tocilizumab for Castleman's disease. J Infect Chemother 2018;24(2): 138–41.
27. Campbell L, Chen C, Bhagat SS, et al. Risk of adverse events including serious infections in rheumatoid arthritis patients treated with tocilizumab: a systematic literature review and meta-analysis of randomized controlled trials. Rheumatology (Oxford) 2011;50(3):552–62.
28. Koike T, Harigai M, Inokuma S, et al. Effectiveness and safety of tocilizumab: postmarketing surveillance of 7901 patients with rheumatoid arthritis in Japan. J Rheumatol 2014;41(1):15–23.
29. Morel J, Constantin A, Baron G, et al. Risk factors of serious infections in patients with rheumatoid arthritis treated with tocilizumab in the French Registry REGATE. Rheumatology (Oxford) 2017;56(10):1746–54.
30. Moots RJ, Sebba A, Rigby W, et al. Effect of tocilizumab on neutrophils in adult patients with rheumatoid arthritis: pooled analysis of data from phase 3 and 4 clinical trials. Rheumatology (Oxford) 2017;56(4):541–9.
31. Frey N, Porter D. Cytokine release syndrome with chimeric antigen receptor T cell therapy. Biol Blood Marrow Transplant 2019;25(4):e123–7.
32. Amarilyo G, Tarp S, Foeldvari I, et al. Biological agents in polyarticular juvenile idiopathic arthritis: a meta-analysis of randomized withdrawal trials. Semin Arthritis Rheum 2016;46(3):312–8.
33. Brunner HI, Ruperto N, Zuber Z, et al. Efficacy and safety of tocilizumab in patients with polyarticular-course juvenile idiopathic arthritis: results from a phase 3, randomised, double-blind withdrawal trial. Ann Rheum Dis 2015;74(6): 1110–7.
34. Ilowite NT, Prather K, Lokhnygina Y, et al. Randomized, double-blind, placebo-controlled trial of the efficacy and safety of rilonacept in the treatment of systemic juvenile idiopathic arthritis. Arthritis Rheumatol 2014;66(9):2570–9.
35. Dumaine C, Bekkar S, Belot A, et al. Infectious adverse events in children with Juvenile idiopathic arthritis treated with biological agents in a real-life setting: data from the JIR cohort. Joint Bone Spine 2019. https://doi.org/10.1016/j.jbspin.2019.07.011.
36. Souto A, Maneiro JR, Salgado E, et al. Risk of tuberculosis in patients with chronic immune-mediated inflammatory diseases treated with biologics and tofacitinib: a systematic review and meta-analysis of randomized controlled trials and long-term extension studies. Rheumatology (Oxford) 2014;53(10):1872–85.
37. Khanna D, Denton CP, Lin CJF, et al. Safety and efficacy of subcutaneous tocilizumab in systemic sclerosis: results from the open-label period of a phase II randomised controlled trial (faSScinate). Ann Rheum Dis 2018;77(2):212–20.
38. Cuomo G, D'Abrosca V, Iacono D, et al. The conversion rate of tuberculosis screening tests during biological therapies in patients with rheumatoid arthritis. Clin Rheumatol 2017;36(2):457–61.
39. Mori S, Fujiyama S. Hepatitis B virus reactivation associated with antirheumatic therapy: risk and prophylaxis recommendations. World J Gastroenterol 2015; 21(36):10274–89.
40. Chen L-F, Mo Y-Q, Jing J, et al. Short-course tocilizumab increases risk of hepatitis B virus reactivation in patients with rheumatoid arthritis: a prospective clinical observation. Int J Rheum Dis 2017;20(7):859–69.

41. Ahn SS, Jung SM, Song JJ, et al. Safety of tocilizumab in rheumatoid arthritis patients with resolved hepatitis B virus infection: data from real-world experience. Yonsei Med J 2018;59(3):452–6.

42. Genovese MC, Fleischmann R, Kivitz AJ, et al. Sarilumab plus methotrexate in patients with active rheumatoid arthritis and inadequate response to methotrexate: results of a phase III study. Arthritis Rheumatol 2015;67(6):1424–37.

43. Genovese MC, van Adelsberg J, Fan C, et al. Two years of sarilumab in patients with rheumatoid arthritis and an inadequate response to MTX: safety, efficacy and radiographic outcomes. Rheumatology (Oxford) 2018;57(8):1423–31.

44. Genovese MC, van der Heijde D, Lin Y, et al. Long-term safety and efficacy of sarilumab plus methotrexate on disease activity, physical function and radiographic progression: 5 years of sarilumab plus methotrexate treatment. RMD Open 2019;5(2):e000887.

45. Kameda H, Wada K, Takahashi Y, et al. Sarilumab monotherapy or in combination with non-methotrexate disease-modifying antirheumatic drugs in active rheumatoid arthritis: A Japan phase 3 trial (HARUKA). Mod Rheumatol 2019;1–10. https://doi.org/10.1080/14397595.2019.1639939.

46. Tanaka Y, Wada K, Takahashi Y, et al. Sarilumab plus methotrexate in patients with active rheumatoid arthritis and inadequate response to methotrexate: results of a randomized, placebo-controlled phase III trial in Japan. Arthritis Res Ther 2019;21(1):79.

47. Fleischmann R, Genovese MC, Lin Y, et al. Long-term safety of sarilumab in rheumatoid arthritis: an integrated analysis with up to 7 years' follow-up. Rheumatology (Oxford) 2019. https://doi.org/10.1093/rheumatology/kez265.

48. Burmester GR, Lin Y, Patel R, et al. Efficacy and safety of sarilumab monotherapy versus adalimumab monotherapy for the treatment of patients with active rheumatoid arthritis (MONARCH): a randomised, double-blind, parallel-group phase III trial. Ann Rheum Dis 2017;76(5):840–7.

49. Fleischmann R, van Adelsberg J, Lin Y, et al. Sarilumab and nonbiologic disease-modifying antirheumatic drugs in patients with active rheumatoid arthritis and inadequate response or intolerance to tumor necrosis factor inhibitors. Arthritis Rheumatol 2017;69(2):277–90.

50. Dos Santos Sobrín R, Pérez Gómez N, Vilas AS, et al. Infection by *Mycobacterium chelonae* at the site of administration of sarilumab for rheumatoid arthritis. Rheumatology (Oxford) 2019. https://doi.org/10.1093/rheumatology/kez186.

51. van Rhee F, Wong RS, Munshi N, et al. Siltuximab for multicentric Castleman's disease: a randomised, double-blind, placebo-controlled trial. Lancet Oncol 2014;15(9):966–74.

52. van Rhee F, Stone K, Szmania S, et al. Castleman disease in the 21st century: an update on diagnosis, assessment, and therapy. Clin Adv Hematol Oncol 2010; 8(7):486–98.

53. van Rhee F, Casper C, Voorhees PM, et al. A phase 2, open-label, multicenter study of the long-term safety of siltuximab (an anti-interleukin-6 monoclonal antibody) in patients with multicentric Castleman disease. Oncotarget 2015;6(30):30408–19.

54. Garcia-Manero G, Gartenberg G, Steensma DP, et al. A phase 2, randomized, double-blind, multicenter study comparing siltuximab plus best supportive care (BSC) with placebo plus BSC in anemic patients with International Prognostic Scoring System low- or intermediate-1-risk myelodysplastic syndrome. Am J Hematol 2014;89(9):E156–62.

55. Fizazi K, De Bono JS, Flechon A, et al. Randomised phase II study of siltuximab (CNTO 328), an anti-IL-6 monoclonal antibody, in combination with mitoxantrone/prednisone versus mitoxantrone/prednisone alone in metastatic castration-resistant prostate cancer. Eur J Cancer 2012;48(1):85–93.

56. Orlowski RZ, Gercheva L, Williams C, et al. A phase 2, randomized, double-blind, placebo-controlled study of siltuximab (anti-IL-6 mAb) and bortezomib versus bortezomib alone in patients with relapsed or refractory multiple myeloma. Am J Hematol 2015;90(1):42–9.

57. Netea MG, van de Veerdonk FL, van der Meer JWM, et al. Inflammasome-independent regulation of IL-1-family cytokines. Annu Rev Immunol 2015;33:49–77.

58. Cavalli G, Dinarello CA. Anakinra therapy for non-cancer inflammatory diseases. Front Pharmacol 2018;9:1157.

59. Martinon F, Mayor A, Tschopp J. The inflammasomes: guardians of the body. Annu Rev Immunol 2009;27:229–65.

60. Lamkanfi M, Dixit VM. Mechanisms and functions of inflammasomes. Cell 2014; 157(5):1013–22.

61. Molgora M, Supino D, Mantovani A, et al. Tuning inflammation and immunity by the negative regulators IL-1R2 and IL-1R8. Immunol Rev 2018;281(1):233–47.

62. Mayer-Barber KD, Andrade BB, Oland SD, et al. Host-directed therapy of tuberculosis based on interleukin-1 and type I interferon crosstalk. Nature 2014; 511(7507):99–103.

63. Di Paolo NC, Shayakhmetov DM. Interleukin 1α and the inflammatory process. Nat Immunol 2016;17(8):906–13.

64. Ji DX, Yamashiro LH, Chen KJ, et al. Type I interferon-driven susceptibility to Mycobacterium tuberculosis is mediated by IL-1Ra. Nat Microbiol 2019. https://doi.org/10.1038/s41564-019-0578-3.

65. Zuñiga J, Torres-García D, Santos-Mendoza T, et al. Cellular and humoral mechanisms involved in the control of tuberculosis. Clin Dev Immunol 2012;2012: 193923.

66. Cavalli G, Dinarello CA. Treating rheumatological diseases and co-morbidities with interleukin-1 blocking therapies. Rheumatology (Oxford) 2015;54(12): 2134–44.

67. Fleischmann RM, Schechtman J, Bennett R, et al. Anakinra, a recombinant human interleukin-1 receptor antagonist (r-metHuIL-1ra), in patients with rheumatoid arthritis: a large, international, multicenter, placebo-controlled trial. Arthritis Rheum 2003;48(4):927–34.

68. Schiff MH, DiVittorio G, Tesser J, et al. The safety of anakinra in high-risk patients with active rheumatoid arthritis: six-month observations of patients with comorbid conditions. Arthritis Rheum 2004;50(6):1752–60.

69. Fleischmann RM, Tesser J, Schiff MH, et al. Safety of extended treatment with anakinra in patients with rheumatoid arthritis. Ann Rheum Dis 2006;65(8): 1006–12.

70. Genovese MC, Cohen S, Moreland L, et al. Combination therapy with etanercept and anakinra in the treatment of patients with rheumatoid arthritis who have been treated unsuccessfully with methotrexate. Arthritis Rheum 2004;50(5): 1412–9.

71. Sibley CH, Plass N, Snow J, et al. Sustained response and prevention of damage progression in patients with neonatal-onset multisystem inflammatory disease treated with anakinra: a cohort study to determine three- and five-year outcomes. Arthritis Rheum 2012;64(7):2375–86.

72. Kullenberg T, Löfqvist M, Leinonen M, et al. Long-term safety profile of anakinra in patients with severe cryopyrin-associated periodic syndromes. Rheumatology (Oxford) 2016;55(8):1499–506.
73. Galloway JB, Hyrich KL, Mercer LK, et al. The risk of serious infections in patients receiving anakinra for rheumatoid arthritis: results from the British Society for Rheumatology Biologics Register. Rheumatology (Oxford) 2011;50(7):1341–2.
74. den Broeder AA, de Jong E, Franssen MJ, et al. Observational study on efficacy, safety, and drug survival of anakinra in rheumatoid arthritis patients in clinical practice. Ann Rheum Dis 2006;65(6):760–2.
75. Ottaviani S, Moltó A, Ea H-K, et al. Efficacy of anakinra in gouty arthritis: a retrospective study of 40 cases. Arthritis Res Ther 2013;15(5):R123.
76. Settas LD, Tsimirikas G, Vosvotekas G, et al. Reactivation of pulmonary tuberculosis in a patient with rheumatoid arthritis during treatment with IL-1 receptor antagonists (anakinra). J Clin Rheumatol 2007;13(4):219–20.
77. Migkos MP, Somarakis GA, Markatseli TE, et al. Tuberculous pyomyositis in a rheumatoid arthritis patient treated with anakinra. Clin Exp Rheumatol 2015;33(5):734–6.
78. Lachmann HJ, Kone-Paut I, Kuemmerle-Deschner JB, et al. Use of canakinumab in the cryopyrin-associated periodic syndrome. N Engl J Med 2009;360(23):2416–25.
79. Ruperto N, Brunner HI, Quartier P, et al. Two randomized trials of canakinumab in systemic juvenile idiopathic arthritis. N Engl J Med 2012;367(25):2396–406.
80. De Benedetti F, Gattorno M, Anton J, et al. Canakinumab for the treatment of autoinflammatory recurrent fever syndromes. N Engl J Med 2018;378(20):1908–19.
81. Kuemmerle-Deschner JB, Hachulla E, Cartwright R, et al. Two-year results from an open-label, multicentre, phase III study evaluating the safety and efficacy of canakinumab in patients with cryopyrin-associated periodic syndrome across different severity phenotypes. Ann Rheum Dis 2011;70(12):2095–102.
82. Yokota S, Imagawa T, Nishikomori R, et al. Long-term safety and efficacy of canakinumab in cryopyrin-associated periodic syndrome: results from an open-label, phase III pivotal study in Japanese patients. Clin Exp Rheumatol 2017;35:19–26. Suppl 108(6).
83. Schlesinger N, Alten RE, Bardin T, et al. Canakinumab for acute gouty arthritis in patients with limited treatment options: results from two randomised, multicentre, active-controlled, double-blind trials and their initial extensions. Ann Rheum Dis 2012;71(11):1839–48.
84. Howard C, Noe A, Skerjanec A, et al. Safety and tolerability of canakinumab, an IL-1β inhibitor, in type 2 diabetes mellitus patients: a pooled analysis of three randomised double-blind studies. Cardiovasc Diabetol 2014;13:94.
85. Ridker PM, MacFadyen JG, Thuren T, et al. Effect of interleukin-1β inhibition with canakinumab on incident lung cancer in patients with atherosclerosis: exploratory results from a randomised, double-blind, placebo-controlled trial. Lancet 2017;390(10105):1833–42.
86. Rossi-Semerano L, Fautrel B, Wendling D, et al. Tolerance and efficacy of off-label anti-interleukin-1 treatments in France: a nationwide survey. Orphanet J Rare Dis 2015;10:19.
87. Horneff G, Schulz AC, Klotsche J, et al. Experience with etanercept, tocilizumab and interleukin-1 inhibitors in systemic onset juvenile idiopathic arthritis patients from the BIKER registry. Arthritis Res Ther 2017;19(1):256.

88. Chandrakumaran A, Malik M, Stevens MP, et al. A case report of locally invasive Aspergillus fumigatus infection in a patient on canakinumab. Eur Heart J Case Rep 2018;2(3):yty098.

89. Economides AN, Carpenter I R, Rudge JS, et al. Cytokine traps: multicomponent, high-affinity blockers of cytokine action. Nat Med 2003;9(1):47–52.

90. Dubois EA, Rissmann R, Cohen AF. Rilonacept and canakinumab. Br J Clin Pharmacol 2011;71(5):639–41.

91. Hoffman HM, Throne ML, Amar NJ, et al. Efficacy and safety of rilonacept (interleukin-1 Trap) in patients with cryopyrin-associated periodic syndromes: results from two sequential placebo-controlled studies. Arthritis Rheum 2008;58(8): 2443–52.

92. Schumacher HR, Evans RR, Saag KG, et al. Rilonacept (interleukin-1 trap) for prevention of gout flares during initiation of uric acid-lowering therapy: results from a phase III randomized, double-blind, placebo-controlled, confirmatory efficacy study. Arthritis Care Res 2012;64(10):1462–70.

93. Mitha E, Schumacher HR, Fouche L, et al. Rilonacept for gout flare prevention during initiation of uric acid-lowering therapy: results from the PRESURGE-2 international, phase 3, randomized, placebo-controlled trial. Rheumatology (Oxford) 2013;52(7):1285–92.

94. Sundy JS, Schumacher HR, Kivitz A, et al. Rilonacept for gout flare prevention in patients receiving uric acid-lowering therapy: results of RESURGE, a phase III, international safety study. J Rheumatol 2014;41(8):1703–11.

95. Mantero JC, Kishore N, Ziemek J, et al. Randomised, double-blind, placebo-controlled trial of IL1-trap, rilonacept, in systemic sclerosis. A phase I/II biomarker trial. Clin Exp Rheumatol 2018;36:146–9. Suppl 113(4).

96. Hoffman HM, Throne ML, Amar NJ, et al. Long-term efficacy and safety profile of rilonacept in the treatment of cryopryin-associated periodic syndromes: results of a 72-week open-label extension study. Clin Ther 2012;34(10):2091–103.

97. Lovell DJ, Giannini EH, Reiff AO, et al. Long-term safety and efficacy of rilonacept in patients with systemic juvenile idiopathic arthritis. Arthritis Rheum 2013; 65(9):2486–96.

98. Garg M, de Jesus AA, Chapelle D, et al. Rilonacept maintains long-term inflammatory remission in patients with deficiency of the IL-1 receptor antagonist. JCI Insight 2017;2(16). https://doi.org/10.1172/jci.insight.94838.

99. Allen JE, Maizels RM. Diversity and dialogue in immunity to helminths. Nat Rev Immunol 2011;11(6):375–88.

100. Nakayama T, Hirahara K, Onodera A, et al. Th2 cells in health and disease. Annu Rev Immunol 2017;35:53–84.

101. Rosenberg HF, Dyer KD, Foster PS. Eosinophils: changing perspectives in health and disease. Nat Rev Immunol 2013;13(1):9–22.

102. Harb H, Chatila TA. Mechanisms of dupilumab. Clin Exp Allergy 2019. https://doi.org/10.1111/cea.13491.

103. Eichenfield LF, Bieber T, Beck LA, et al. Infections in dupilumab clinical trials in atopic dermatitis: a comprehensive pooled analysis. Am J Clin Dermatol 2019; 20(3):443–56.

104. Deleuran M, Thaçi D, Beck LA, et al. Dupilumab shows long-term safety and efficacy in moderate-to-severe atopic dermatitis patients enrolled in a phase 3 open-label extension study. J Am Acad Dermatol 2019. https://doi.org/10.1016/j.jaad.2019.07.074.

105. Xiong X-F, Zhu M, Wu H-X, et al. Efficacy and safety of dupilumab for the treatment of uncontrolled asthma: a meta-analysis of randomized clinical trials. Respir Res 2019;20(1):108.

106. Bachert C, Han JK, Desrosiers M, et al. Efficacy and safety of dupilumab in patients with severe chronic rhinosinusitis with nasal polyps (LIBERTY NP SINUS-24 and LIBERTY NP SINUS-52): results from two multicentre, randomised, double-blind, placebo-controlled, parallel-group phase 3 trials. Lancet 2019; 394(10209):1638–50.

107. Schneeweiss MC, Perez-Chada L, Merola JF. Comparative safety of systemic immuno-modulatory medications in adults with atopic dermatitis. J Am Acad Dermatol 2019. https://doi.org/10.1016/j.jaad.2019.05.073.

108. Wenzel S, Castro M, Corren J, et al. Dupilumab efficacy and safety in adults with uncontrolled persistent asthma despite use of medium-to-high-dose inhaled corticosteroids plus a long-acting β2 agonist: a randomised double-blind placebo-controlled pivotal phase 2b dose-ranging trial. Lancet 2016;388(10039): 31–44.

109. Castro M, Corren J, Pavord ID, et al. Dupilumab efficacy and safety in moderate-to-severe uncontrolled asthma. N Engl J Med 2018;378(26):2486–96.

110. Rabe KF, Nair P, Brusselle G, et al. Efficacy and safety of dupilumab in glucocorticoid-dependent severe asthma. N Engl J Med 2018;378(26):2475–85.

111. Hirano I, Dellon ES, Hamilton JD, et al. Efficacy of dupilumab in a phase 2 randomized trial of adults with active eosinophilic esophagitis. Gastroenterology 2019. https://doi.org/10.1053/j.gastro.2019.09.042.

112. Thaçi D, Simpson EL, Beck LA, et al. Efficacy and safety of dupilumab in adults with moderate-to-severe atopic dermatitis inadequately controlled by topical treatments: a randomised, placebo-controlled, dose-ranging phase 2b trial. Lancet 2016;387(10013):40–52.

113. Cork MJ, Thaçi D, Eichenfield LF, et al. Dupilumab in adolescents with uncontrolled moderate-to-severe atopic dermatitis: results from a phase IIa open-label trial and subsequent phase III open-label extension. Br J Dermatol 2019. https://doi.org/10.1111/bjd.18476.

114. Ong PY, Leung DYM. Bacterial and viral infections in atopic dermatitis: a comprehensive review. Clin Rev Allergy Immunol 2016;51(3):329–37.

115. Serrano L, Patel KR, Silverberg JI. Association between atopic dermatitis and extracutaneous bacterial and mycobacterial infections: a systematic review and meta-analysis. J Am Acad Dermatol 2019;80(4):904–12.

116. Callewaert C, Nakatsuji T, Knight R, et al. IL-4Rα blockade by dupilumab decreases staphylococcus aureus colonization and increases microbial diversity in atopic dermatitis. J Invest Dermatol 2019. https://doi.org/10.1016/j.jid.2019.05.024.

117. de Wijs LEM, Bosma AL, Erler NS, et al. Effectiveness of dupilumab treatment in 95 patients with atopic dermatitis: daily practice data. Br J Dermatol 2019. https://doi.org/10.1111/bjd.18179.

118. Ivert LU, Wahlgren C-F, Ivert L, et al. Eye complications during dupilumab treatment for severe atopic dermatitis. Acta Derm Venereol 2019;99(4):375–8.

119. Ly K, Smith MP, Thibodeaux Q, et al. Dupilumab in patients with chronic hepatitis B on concomitant entecavir. JAAD Case Rep 2019;5(7):624–6.

120. Storan ER, Woolf RT, Smith CH, et al. Clearance of molluscum contagiosum virus infection in patients with atopic eczema treated with dupilumab. Br J Dermatol 2019;181(2):385–6.

121. Grubor-Bauk B, Simmons A, Mayrhofer G, et al. Impaired clearance of herpes simplex virus type 1 from mice lacking CD1d or NKT cells expressing the semi-variant V alpha 14-J alpha 281 TCR. J Immunol 2003;170(3):1430–4.
122. Gaya M, Barral P, Burbage M, et al. Initiation of antiviral B cell immunity relies on innate signals from spatially positioned NKT cells. Cell 2018;172(3):517–33.e20.
123. Akinlade B, Guttman-Yassky E, de Bruin-Weller M, et al. Conjunctivitis in dupilumab clinical trials. Br J Dermatol 2019;181(3):459–73.
124. Nahum Y, Mimouni M, Livny E, et al. Dupilumab-induced ocular surface disease (DIOSD) in patients with atopic dermatitis: clinical presentation, risk factors for development and outcomes of treatment with tacrolimus ointment. Br J Ophthalmol 2019. https://doi.org/10.1136/bjophthalmol-2019-315010.
125. Thyssen JP, de Bruin-Weller MS, Paller AS, et al. Conjunctivitis in atopic dermatitis patients with and without dupilumab therapy - international eczema council survey and opinion. J Eur Acad Dermatol Venereol 2019;33(7):1224–31.
126. Blauvelt A, Simpson EL, Tyring SK, et al. Dupilumab does not affect correlates of vaccine-induced immunity: a randomized, placebo-controlled trial in adults with moderate-to-severe atopic dermatitis. J Am Acad Dermatol 2019;80(1):158–67.e1.
127. Bel EH, Wenzel SE, Thompson PJ, et al. Oral glucocorticoid-sparing effect of mepolizumab in eosinophilic asthma. N Engl J Med 2014;371(13):1189–97.
128. Ortega HG, Liu MC, Pavord ID, et al. Mepolizumab treatment in patients with severe eosinophilic asthma. N Engl J Med 2014;371(13):1198–207.
129. Pavord ID, Chanez P, Criner GJ, et al. Mepolizumab for eosinophilic chronic obstructive pulmonary disease. N Engl J Med 2017;377(17):1613–29.
130. Wechsler ME, Akuthota P, Jayne D, et al. Mepolizumab or placebo for eosinophilic granulomatosis with polyangiitis. N Engl J Med 2017;376(20):1921–32.
131. Gupta A, Ikeda M, Geng B, et al. Long-term safety and pharmacodynamics of mepolizumab in children with severe asthma with an eosinophilic phenotype. J Allergy Clin Immunol 2019;144(5):1336–42.e7.
132. Gupta A, Pouliquen I, Austin D, et al. Subcutaneous mepolizumab in children aged 6 to 11 years with severe eosinophilic asthma. Pediatr Pulmonol 2019;54(12):1957–67.
133. Lugogo N, Domingo C, Chanez P, et al. Long-term efficacy and safety of mepolizumab in patients with severe eosinophilic asthma: a multi-center, open-label, phase IIIb study. Clin Ther 2016;38(9):2058–70.e1.
134. Khurana S, Brusselle GG, Bel EH, et al. Long-term safety and clinical benefit of mepolizumab in patients with the most severe eosinophilic asthma: the COSMEX study. Clin Ther 2019;41(10):2041–56.e5.
135. Khatri S, Moore W, Gibson PG, et al. Assessment of the long-term safety of mepolizumab and durability of clinical response in patients with severe eosinophilic asthma. J Allergy Clin Immunol 2019;143(5):1742–51.e7.
136. Pertzov B, Unterman A, Shtraichman O, et al. Efficacy and safety of mepolizumab in a real-world cohort of patients with severe eosinophilic asthma. J Asthma 2019;1–6. https://doi.org/10.1080/02770903.2019.1658208.
137. Rothenberg ME, Klion AD, Roufosse FE, et al. Treatment of patients with the hypereosinophilic syndrome with mepolizumab. N Engl J Med 2008;358(12):1215–28.
138. Roufosse FE, Kahn J-E, Gleich GJ, et al. Long-term safety of mepolizumab for the treatment of hypereosinophilic syndromes. J Allergy Clin Immunol 2013;131(2):461–7.e1-5.

139. Agarwal R, Chakrabarti A, Shah A, et al. Allergic bronchopulmonary aspergillosis: review of literature and proposal of new diagnostic and classification criteria. Clin Exp Allergy 2013;43(8):850–73.

140. Altman MC, Lenington J, Bronson S, et al. Combination omalizumab and mepolizumab therapy for refractory allergic bronchopulmonary aspergillosis. J Allergy Clin Immunol Pract 2017;5(4):1137–9.

141. Terashima T, Shinozaki T, Iwami E, et al. A case of allergic bronchopulmonary aspergillosis successfully treated with mepolizumab. BMC Pulm Med 2018; 18(1):53.

142. Tsubouchi H, Tsuchida S, Yanagi S, et al. Successful treatment with mepolizumab in a case of allergic bronchopulmonary aspergillosis complicated with nontuberculous mycobacterial infection. Respir Med Case Rep 2019;28:100875.

143. Hirota S, Kobayashi Y, Ishiguro T, et al. Allergic bronchopulmonary aspergillosis successfully treated with mepolizumab: case report and review of the literature. Respir Med Case Rep 2019;26:59–62.

144. Spergel JM, Rothenberg ME, Collins MH, et al. Reslizumab in children and adolescents with eosinophilic esophagitis: results of a double-blind, randomized, placebo-controlled trial. J Allergy Clin Immunol 2012;129(2):456–63, 463.e1-3.

145. Markowitz JE, Jobe L, Miller M, et al. Safety and efficacy of reslizumab for children and adolescents with eosinophilic esophagitis treated for 9 years. J Pediatr Gastroenterol Nutr 2018;66(6):893–7.

146. Virchow JC, Katial R, Brusselle GG, et al. Safety of reslizumab in uncontrolled asthma with eosinophilia: a pooled analysis from 6 trials. J Allergy Clin Immunol Pract 2019. https://doi.org/10.1016/j.jaip.2019.07.038.

147. Kolbeck R, Kozhich A, Koike M, et al. MEDI-563, a humanized anti-IL-5 receptor alpha mAb with enhanced antibody-dependent cell-mediated cytotoxicity function. J Allergy Clin Immunol 2010;125(6):1344–53.e2.

148. Brightling CE, Bleecker ER, Panettieri RA, et al. Benralizumab for chronic obstructive pulmonary disease and sputum eosinophilia: a randomised, double-blind, placebo-controlled, phase 2a study. Lancet Respir Med 2014; 2(11):891–901.

149. Bleecker ER, FitzGerald JM, Chanez P, et al. Efficacy and safety of benralizumab for patients with severe asthma uncontrolled with high-dosage inhaled corticosteroids and long-acting β2-agonists (SIROCCO): a randomised, multicentre, placebo-controlled phase 3 trial. Lancet 2016;388(10056):2115–27.

150. FitzGerald JM, Bleecker ER, Nair P, et al. Benralizumab, an anti-interleukin-5 receptor α monoclonal antibody, as add-on treatment for patients with severe, uncontrolled, eosinophilic asthma (CALIMA): a randomised, double-blind, placebo-controlled phase 3 trial. Lancet 2016;388(10056):2128–41.

151. Nair P, Wenzel S, Rabe KF, et al. Oral glucocorticoid-sparing effect of benralizumab in severe asthma. N Engl J Med 2017;376(25):2448–58.

152. Ferguson GT, FitzGerald JM, Bleecker ER, et al. Benralizumab for patients with mild to moderate, persistent asthma (BISE): a randomised, double-blind, placebo-controlled, phase 3 trial. Lancet Respir Med 2017;5(7):568–76.

153. Busse WW, Bleecker ER, FitzGerald JM, et al. Long-term safety and efficacy of benralizumab in patients with severe, uncontrolled asthma: 1-year results from the BORA phase 3 extension trial. Lancet Respir Med 2019;7(1):46–59.

154. Criner GJ, Celli BR, Brightling CE, et al. Benralizumab for the prevention of COPD exacerbations. N Engl J Med 2019;381(11):1023–34.

155. Tian B-P, Zhang G-S, Lou J, et al. Efficacy and safety of benralizumab for eosinophilic asthma: a systematic review and meta-analysis of randomized controlled trials. J Asthma 2018;55(9):956–65.

156. Liu W, Ma X, Zhou W. Adverse events of benralizumab in moderate to severe eosinophilic asthma: a meta-analysis. Medicine (Baltimore) 2019;98(22): e15868.

157. Mishra AK, Sahu KK, James A. Disseminated herpes zoster following treatment with benralizumab. Clin Respir J 2019;13(3):189–91.

158. Zeitlin PL, Leong M, Cole J, et al. Benralizumab does not impair antibody response to seasonal influenza vaccination in adolescent and young adult patients with moderate to severe asthma: results from the Phase IIIb ALIZE trial. J Asthma Allergy 2018;11:181–92.

159. Davies AM, Allan EG, Keeble AH, et al. Allosteric mechanism of action of the therapeutic anti-IgE antibody omalizumab. J Biol Chem 2017;292(24):9975–87.

160. Boulet LP, Chapman KR, Côté J, et al. Inhibitory effects of an anti-IgE antibody E25 on allergen-induced early asthmatic response. Am J Respir Crit Care Med 1997;155(6):1835–40.

161. Fahy JV, Fleming HE, Wong HH, et al. The effect of an anti-IgE monoclonal antibody on the early- and late-phase responses to allergen inhalation in asthmatic subjects. Am J Respir Crit Care Med 1997;155(6):1828–34.

162. Humbert M, Busse W, Hanania NA, et al. Omalizumab in asthma: an update on recent developments. J Allergy Clin Immunol Pract 2014;2(5):525–36.e1.

163. Milgrom H, Fowler-Taylor A, Vidaurre CF, et al. Safety and tolerability of omalizumab in children with allergic (IgE-mediated) asthma. Curr Med Res Opin 2011; 27(1):163–9.

164. Corren J, Casale TB, Lanier B, et al. Safety and tolerability of omalizumab. Clin Exp Allergy 2009;39(6):788–97.

165. McCormack PL. Omalizumab: a review of its use in patients with chronic spontaneous urticaria. Drugs 2014;74(14):1693–9.

166. Teach SJ, Gill MA, Togias A, et al. Preseasonal treatment with either omalizumab or an inhaled corticosteroid boost to prevent fall asthma exacerbations. J Allergy Clin Immunol 2015;136(6):1476–85.

167. Gern JE. The ABCs of rhinoviruses, wheezing, and asthma. J Virol 2010;84(15): 7418–26.

168. Jartti T, Gern JE. Role of viral infections in the development and exacerbation of asthma in children. J Allergy Clin Immunol 2017;140(4):895–906.

169. Busse WW, Morgan WJ, Gergen PJ, et al. Randomized trial of omalizumab (anti-IgE) for asthma in inner-city children. N Engl J Med 2011;364(11):1005–15.

170. Esquivel A, Busse WW, Calatroni A, et al. Effects of omalizumab on rhinovirus infections, illnesses, and exacerbations of asthma. Am J Respir Crit Care Med 2017;196(8):985–92.

171. Gill MA, Liu AH, Calatroni A, et al. Enhanced plasmacytoid dendritic cell antiviral responses after omalizumab. J Allergy Clin Immunol 2018;141(5):1735–43.e9.

172. Voskamp AL, Gillman A, Symons K, et al. Clinical efficacy and immunologic effects of omalizumab in allergic bronchopulmonary aspergillosis. J Allergy Clin Immunol Pract 2015;3(2):192–9.

173. Perisson C, Destruys L, Grenet D, et al. Omalizumab treatment for allergic bronchopulmonary aspergillosis in young patients with cystic fibrosis. Respir Med 2017;133:12–5.

174. Li J-X, Fan L-C, Li M-H, et al. Beneficial effects of omalizumab therapy in allergic bronchopulmonary aspergillosis: a synthesis review of published literature. Respir Med 2017;122:33–42.
175. Cooper PJ, Ayre G, Martin C, et al. Geohelminth infections: a review of the role of IgE and assessment of potential risks of anti-IgE treatment. Allergy 2008;63(4): 409–17.
176. Gurish MF, Bryce PJ, Tao H, et al. IgE enhances parasite clearance and regulates mast cell responses in mice infected with Trichinella spiralis. J Immunol 2004;172(2):1139–45.
177. Finkelman FD, Shea-Donohue T, Morris SC, et al. Interleukin-4- and interleukin-13-mediated host protection against intestinal nematode parasites. Immunol Rev 2004;201:139–55.
178. Savioli L, Albonico M. Soil-transmitted helminthiasis. Nat Rev Microbiol 2004; 2(8):618–9.
179. Cruz AA, Lima F, Sarinho E, et al. Safety of anti-immunoglobulin E therapy with omalizumab in allergic patients at risk of geohelminth infection. Clin Exp Allergy 2007;37(2):197–207.
180. Skiepko R, Zietkowski Z, Skiepko U, et al. Echinococcus multilocularis infection in a patient treated with omalizumab. J Investig Allergol Clin Immunol 2013; 23(3):199–200.

Infectious Complications of Immune Checkpoint Inhibitors

Michael S. Abers, MD[a], Michail S. Lionakis, MD, ScD[b],*

KEYWORDS

- Checkpoint inhibitors • Infection • Infectious diseases • Immunosuppression
- Immunotherapy • Immune checkpoint

KEY POINTS

- The clearance of both tumors and microbes depends on highly coordinated immune responses that are sufficiently potent to kill malignant or microbial cells while avoiding immunopathology from an overly exuberant inflammatory response.
- A molecular understanding of the immune pathways that regulate these immune responses paved the way for the development of checkpoint inhibitors (CPIs) as a therapeutic strategy to boost endogenous antitumor immunity.
- CPIs have demonstrated survival benefits across a wide spectrum of human cancers.
- Immune-related adverse events (irAEs) have emerged as a major source of morbidity and even mortality in patients who receive CPIs.
- Importantly, irAEs frequently require immunosuppressive therapies, such as corticosteroids and infliximab, which predispose to subsequent infection.

INTRODUCTION

Increasingly, basic discoveries in cancer biology have revealed a critical role for the immune system in controlling tumor development, persistence, and progression. A deeper understanding of the mechanisms responsible for antitumor host defense has led to the discovery of the immunologic checkpoint molecules cytotoxic T-lymphocyte associated protein 4 (CTLA-4), programmed cell death protein

Funding source: This work was supported in part by the Division of Intramural Research (DIR) of the National Institute of Allergy and Infectious Diseases (NIAID).
[a] Fungal Pathogenesis Section, Laboratory of Clinical Immunology and Microbiology (LCIM), National Institute of Allergy and Infectious Diseases (NIAID), National Institutes of Health (NIH), 9000 Rockville Pike, Building 10/Room 11C116, Bethesda, MD 20892, USA; [b] Fungal Pathogenesis Section, Laboratory of Clinical Immunology and Microbiology (LCIM), National Institute of Allergy and Infectious Diseases (NIAID), National Institutes of Health (NIH), 9000 Rockville Pike, Building 10/Room 12C103A, Bethesda, MD 20892, USA
* Corresponding author.
E-mail address: lionakism@mail.nih.gov

1 (PD-1), and PD-1 ligand (PD-L1). The signaling pathways triggered by these molecules play a key role in modulating T-cell activity. Upon host recognition of cancer cells and microbes, the immune response must be finely regulated to promote the clearance of malignant or microbial cells while avoiding damage to host tissues. The risk of immune-mediated damage to the host is particularly heightened when the inciting event is slowly cleared, thus exposing host tissues to a greater risk of inflammatory injury. In this context, host cells increase their expression of checkpoint molecules, which can serve as a "brake" on T-cell activity, protecting the host against an overly exuberant, unchecked immune response. Experimental and clinical studies have demonstrated that tumors are able to increase the expression of CTLA-4 and/or PD-1/PD-L1, thereby evading immune clearance. Monoclonal antibodies that inhibit these checkpoint molecules increase T-cell activity, which promotes tumor clearance. The therapeutic efficacy of checkpoint inhibitors (CPIs) in oncologic patients is now well established with evidence of prolonged survival in numerous randomized clinical trials that span a wide spectrum of malignancies and patient populations. More recently, concern has been raised by a growing recognition of potential adverse effects associated with immune checkpoint blockade. Indeed, the consequences of unleashing T-cell activity in an antigen-nonspecific manner are evident by an approximately 40% risk of immune-related adverse events (irAEs) in CPI-treated individuals.

From an infectious disease standpoint, the treatment of irAEs with systemic immunosuppressive therapies raises the risk of subsequent infection development. In addition, emerging data support a potential direct link between administration of CPIs and increased risk of certain infections. In this mini-review, the authors outline how CPIs may heighten the risk of infection, via either direct CPI effects on immune pathways that are critical for infection surveillance or indirect causes by the immunosuppressive effects of therapies administered to treat CPI-associated irAEs. A better understanding of the interplay between CPIs and infection risk may help devise strategies for better recognition, diagnosis, and treatment of infections in CPI-treated patients with cancer.

MECHANISM OF ACTION OF CHECKPOINT INHIBITORS

In the peripheral tissues, foreign antigen is taken up and processed by antigen-presenting cells (APCs), which load antigen onto major histocompatibility complex (MHC) molecules. T-cell activation occurs when a naïve T cell recognizes its specific antigen complexed with an MHC molecule on the surface of an APC (signal 1). In addition to signal 1, further stimulatory input to T cells is provided by the engagement of CD28 on T cells with CD80 (B7-1) or CD86 (B7-2) on APCs.[1,2] This interaction is often referred to as "costimulation" or signal 2. Importantly, costimulation is modulated by a regulatory process that prevents the detrimental consequences that would result from uncontrolled T-cell activation. Specifically, CD28 signaling, in addition to providing stimulatory input to T cells, simultaneously triggers the expression of CTLA-4 on the surface of T cells. CTLA-4 is antagonistic to CD28 by competing for CD80 and CD86 binding sites.[2] The balance between T-cell activation via CD28 and inhibition through CTLA-4 provides T cells with the capacity to self-control their own activity. Blockade of CTLA-4 with the monoclonal antibody ipilimumab removes this "brake" on T-cell activity, unleashing T cells to kill cancer cells. Importantly, ipilimumab boosts not only the activation of tumor-specific T cells but also T cells that target other antigens, including self-antigens. Thus, autoimmunity in a variety of host tissues can develop as an off-target consequence of CTLA-4 blockade.

Distinct from the CTLA-4 pathway, signaling can be triggered by the interaction of PD-1 on T cells with PD-L1 on host tissues. This pathway is triggered when T cells at the site of infection or cancer release proinflammatory cytokines, which trigger the expression of PD-L1 by host tissues.[3] Ligation of PD-1 by PD-L1 down-modulates T-cell activity, thereby protecting host tissues from immune-mediated damage. Inhibitors of PD-1 (ie, nivolumab, pembrolizumab) and PD-L1 (ie, atezolizumab, avelumab, durvalumab) have been shown to prolong survival in a variety of human malignancies. Similar to CTLA-4 inhibitors, the use of PD-1/PD-L1 blockers has also been associated with an expanding number of autoimmune toxicities.

ROLE OF TARGETING THE CYTOTOXIC T-LYMPHOCYTE ASSOCIATED PROTEIN4 AND PROGRAMMED CELL DEATH PROTEIN 1/PROGRAMMED CELL DEATH PROTEIN 1 LIGAND PATHWAYS IN HOST DEFENSE AGAINST INFECTION

Both the CTLA-4 and the PD-1/PD-L1 pathways have been extensively studied in animal models of acute and chronic infection. Although the role of these signaling pathways varies depending on pathogen-, host-, cell-, organ-, and context-specific factors, checkpoint blockade generally promotes pathogen clearance and, in many experimental models, improves host survival. The authors have recently critically reviewed the literature on the therapeutic potential of CPIs in the management of infections (especially those that are chronic).[4] Although recent reports have ignited enthusiasm for developing CPIs as adjunctive immunotherapies to treat infection,[5,6] a cautious approach is warranted given the evidence to suggest that checkpoint blockade may worsen outcomes in a subset of infections. The authors summarize their current understanding of the infectious complications associated with the use of CPIs in later discussion.

THE SPECTRUM OF INFECTIOUS COMPLICATIONS DURING CHECKPOINT INHIBITORS THERAPY

Few studies to date have comprehensively investigated the risk of infection in CPI-treated patients, and much of the available literature is limited by uncontrolled study designs and lack of details regarding microbiologic cause, diagnostic methods used to diagnose infection, timing of infection relative to CPI use, and the frequency of concomitant risk factors for infection. The largest and most informative study to date reported the experience at Memorial Sloan Kettering Cancer Center (MSKCC) in treating 740 patients with melanoma with CPIs.[7] This study evaluated the incidence of serious infectious complications, defined as infection requiring hospitalization and/or the use of parenteral antimicrobials that occurred during or within 1 year following the use CPIs. Overall, serious infections occurred in 7% of patients. The time interval between CPI exposure and the onset of infection ranged from 6 to 491 days with 80% of cases occurring during the first 6 months of therapy. Infectious episodes were fatal in 17% of patients. Most infections (85%) were caused by bacteria, with bacteremia reported in 28% of cases. Pneumonia and intraabdominal infections were the most common infectious syndromes. Most of the remaining infections were caused by herpesviruses (varicella zoster virus [VZV], cytomegalovirus [CMV], and Epstein-Barr virus) or opportunistic fungi (*Pneumocystis jirovecii*, *Aspergillus*, and *Candida*). A single case of *Strongyloides* hyperinfection syndrome was also reported. Corticosteroid exposure, defined as ≥10 mg/d of prednisone for ≥10 days, was identified in 85% of patients who experienced serious infectious complications. Of note, despite a median dose of 40 mg administered for a median duration of 60 days, only 42% of corticosteroid-treated patients had received prophylaxis against *P jirovecii* infection. Differences in the incidence of infection between the various CPI regimens were largely explained by their propensity to cause irAEs requiring immunosuppressive therapy.[7]

In another study of 167 Japanese patients who received the PD-1 inhibitor nivolumab for the management of non–small cell lung cancer, infections occurred in 19% of patients, developing a mean of 90 days after the administration of nivolumab.[8] No infection-related deaths were reported. Pulmonary infections accounted for most cases and were typically caused by community-acquired bacterial (*Streptococcus pneumoniae, Haemophilus influenzae, Staphylococcus aureus*) or viral (influenza) pathogens. Two patients developed VZV infections, including 1 case of disseminated infection. Opportunistic fungal infections occurred in 2 patients, including 1 with esophageal candidiasis and another with presumed invasive pulmonary aspergillosis (IPA) diagnosed by the growth of *Aspergillus* in bronchoalveolar lavage (BAL) fluid. Because of substantial challenges in the diagnosis of IPA, the possibility remains that *Aspergillus* growth reflected colonization or contamination of BAL fluid rather than invasive infection. In multivariate analysis, diabetes was the only host factor associated with the development of infection. Corticosteroid exposure, defined as $\geq$5 mg/d, was noted in half of patients and was not associated with the development of infection. Of note, in 11 patients with pneumonia, no pathogen was identified, and the diagnosis of infection was based on clinical grounds alone. In these cases, the investigators could not rule out the possibility of CPI-induced pneumonitis, a well-described complication of CPI reported in approximately 5% of patients with lung cancer who receive nivolumab.[9–11] This observation raises a broader clinical challenge that may be encountered in the setting of CPI treatment. It is often difficult to differentiate between a pulmonary (or intestinal) CPI-associated irAE and an infection in the lungs (or the colon); occasionally both may coexist. Because treatments of the aforementioned pathologic conditions are different, a thorough diagnostic workup and a high index of clinical suspicion are warranted in such scenarios.

Another important clinical lesson that emerges from these studies is that most life-threatening and opportunistic infectious complications that arise during CPI therapy are likely attributable to immunosuppressive agents used in the management of irAEs. Indeed, in the MSKCC study, both corticosteroids and infliximab were associated with an increased risk of infection. Importantly, irAEs develop in ~40% of CPI-treated patients, many of whom require immunosuppressive therapy. Numerous professional societies have issued guidelines to facilitate the management of irAEs.[12–15] The mainstay of therapy for irAEs involves the use of high-dose corticosteroids (ie, equivalent of 0.5 mg/kg/d of prednisone for mild irAEs and 1–2 mg/kg/d for severe irAEs). Patients who fail to respond to corticosteroids within 1 week of therapy typically receive tumor necrosis factor-α inhibition with infliximab. It is important for clinicians to recognize the substantial burden of infectious complications that can complicate therapy with corticosteroids and infliximab, which impair key immune surveillance pathways (reviewed elsewhere[16,17]). The recent reports of using other immunosuppressive treatments for severe irAEs (ie, alemtuzumab, abatacept), which can independently increase the risk of certain opportunistic infections, warrants surveillance and awareness by clinicians in this rapidly moving field.[18,19] Collectively, appropriate use of antimicrobial prophylaxis and monitoring for infectious complications are critically important in the management of these patients.

SPECIFIC INFECTIOUS COMPLICATIONS THAT MAY RELATE TO CHECKPOINT INHIBITORS
Human Immunodeficiency Virus

There is strong evidence that human immunodeficiency virus (HIV) infection upregulates the expression of coinhibitory molecules, thereby promoting T-cell exhaustion.[20–23] Interestingly, PD-1$^+$ CD4$^+$ cells represent the greatest virologic reservoir in patients who achieve virologic control on antiretrovirals.[24] Although experimental studies in nonhuman primates have suggested a potential role for PD-1 blockade in boosting virologic clearance,[25] this hypothesis has not been tested in appropriately powered clinical studies of HIV-infected patients. Notably, HIV infection does not appear to compromise the antitumor efficacy of CPIs, and the incidence of CPI-related irAEs in HIV-infected patients is comparable to that observed in HIV-uninfected patients.[26] Furthermore, CPIs do not appear to have detrimental effects on virologic control when administered to HIV-infected patients.[27]

Hepatitis B Virus

During chronic infection with hepatitis B virus (HBV), PD-1 expression is upregulated on T and B cells.[28,29] Ex vivo studies have demonstrated that inhibition of either CTLA-4 or PD-1/PD-L1 signaling enhances the function HBV-specific cytotoxic T cells (CTLs) and promotes humoral immunity.[29–31] These studies have suggested that CPI therapy might improve virologic clearance in chronically infected patients. However, enthusiasm for the therapeutic potential of CPIs against HBV has been tempered by recent evidence of an inverse relationship between PD-1 expression on CTLs and the risk of subsequent flares of hepatitis in patients with chronic HBV infection.[32] Nonetheless, studies of HBV-infected patients who received nivolumab for the management of hepatocellular carcinoma have not reported clinically significant hepatitis flares as a complication of nivolumab therapy.[33,34] Although 1 study found that nivolumab increased HBV viral load in 9% of patients, these changes were not associated with biochemical or clinical evidence of liver injury.[34] Future efforts to identify the subset of patients in whom CPIs might predispose to hepatitis flares are critically needed.

Cytomegalovirus

CMV infection has been reported in patients with CPI-induced colitis that is refractory to corticosteroids and infliximab. In 1 report of 5 patients with ipilimumab-induced colitis refractory to corticosteroids, 4 of whom also received infliximab, CMV was identified by polymerase chain reaction in blood or colonic biopsy specimens in all 5 patients. Immunohistochemistry performed on colonic biopsy specimens demonstrated strong immunoreactivity in 2 patients and absence of reactivity in the remaining 3 cases.[35] An additional case of CMV hepatitis has been reported in an ipilimumab-treated patient who developed hepatitis in the context of receiving corticosteroids and infliximab for CPI-associated autoimmune colitis.[36]

Bacterial Infections

In addition to 10 cases of Clostridioidesdifficile–associated diarrhea (CDAD) reported in the MSKCC study,[7] a potential association between CPI therapy and CDAD was recently suggested by a case series of 5 patients who developed CDAD while undergoing treatment of CPI-induced colitis.[37] Notably, CDAD occurred in the absence of prior antibiotic exposure in 4 of these 5 patients. Future studies are necessary to examine the direct impact of CPI therapy on CDAD risk however, especially in light of the high burden of CDAD in patients with cancer.[38] An additional layer of complexity to this potential association is the observation that colitis itself (ie, independent of immunosuppressive therapy) predisposes to CDAD, analogous to the risk of CDAD in patients with inflammatory bowel disease.[39]

Preclinical models have suggested that PD-L1 blockade may worsen clinical outcomes during Listeria infections.[40] The relevance of this finding to human patients is currently unclear given the rarity of listeriosis in patients with cancer. However, Listeria infections should be considered in patients who develop meningitis and/or encephalitis in the context of CPI treatment.

Mycobacterial Infections

In preclinical models of tuberculosis, PD-1–deficient animals are highly susceptible to infection with *Mycobacterium tuberculosis*. The increased mortality in these animals is driven by excessive interferon-γ production by type 1 helper T (Th1) cells.. The observation that these mice can be rescued by depletion of CD4+ T cells combined with the established importance of Th1 cells in controlling *M tuberculosis* highlights the importance of striking a fine balance in T-cell reactivity to promote pathogen clearance while avoiding tissue immunopathology.[41–43] The hypothesis that the PD-1 pathway is protective against tuberculosis and that inhibition of PD-1/PD-L1 signaling may be detrimental has been suggested by several case reports of tuberculosis developing in temporal association with the initiation of CPIs.[44] Furthermore, preliminary evidence suggests that previous observations in PD-1–deficient mice may be relevant to human patients treated with PD-1/PD-L1 blockers. In a recent report by Barber and colleagues,[43] administration of the PD-1 inhibitor pembrolizumab to a patient with Merkel cell carcinoma led to an increased frequency of tuberculosis-specific Th1 cells in the peripheral blood, which was temporally associated with the onset of reactivation pulmonary tuberculosis. Although rare cases of tuberculosis reactivation have been reported in patients who receive CPIs, the magnitude of this risk is likely quite small. Indeed, in a French study of 908 patients who received PD-1 or PD-L1 inhibitors between 2013 and 2017, only 2 cases of tuberculosis were identified.[45] Moreover, a recent systematic review of the literature identified only 14 cases of CPI-related tuberculosis.[44] In most cases, reactivation tuberculosis developed within 3 to 6 months of CPI initiation and was limited to pulmonary involvement. Nearly half of all patients were asymptomatic at the time of diagnosis with tuberculosis. Considerable heterogeneity in the management of these patients makes it challenging to draw conclusions about the optimal management of CPI-related tuberculosis. Of note, however, CPI therapy was continued following the onset of tuberculosis in 4 patients, none of whom developed progressive or uncontrolled infection. In an additional 3 patients, CPIs were temporarily held but later restarted after several weeks of tuberculosis therapy without recurrence of infection.[44] Thus, the diagnosis of tuberculosis in CPI-treated patients should not necessarily preclude future use of CPIs assuming microbiologic control with the use of antimycobacterial agents. In summary, PD-1/PD-L1 blockade may enhance host susceptibility to reactivation tuberculosis. Although further studies evaluating the PD-1/PD-L1 pathway in human antituberculous immunity are necessary, it is reasonable to consider screening for latent tuberculosis before the initiation of CPIs. Management decisions in patients who test positive should involve collaboration between infectious disease specialists and oncologists.

COMPLICATIONS OF CHECKPOINT INHIBITORS–INDUCED NEUTROPENIA

In addition to concerns about "on-target" effects of CPIs on host immunity, concern has also arisen regarding indirect effect of CPIs on susceptibility to infection. To that end, CPI-induced neutropenia has been reported in 11 patients.[46] Neutropenia is typically profound, and the median duration of time with an absolute neutrophil count less than 500/mm^3 is 17 days. In 55% of these cases, neutropenia was complicated by infection. Granulocyte colony-stimulating factor (G-CSF) therapy was the mainstay of treatment, and complete neutrophil recovery was generally observed.[46]

Further studies with prospective monitoring are critically needed to capture the full spectrum of infectious complications that arise during the course of CPI therapy.

Efforts to determine tumor- and drug-specific patterns of infectious complications will likely require large multicenter studies.

SUMMARY

Although CPIs have exhibited the capacity to substantially prolong survival in patients with advanced malignancy, CPI-associated toxicity is frequently encountered and often requires immunosuppressive therapy with corticosteroids and/or infliximab, and/or other biologics. Similar to the use of these agents in other clinical settings, their use is associated with an increased risk of infection. When clinically indicated, antimicrobial prophylaxis and careful monitoring may improve clinical outcomes. In addition to infections that arise during immunosuppression given for CPI-associated irAEs, CPIs may also directly predispose to certain infections in a subset of patients, such as tuberculosis. Surveillance to detect infections in CPI-treated patients and systematic reporting of these cases will play a critical role in uncovering the clinical settings in which CPIs may lead to adverse patient outcomes.

DISCLOSURE

The authors have no conflicts of interests to disclose.

REFERENCES

1. Teft WA, Kirchhof MG, Madrenas J. A molecular perspective of CTLA-4 function. Annu Rev Immunol 2006;24:65–97.
2. Callahan MK, Wolchok JD, Allison JP. Anti-CTLA-4 antibody therapy: immune monitoring during clinical development of a novel immunotherapy. Semin Oncol 2010;37:473–84.
3. Keir ME, Liang SC, Guleria I, et al. Tissue expression of PD-L1 mediates peripheral T cell tolerance. J Exp Med 2006;203:883–95.
4. Abers MS, Lionakis MS, Kontoyiannis DP. Checkpoint inhibition and infectious diseases: a good thing? Trends Mol Med 2019;25(12):1080–93.
5. Cortese I, Muranski P, Enose-Akahata Y, et al. Pembrolizumab treatment for progressive multifocal leukoencephalopathy. N Engl J Med 2019;380:1597–605.
6. Hoang E, Bartlett NL, Goyal MS, et al. Progressive multifocal leukoencephalopathy treated with nivolumab. J Neurovirol 2019;25:284–7.
7. Del Castillo M, Romero FA, Argüello E, et al. The spectrum of serious infections among patients receiving immune checkpoint blockade for the treatment of melanoma. Clin Infect Dis 2016;63:1490–3.
8. Fujita K, Kim YH, Kanai O, et al. Emerging concerns of infectious diseases in lung cancer patients receiving immune checkpoint inhibitor therapy. Respir Med 2019; 146:66–70.
9. Cadranel J, Canellas A, Matton L, et al. Pulmonary complications of immune checkpoint inhibitors in patients with nonsmall cell lung cancer. Eur Respir Rev 2019;28 [pii:190058].
10. Nishino M, Giobbie-Hurder A, Hatabu H, et al. Incidence of programmed cell death 1 inhibitor-related pneumonitis in patients with advanced cancer: a systematic review and meta-analysis. JAMA Oncol 2016;2:1607–16.
11. Sears CR, Peikert T, Possick JD, et al. Knowledge gaps and research priorities in immune checkpoint inhibitor-related pneumonitis. An official American Thoracic Society research statement. Am J Respir Crit Care Med 2019;200:e31–43.

12. Champiat S, Lambotte O, Barreau E, et al. Management of immune checkpoint blockade dysimmune toxicities: a collaborative position paper. Ann Oncol 2016;27:559–74.
13. Haanen JBAG, Carbonnel F, Robert C, et al. Management of toxicities from immunotherapy: ESMO clinical practice guidelines for diagnosis, treatment and follow-up. Ann Oncol 2017;28:iv119–42.
14. Brahmer JR, Lacchetti C, Schneider BJ, et al. Management of immune-related adverse events in patients treated with immune checkpoint inhibitor therapy: American Society of Clinical Oncology clinical practice guideline. J Clin Oncol 2018;36:1714–68.
15. Puzanov I, Diab A, Abdallah K, et al. Managing toxicities associated with immune checkpoint inhibitors: consensus recommendations from the Society for Immunotherapy of Cancer (SITC) Toxicity Management Working Group. J Immunother Cancer 2017;5:95.
16. Lionakis MS, Kontoyiannis DP. Glucocorticoids and invasive fungal infections. Lancet 2003;362:1828–38.
17. Winthrop KL. Risk and prevention of tuberculosis and other serious opportunistic infections associated with the inhibition of tumor necrosis factor. Nat Clin Pract Rheumatol 2006;2:602–10.
18. Salem J-E, Allenbach Y, Vozy A, et al. Abatacept for severe immune checkpoint inhibitor-associated myocarditis. N Engl J Med 2019;380:2377–9.
19. Esfahani K, Buhlaiga N, Thébault P, et al. Alemtuzumab for immune-related myocarditis due to PD-1 therapy. N Engl J Med 2019;380:2375–6.
20. Day CL, Kaufmann DE, Kiepiela P, et al. PD-1 expression on HIV-specific T cells is associated with T-cell exhaustion and disease progression. Nature 2006;443: 350–4.
21. Trautmann L, Janbazian L, Chomont N, et al. Upregulation of PD-1 expression on HIV-specific CD8+ T cells leads to reversible immune dysfunction. Nat Med 2006;12:1198–202.
22. Trabattoni D, Saresella M, Biasin M, et al. B7-H1 is up-regulated in HIV infection and is a novel surrogate marker of disease progression. Blood 2003;101: 2514–20.
23. Grabmeier-Pfistershammer K, Steinberger P, Rieger A, et al. Identification of PD-1 as a unique marker for failing immune reconstitution in HIV-1-infected patients on treatment. J Acquir Immune Defic Syndr 2011;56:118–24.
24. Banga R, Procopio FA, Noto A, et al. PD-1(+) and follicular helper T cells are responsible for persistent HIV-1 transcription in treated aviremic individuals. Nat Med 2016;22:754–61.
25. Mylvaganam GH, Chea LS, Tharp GK, et al. Combination anti-PD-1 and antiretroviral therapy provides therapeutic benefit against SIV. JCI Insight 2018;3 [pii: 122940].
26. Cook MR, Kim C. Safety and efficacy of immune checkpoint inhibitor therapy in patients with HIV infection and advanced-stage cancer: a systematic review. JAMA Oncol 2019;5:1049–54.
27. Abbar B, Baron M, Katlama C, et al. Immune checkpoint inhibitors in people living with HIV: what about anti-HIV effects? AIDS 2020;34(2):167–75.
28. Boni C, Fisicaro P, Valdatta C, et al. Characterization of hepatitis B virus (HBV)-specific T-cell dysfunction in chronic HBV infection. J Virol 2007;81:4215–25.
29. Salimzadeh L, Le Bert N, Dutertre C-A, et al. PD-1 blockade partially recovers dysfunctional virus-specific B cells in chronic hepatitis B infection. J Clin Invest 2018;128:4573–87.

30. Fisicaro P, Valdatta C, Massari M, et al. Antiviral intrahepatic T-cell responses can be restored by blocking programmed death-1 pathway in chronic hepatitis B. Gastroenterology 2010;138:682–93, 693.e1.
31. Schurich A, Khanna P, Lopes AR, et al. Role of the coinhibitory receptor cytotoxic T lymphocyte antigen-4 on apoptosis-prone CD8 T cells in persistent hepatitis B virus infection. Hepatology 2011;53:1494–503.
32. Rivino L, Le Bert N, Gill US, et al. Hepatitis B virus-specific T cells associate with viral control upon nucleos(t)ide-analogue therapy discontinuation. J Clin Invest 2018;128:668–81.
33. El-Khoueiry AB, Sangro B, Yau T, et al. Nivolumab in patients with advanced hepatocellular carcinoma (CheckMate 040): an open-label, non-comparative, phase 1/2 dose escalation and expansion trial. Lancet 2017;389:2492–502.
34. Yau T, Hsu C, Kim T-Y, et al. Nivolumab in advanced hepatocellular carcinoma: sorafenib-experienced Asian cohort analysis. J Hepatol 2019;71:543–52.
35. Franklin C, Rooms I, Fiedler M, et al. Cytomegalovirus reactivation in patients with refractory checkpoint inhibitor-induced colitis. Eur J Cancer 2017;86:248–56.
36. Uslu U, Agaimy A, Hundorfean G, et al. Autoimmune colitis and subsequent CMV-induced hepatitis after treatment with ipilimumab. J Immunother 2015;38:212–5.
37. Babacan NA, Tanvetyanon T. Superimposed Clostridium difficile infection during checkpoint inhibitor immunotherapy-induced colitis. J Immunother 2019;42:350–3.
38. Gupta A, Tariq R, Frank RD, et al. Trends in the incidence and outcomes of hospitalized cancer patients with Clostridium difficile infection: a nationwide analysis. J Natl Compr Canc Netw 2017;15:466–72.
39. Khanna S, Shin A, Kelly CP. Management of Clostridium difficile infection in inflammatory bowel disease: expert review from the clinical practice updates committee of the AGA Institute. Clin Gastroenterol Hepatol 2017;15:166–74.
40. Seo S-K, Jeong H-Y, Park S-G, et al. Blockade of endogenous B7-H1 suppresses antibacterial protection after primary Listeria monocytogenes infection. Immunology 2008;123:90–9.
41. Barber DL, Mayer-Barber KD, Feng CG, et al. CD4 T cells promote rather than control tuberculosis in the absence of PD-1-mediated inhibition. J Immunol 2011;186:1598–607.
42. Sakai S, Kauffman KD, Sallin MA, et al. CD4 T cell-derived IFN-γ plays a minimal role in control of pulmonary Mycobacterium tuberculosis infection and must be actively repressed by PD-1 to prevent lethal disease. PLoS Pathog 2016;12:e1005667.
43. Barber DL, Sakai S, Kudchadkar RR, et al. Tuberculosis following PD-1 blockade for cancer immunotherapy. Sci Transl Med 2019;11.
44. Anastasopoulou A, Ziogas DC, Samarkos M, et al. Reactivation of tuberculosis in cancer patients following administration of immune checkpoint inhibitors: current evidence and clinical practice recommendations. J Immunother Cancer 2019;7:239.
45. Picchi H, Mateus C, Chouaid C, et al. Infectious complications associated with the use of immune checkpoint inhibitors in oncology: reactivation of tuberculosis after anti PD-1 treatment. Clin Microbiol Infect 2018;24:216–8.
46. Michot JM, Lazarovici J, Tieu A, et al. Haematological immune-related adverse events with immune checkpoint inhibitors, how to manage? Eur J Cancer 2019;122:72–90.

Infectious Complications of Tyrosine Kinase Inhibitors in Hematological Malignancies

Andrew Kin, MD[a],*, Charles A. Schiffer, MD[b]

KEYWORDS

- TKI • BCR-ABL • CML • BTK • CLL • Ibrutinib • Infection • Prophylaxis

KEY POINTS

- Molecularly targeted tyrosine kinase inhibitors are remarkably effective in many hematologic diseases.
- BCR-ABL1 targeted inhibitors for chronic myeloid leukemia, including imatinib, are well tolerated with at least 15 years of follow-up.
- Bruton tyrosine kinase (BTK) inhibitors, including ibrutinib, produce less neutropenia and fewer infections compared with chemoimmunotherapy for lymphoproliferative disorders.
- Universal prophylaxis is not recommended with the use of BCR-ABL or BTK inhibitors.

INTRODUCTION

Tyrosine kinases are a family of molecules that regulate a variety of integral cellular functions. They can be membrane-bound receptors or intracellular. Many tyrosine kinase inhibitors (TKIs) play a key role in cell-cycle regulation and, therefore, carry significant potential for oncogenesis if mutated. The approval of imatinib mesylate in 2001 for chronic myeloid leukemia (CML) represented the first agent targeting a specific mutation in hematologic malignances and subsequently spawned a new class of targeted therapies. There are now many other approved TKIs for patients with hematologic malignancies, including ibrutinib for chronic lymphocytic leukemia (CLL) and other B-cell malignancies, and some now approved for acute myeloid leukemia (AML), each agent with its own side-effect profile.

Although they are considered targeted therapy, kinase inhibitors inhibit several different enzymes with variable affinity.[1] Imatinib, for example, initially was approved as a BCR-ABL1 inhibitor but inhibits a broad range of kinases in vitro across many

[a] Department of Oncology, Wayne State University School of Medicine, Karmanos Cancer Institute, HWCRC – 4th Floor, 4100 John R, Detroit, MI 48201, USA; [b] Department of Oncology, Wayne State University School of Medicine, Karmanos Cancer Institute, HWCRC – 4th Floor, 4100 John R, Detroit, MI 48201, USA
* Corresponding author.
E-mail address: kina@karmanos.org

Infect Dis Clin N Am 34 (2020) 245–256
https://doi.org/10.1016/j.idc.2020.02.008
0891-5520/20/© 2020 Elsevier Inc. All rights reserved.

kinase families. As a result, it also is clinically useful for diseases driven by c-kit mutations, such as gastrointestinal stromal tumors and systemic mastocytosis, as well as diseases related to PDGFRA mutations, such as hypereosinophilic syndromes, and in some patients with chronic myelomonocytic leukemia. The promiscuity of interactions with other kinases can produce off-target side effects and in some cases may even enhance the therapeutic effect by inhibiting other kinases.

BCR-ABL

The Philadelphia chromosome is created by a translocation between chromosomes 9 and 22 (t9;22) in CML. This places the Abelson tyrosine kinase (ABL1) gene downstream from the breakpoint cluster region (BCR) and creates a fusion protein in which the kinase function of ABL1 is constitutively active. This provides a growth and survival signal that in CML is both necessary and sufficient for leukemogenesis. There are 5 tyrosine kinase inhibitors (TKIs) currently approved for the treatment of CML: imatinib, dasatinib, nilotinib, bosutinib, and ponatinib. These all share a common mechanism of binding to the ATP binding site of the mutant BCR-ABL fusion protein with high affinity.

There are few infectious issues in patients with CML in chronic phase given the universal presence of elevated neutrophil counts with normal humoral and cellular immune function. Infectious complications associated with these agents are a result of neutropenia, which occurs within the first couple months of treatment, rather than a direct effect of these drugs on different tissues or immune dysregulation. Second-generation TKIs are more potent inhibitors, which can produce deeper neutropenia until polyclonal nonmalignant stem cell clones can recover. That said, in comparison to cytotoxic therapies, it is unusual to require adjunctive therapy with myeloid growth factors; temporary cessation of treatment and/or dose reduction is adequate in the event severe neutropenia develops. As a result, prophylaxis with antibacterial, antifungal, or antiviral agents is unnecessary in chronic-phase CML.

Although each agent has its own unique side effects, they generally are well tolerated and more than 85% of chronic-phase patients treated with TKIs enjoy long-term response and have an overall survival equivalent to that of age-matched controls. Most such patients continue TKI treatment indefinitely and neutropenia is exceedingly rare in patients in long-term follow-up.

Severe neutropenia is more common in patients either presenting with or progressing to either lymphoid or myeloid blast crisis or those diagnosed initially with Philadelphia chromosome–positive acute lymphoblastic leukemia. Such individuals usually are treated with second-generation TKIs in combination with chemotherapy and can experience episodes of neutropenic fever with the clinical spectrum of infections similar to that seen in patients treated for acute leukemia. The established principles of infectious prophylaxis and treatment should be used in such patients.

This review focuses on patients in chronic phase, relying primarily on data from large randomized registration trials in which toxicity endpoints are collected carefully. The results of these studies and neutropenia rates are summarized in **Table 1** and are consistent with other large trials of TKIs which have been reported.

Imatinib

Imatinib was the first TKI approved in CML. The data from the phase 3 IRIS study reported in 2003, using imatinib as initial treatment of newly diagnosed chronic-phase CML, showed 60.8% all-grade neutropenia with imatinib, of which only 14.3% were grades 3 and 4.[2] The most common infections noted were nasopharyngitis (22%)

Table 1
Infectious adverse events—frontline, randomized, chronic-phase chronic myelocytic leukemia trials

	Number of Patients Treated	Neutropenia (All Grade), %	Neutropenia (Grades 3 and 4), %	Upper Respiratory Infection, %
Imatinib (IRIS)[2,3]	551	60.8	14.3	14.5
Dasatinib (DASISION)[4,5]	258	65	29	Not reported
Nilotinib (ENESTnd)[7]	556	40.6	10.8	Not reported
Bosutinib (BELA)[8]	248	28	11	10
Bosutinib (BFORE)[9]	268	11.2	6.7	8.6

and upper respiratory infection (14.5%), virtually all low grade and most of which were likely viral in origin. These were marginally higher than the comparator with interferon and cytarabine. Long-term results were published in 2017 with a median follow-up of approximately 11 years.[3] Safety data for serious adverse events were compiled by year, and those that were deemed likely related to imatinib were reported. Nearly all infectious complications occurred within the first year of use. Only 1 patient each was reported as having treatment-related neutropenia, febrile neutropenia, and an anorectal infection in the first year of treatment, whereas 1 patient each developed appendicitis and cellulitis in years 6 and 11, respectively.

Dasatinib

Dasatinib is a second-generation TKI and produces stronger inhibition of BCR-ABL. The randomized DASISION trial using dasatinib in newly diagnosed chronic-phase patients showed grade 3 and 4 neutropenia of 21% compared with 20% with imatinib, which increased to 29% and 24%, respectively, in the final analysis.[4,5] Infectious complications in newly diagnosed chronic-phase patients were uncommon; no serious infectious adverse events were reported. There was some initial concern that dasatinib used continuously may be more permissive of infection due to its potent inhibition of other tyrosine kinase families.[6] Five-year safety follow-up of the DASISION trial showed a total of 11 patients died of infection, only 4 within 30 days of their last dose of dasatinib: 1 each of *Klebsiella* meningoencephalitis, sepsis, pneumonia, and an unknown infection. Only 1 patient also had neutropenia, and that individual died 4 years after stopping dasatinib.

Of the TKIs, dasatinib is uniquely associated with the development of pleural effusions in as many as 30% of patients, either unilateral or bilateral. Most occur within the first few months of treatment although effusions can develop months to years afterward in patients on long-term dasatinib. Although occasionally presenting with acute onset of dyspnea, most patients experience gradual onset of shortness of breath without fever or productive cough. The effusions can be exudative in character although cultures invariably are negative. The pathophysiology is poorly understood. In the absence of signs of infection, thoracentesis is not mandatory, although some patients with significant dyspnea can benefit from therapeutic removal of fluid. The effusions resolve with cessation of dasatinib and many patients can be retreated successfully at lower doses.

Nilotinib

Nilotinib is a second-generation BCR-ABL inhibitor, which was approved shortly after dasatinib, initially in the relapsed or refractory setting, and then front line. The

ENESTnd trial randomized newly diagnosed patients to receive either imatinib or 2 different doses of nilotinib.[7] The incidence of neutropenia was somewhat less than for the comparator imatinib, at 43% for nilotinib, 300 mg, and 38% for nilotinib, 400 mg, compared with 68% all-grade neutropenia for imatinib. Grade 3 and4 neutropenia also was lower, at 12% and 10%, respectively, compared with 20% in the imatinib arm. Serious adverse events were reported by organ system only: 1 low-grade infection and 3 respiratory adverse events not specifically characterized as infection.

Bosutinib

Bosutinib was the latest BCR-ABL inhibitor approved for use in newly diagnosed chronic-phase CML. It was first approved in 2012 and expanded to include initial treatment of chronic phase in December 2017. The BELA trial showed 28% all-grade neutropenia versus 54% with imatinib, grade 3 and 4, 11% and 24%, respectively.[8] In the BFORE trial frontline, all-grade neutropenia was 11.2% versus 20.8% with imatinib and grade 3 and 4 were 6.7% versus 12.1% with imatinib.[9] Respiratory infections were no different from imatinib at 8.6%, nearly all low grade.

The second-generation inhibitors also are associated with an increased risk of pancreatitis and transaminitis. In the ENESTnd trial, grade 3 and 4 events occurred in 6.5% and 5.7%, respectively, of patients treated with nilotinib compared with 3% each with imatinib. The BFORE trial reported 9.7% high-grade pancreatitis and 24.3% transaminitis. These too are noninfectious and resolve with temporary cessation of the TKI.

Ponatinib

Ponatinib is the most potent BCR-ABL inhibitor approved by the Food and Drug Administration (FDA), first in 2012 and expanded in 2016 for all indications in which other BCR-ABL inhibitors are no longer effective, including the T315I mutation, which is resistant to all other TKIs. The phase 2 PACE trial, which included patients in all stages of CML, has reported 5-year safety and survival data.[10] The rates of neutropenia and infection, shown in **Table 2**, are considerably higher in patients in advanced-stage disease than those in newly diagnosed patients. There also were separately reported rates of grade 3/4 pneumonia, approximately 7% in the whole group. Fatal infectious events were noted: 1 pneumonia in the chronic-phase group and 1 fungal pneumonia in the accelerated-phase group.

Table 2
Select infectious adverse events with single-agent ponatinib across all indications

Infectious Adverse Events	Chronic-Phase–Chronic Myeloid Leukemia, n = 270		Blast-Phase–Chronic Myeloid Leukemia, n = 62		Philadelphia Chromosome–Positive Acute Lymphoblastic Leukemia, n = 32	
	Any Grade	Grade 3 and 4	Any Grade	Grade 3 and 4	Any Grade	Grade 3 and 4
Neutropenia	20%	17%	35%	29%	25%	22%
Febrile neutropenia	<1%	<1%	3%	3%	6%	6%
Death due to sepsis	—	1 (<1%)	—	1 (2%)	—	2 (3%)

Data from Cortes JE, Kim DW, Pinilla-Ibarz J, et al. Ponatinib efficacy and safety in Philadelphia chromosome-positive leukemia: final 5-year results of the phase 2 PACE trial. *Blood.* 2018;132(4):393-404.

Hepatitis B

The hepatitis B virus (HBV) merits special mention. Some data have been presented suggesting an increased risk of HBV reactivation. Of 702 South Korean patients, 43 had positive HBV surface antigen and 15 of those had disease reactivation.[11] Nine patients received prophylaxis and none of them experienced relapse. Another report from Israel reviewed 181 patients at their center, of whom 11 patients had a history of HBV with core antibody positive although surface antibody was negative. Only 1 patient had a positive surface antigen and 2 patients were treated with lamivudine prophylaxis. Over 1195 patient-years on treatment, no patients experienced HBV reactivation.[12]

In general, the incidence of reactivation is very low but has been well documented in case reports. Prescreening for HBV is not necessary; however, if a patient is at risk or from an area endemic for HBV then serology should be determined. Prophylaxis is effective and can be considered, especially in those with preexisting liver dysfunction in whom reactivation may be life-threatening. Please see Eiichi Ogawa and colleagues' article "Hepatitis B Virus Reactivation Potentiated by Biologics," in this issue, for further information on this topic.

BRUTON TYROSINE KINASE

Bruton tyrosine kinase (BTK) inhibitors interfere with B-cell receptor signaling. Initial observations of the potential therapeutic benefit of this target were extrapolated from clinical observations of patients with Bruton agammaglobulinemia, an X-chromosome linked congenital disorder in which BTK is mutated. The disease phenotype is characterized by a lack of mature B cells and severe hypogammaglobulinemia, with an increased susceptibility to bacterial infections. Targeted inhibitors of BTK have proved highly effective in several diseases involving B lymphocytes.

Given this mechanism of action, particularly when used in combination with monoclonal antibodies targeting CD20, a significant risk of infectious complications associated with hypogammaglobulinemia in diseases, such as CLL, in which hypogammaglobulinemia is common and antibody response to neoantigens is already impaired, might be hypothesized. Despite this, these agents have proved remarkably well tolerated with regard to infection.

In general, ibrutinib therapy is continued indefinitely in patients responding to treatment and hematologic and infectious complications from ibrutinib therapy are different during the initial induction phases of treatment, in part because of cytopenias and other comorbidities in patients with active leukemia/lymphoma. Long-term therapy in responders, who usually have normal blood counts and normal performance status, is generally well tolerated with infrequent infectious issues, although other side effects, such as atrial fibrillation, increased risk of bleeding, and musculoskeletal complaints, sometimes require dose reduction or drug discontinuation. This article focuses on the infectious issues encountered during the earlier weeks of ibrutinib therapy.

Chronic Lymphocytic Leukemia

Ibrutinib

Ibrutinib is an oral, irreversible inhibitor of the BTK receptor, covalently binding to the cysteine-481 residue of the BTK molecule. The RESONATE trial was the first to demonstrate its remarkable efficacy in a previously heavily treated CLL population.[13] As a consequence of prior treatment and bone marrow involvement by CLL, 41% of patients had neutropenia prior to treatment; 75% of those patients achieved sustained hematologic improvement with ongoing response of their CLL, and grade 3 or grade 4 neutropenia declined from 18% the first year to less than 5% after 3 years. The incidence of high-grade pneumonias and other infections likewise markedly improved from 14% and 28%, respectively, during the first year of treatment to 4% and 11%, respectively, after the third year.[14] Responders continued on daily therapy indefinitely.

Three-year follow-up of the first phase 1b/2 study of ibrutinib provided additional specific insights[15]; 31 treatment-naïve patients deemed not eligible for upfront cytotoxic therapy were treated in whom the incidence of grade 3 neutropenia was 3%, compared with 18% grade 3 and 4 in the 85 previously treated patients. High-grade infections occurred in 13% of treatment-naïve patients compared with 51% of previously treated patients. A majority of previously treated patients received prophylactic immunoglobulin, which was continued during the study. Some patients were able to recover their immunoglobulin levels with sustained BTK inhibition. Varicella zoster infections, known to be common in patients previously treated with fludarabine-based chemotherapy regimens, occurred in 5 patients despite prophylaxis.

Phosphoinositide-3 kinase inhibitors

Idelalisib, a phosphoinositide 3-kinase (PI3K) inhibitor also FDA approved for relapsed CLL, merits discussion because it works downstream of the BCR pathway. Despite acting on a common pathway, many of the shared side effects occur much more frequently with PI3K inhibitors. A study comparing idelalisib with rituximab to rituximab alone in previously treated CLL patients showed a high rate of noninfectious colitis or diarrhea in more than 30% of patients, 10% high grade.[16] Noninfectious pneumonitis can result in hypoxia and impressive infiltrates on radiograph that often require bronchoscopy to effectively rule out infectious organisms. In contrast, pneumonitis with ibrutinib occurs in approximately 1% or less of patients in large randomized studies.

There also was a high rate of *Pneumocystis jirovecii* pneumonia (PJP) at 3.6%, including 2 deaths with idelalisib. An early case series of ibrutinib identified 5 cases of pneumonia (PJP) out of 96 patients treated.[17] As with zoster, patients treated previously with fludarabine-based regimens were felt to be at higher risk for these infections. Viral infections, especially cytomegalovirus (CMV) infections, also are more common with idelalisib. Two patients (1.8%) were diagnosed with CMV, and 1 patient had progressive multifocal leukoencephalopathy as a result of JC virus infection. There have been a few case reports of progressive multifocal leukoencephalopathy in patients treated with ibrutinib.[18]

Infectious and inflammatory side effects appear to be a class effect as duvelisib, another PI3K inhibitor more recently approved for relapsed CLL, shows many of the same side effects.[19] PJP prophylaxis was required on this trial, although CMV prophylaxis was optional. Severe colitis occurred in 12% of patients, although only 3% of patients had pneumonitis. Three patients (1.9%) developed PJP, all of whom had stopped prophylaxis due to intolerance. As a result, the package label recommends prophylaxis against PJP for both agents until the absolute $CD4^+$ T-cell count is greater than 200 cells/μL. Prophylaxis against CMV should be considered, although dual prophylaxis can compound cytopenias.

Ibrutinib—newly diagnosed chronic lymphocytic leukemia

Given the high efficacy and tolerability in patients with advanced CLL, ibrutinib was then studied in newly diagnosed CLL, first in older patients not suitable for cytotoxic therapy and then to include all populations. Results of the ibrutinib-containing arms for the following trials are noted in **Table 3**.

RESONATE 2 was conducted in a first-line setting in an older population felt to be unsuitable for cytotoxic chemotherapy.[20] Only 7% of patients were neutropenic at

Table 3
Infectious adverse events—frontline, randomized trials of ibrutinib for chronic lymphocytic leukemia

	Number of Patients Treated	Neutropenia (Grade 3 and 4), %	Infection (Grade 3 and 4), %	Pneumonia (Grade 3 and 4), %
RESONATE 2[20]	136	10	8	4
A041202 (ibrutinib only)[21]	180	15	20.6	6.7
A041202 (+ rituximab)[21]	181	21.5	20.4	9.4
E1912 (+ rituximab)[22]	352	25.6	9.4	2.6

the beginning of the study. All-grade neutropenia occurred in 16% of patients compared with 23% in the chlorambucil control group. Grade 3 or higher neutropenia occurred in just 14 patients (10%). Serious infectious complications on the ibrutinib arm of this study included 5 patients (4%) with pneumonia, 3 patients (2%) each with febrile neutropenia, upper respiratory infection, and cellulitis.

The A041202 trial in untreated older patients compared ibrutinib alone (I), ibrutinib combined with rituximab (IR), and bendamustine and rituximab (BR), a standard chemoimmunotherapy regimen in older patients.[21] The addition of rituximab slightly increased grades 3and 4 neutropenia (22% IR v 15% I), with similar rates of high-grade infections, whereas both neutropenia and febrile neutropenia were higher in the chemoimmunotherapy arm. The addition of rituximab did not improve response rates or progression-free survival.

Respiratory tract infections were the most common infectious side effect, with 1 fatality in the ibrutinib monotherapy group. There were few deaths due to sepsis in each arm (1% I, 1% IR, and 2% BR), and few serious central nervous system (CNS) infections (1% I, 1% IR, and 1% BR). Other serious infections, including skin and soft tissue and urinary infections, also were uncommon (2% I, 3% IR, and 2% BR).

The E1912 trial compared ibrutinib plus rituximab with standard chemoimmunotherapy fludarabine, cyclophosphamide, and rituximab in younger patients, including those less than 70 years of age not included in the other trials.[22] The protocol specified prophylactic medications with trimethoprim-sulfamethoxazole, 3 times weekly, and twice-daily acyclovir.

Comparable to other trials, there was a lower incidence of grade 3 and 4 neutropenia at 25.6% using ibrutinib compared with 44.9% from chemotherapy and approximately half the rate of febrile neutropenia (10.5% vs 20.3%). There was 1 fatality from respiratory infection reported in the ibrutinib arm and 2 infectious fatalities on the chemotherapy arm. There was 1 additional death due to sepsis. Other high-grade infections include occasional urinary tract infections and various skin and soft tissue infections, at 1.1% each.

Overall, it is clear that ibrutinib used in a treatment-naïve population has far fewer infectious complications than when used in advanced or refractory disease. This is due partly to less neutropenia prior to and during treatment and also may reflect immunoglobulin levels, particularly in patients pretreated with purine analogs. There is some evidence to suggest immunoglobulin levels can improve with sustained treatment, and, unless patients have repeated infections, there is no role for prophylactic IVIG. Due to low incidence of infections, the official package label advises monitoring only. Infectious prophylaxis is not universally recommended for patients taking ibrutinib although some experts do advocate for prophylaxis against herpes zoster.

Non-Hodgkin Lymphomas

Ibrutinib was approved in 2013 for relapsed mantle cell lymphoma on the basis of a phase 2 trial. A 3-year follow-up of this trial showed grades 3 and 4 neutropenia in 17% of patients and 3% febrile neutropenia.[23] Over the study period, 78% of patients had some infectious complication, with 20% being a serious adverse event. The most common infections were low-grade respiratory infections at 28%, 16% urinary tract infections, and 15% sinusitis. Pneumonia was the most common serious adverse event (SAE) at 8%, with 1 (PJP) infection. Other unusual infections included 1 case of histoplasmosis and 1 case of cryptococcosis. There was no reported effect on immunoglobulin levels.

Ibrutinib was first approved in 2015 for Waldenström macroglobulinemia, also known as lymphoplasmacytic lymphoma, and is now approved in combination with rituximab as well. This is a disease in which malignant B cells produce excess IgM, with concomitant reductions in IgA and IgG, thus leaving patients potentially at increased risk of infection. Mutations in the MYD88 gene are common, affecting pathways just downstream of the BCR. Ibrutinib was first used in 68 patients with refractory disease.[24] Grade 2 through 4 neutropenia was 22%, with only 1 episode of febrile neutropenia. Infections were sparse, with a handful of grade 3, including zoster, pneumonia, and 1 streptococcal endocarditis. Combination therapy with rituximab versus rituximab alone was used in 150 patients in the iNNOVATE trial.[25] Pneumonia was the most common serious adverse event in 6 patients (8%) compared with 2 pneumonias in the rituximab arm.

Single-agent ibrutinib has been explored in primary CNS lymphoma, a rare disorder that has been shown to harbor mutations activating the BCR. A phase 1b trial used ibrutinib alone as a monotherapy run-in, followed by a combination phase with chemotherapy.[26] The dose of ibrutinib needed to meaningfully overcome blood-brain barrier limitations was 840 mg, double that used in the CLL trials; 7 of 18 patients treated developed infections with aspergillus, 2 of which occurred in the ibrutinib monotherapy run-in phase, involved both the brain and lungs and were fatal. In CNS lymphoma, it is common for patients to be on prolonged high-dose steroids to address brain edema, and both cases of fatal CNS aspergillosis in this trial had received 2 weeks to 4 weeks of dexamethasone.

Invasive Fungal Infection

After these events, the investigators instituted pulmonary computed tomography screening to identify and initiate early treatment of probable aspergillus. The investigators performed additional correlative studies to try to explain the high rates of fungal infection. There was no significant difference between B-lymphocyte or T-lymphocyte function in these patients. They were able to show in a murine model that knocking out BTK in macrophages likely plays a significant role in innate immunity, particularly against aspergillus.[26]

The question of increased risk of invasive fungal infection (IFI) has been examined in a few retrospective studies. A study from 15 institutions across 6 countries described 28 patients identified with IFI.[27] These were mostly aspergillosis, but other fungal species included 3 patients with mucormycosis, 7 patients with cryptococcosis, and 1 patient with PJP; 61% of these infections were fatal. Memorial Sloan Kettering Cancer Center experience showed 11% of patients on ibrutinib experienced grade 3 or higher infections.[28] Of these, 37% were IFI. This included 8 aspergillus, 3 (PJP), 3 cryptococcosis, and 1 Candida albicans fungemia.

It is perhaps most informative in terms of overall risk that further studies in CNS lymphoma have not shown these same high rates of IFI; 15 patients with relapsed or refractory CNS lymphoma were treated on a phase 1b trial using ibrutinib in combination with high dose methotrexate and rituximab.[29] There were four grade 3 infections reported, none of which was fungal. A phase 2 trial in relapsed or refractory CNS lymphoma treated 44 patients with ibrutinib monotherapy.[30] There were three grade 3 urinary infections, three grade 3 and 4 pneumonias, and one infectious encephalitis. There was one aspergillus infection reported in a patient on chronic steroids.

Thus, although there are several reports of ibrutinib use associated with the occurrence of IFI and other atypical infections, it is unclear to what extent this is attributable solely to ibrutinib. In particular, the high rates of fungal infection seen in some CNS lymphoma trials occurred in patients receiving prolonged treatment with corticosteroids, with some undergoing very-high-intensity chemotherapy in combination with the ibrutinib. A caution with retrospective studies and case reports is that they may not necessarily capture a representative population. Long-term follow-up of the earlier CLL trials demonstrate that IFI occur rarely, if at all, in the absence of the use of other immunosuppressive or myelosuppressive treatment.

A final note about ibrutinib regarding vaccination: there have been some small studies to suggest that seroconversion after vaccination for influenza and pneumococcus is low; in some reports, no patients responded to vaccination.[31] It is difficult to attribute this entirely to ibrutinib because CLL patients inherently have lower response rates to vaccination. Generally, if a patient requires vaccination, it should be done earlier in the disease course and preferably pretreatment, before immunoparesis worsens.

Second-Generation Bruton Tyrosine Kinase Inhibitors

Acalabrutinib is a second-generation, high-affinity, irreversible BTK inhibitor that recently was approved for patients with relapsed/refractory mantle cell lymphoma and advanced CLL. There is a lower incidence of side effects, such as atrial fibrillation and hemorrhage, and comparative studies with ibrutinib are in progress.

A phase 1 to phase 2 study was done in relapsed or refractory CLL patients, of whom 25% were neutropenic at baseline.[32] Among SAEs, there were 6 cases of pneumonia, including 1 fatal case. Other SAEs include 1 event each of febrile neutropenia, cellulitis, wound infection, lymphangitis, sepsis, and a viral myocarditis. Correlative studies explored natural killer function, which showed an early decline, but appeared to recover numbers and function quickly; immunoglobulins, at least over the relatively short time period of this study, did not seem to be adversely impacted.

In mantle cell lymphoma, the first approved indication for acalabrutinib, the key study was the ACE-LY-004 study.[33] From an infectious standpoint, this was very well tolerated; only 10% of patients developed high-grade neutropenia, and just 5% had a pneumonia, although 1 case of PJP also was reported. Other side effects of interest included 2 SAEs due to sepsis, and 2 reports of pneumonitis; longer follow-up did not identify additional significant infectious complications.

Finally, a pooled analysis was presented in abstract form with 3-year follow-up on the use of acalabrutinib in several phase 1 and phase 2 studies across all diseases.[34] Similar to prior experience, neutropenia was the most common high-grade finding at 9.9%, although only 6.6% attributed to drug. Grade 3 or higher infection occurred in 16.2% of patients, with pneumonia the most common. There were 4 reports of fungal infection, including 2 aspergillosis, 1 low-grade PJP, and 1 cryptococcosis.

OTHER TYROSINE KINASE INHIBITORS

FMS-like tyrosine kinase 3 (FLT3) is a tyrosine kinase mutated in approximately 30% of AML patients that typically portends a higher relapse rate and poorer overall survival.

Midostaurin and gilteritinib recently have been FDA approved for use in FLT3-mutated AML, and others are under investigation. These agents are broad-acting, multikinase inhibitors. Infectious complications with these agents are difficult to separate from those of the underlying disease state or treatment with high-dose cytotoxic chemotherapy.

SUMMARY

TKIs are oral medications that are used to inhibit pathways contributing to oncogenesis and tumor growth. They often inhibit multiple kinase pathways, which may be responsible for a wide range of side effects. The advent of these targeted therapies has had a dramatic impact on survival in many diseases, especially CML and CLL. The limited side-effect profile means patients can continue on these therapies potentially for years. In terms of infectious complications, the risk can vary greatly with the underlying disease and prior or concurrent therapy. As a class, TKIs targeting BCR-ABL are well tolerated with few infectious issues. Infectious complications related to BTK inhibitors, such as ibrutinib, were more common in early trials in advanced and refractory disease. Now approved in treatment-naïve patients, there is low infectious risk with years of continuous follow-up, suggesting prophylaxis may be safely omitted. PI3K inhibitors are a notable exception, with high rates of PJP and CMV infection, and prophylaxis is highly recommended with these agents. Several other agents are making their way to market in other diseases, because the development of TKIs remain an active and exciting area of investigation.

DISCLOSURE

A. Kin has nothing to disclose. C.A. Schiffer discloses the following: DSMB—Pharmacyclics; Advisory Board—Abbvie; and Research Support for Clinical Trials—Pharmacyclics and Takeda.

REFERENCES

1. Kitagawa D, Yokota K, Gouda M, et al. Activity-based kinase profiling of approved tyrosine kinase inhibitors. Genes Cells 2013;18(2):110–22.
2. O'Brien SG, Guilhot F, Larson RA, et al. Imatinib compared with interferon and low-dose cytarabine for newly diagnosed chronic-phase chronic myeloid leukemia. N Engl J Med 2003;348(11):994–1004.
3. Hochhaus A, Larson RA, Guilhot F, et al. Long-term outcomes of imatinib treatment for chronic myeloid leukemia. N Engl J Med 2017;376(10):917–27.
4. Kantarjian H, Shah NP, Hochhaus A, et al. Dasatinib versus imatinib in newly diagnosed chronic-phase chronic myeloid leukemia. N Engl J Med 2010; 362(24):2260–70.
5. Cortes JE, Saglio G, Kantarjian HM, et al. Final 5-year study results of dasision: the dasatinib versus imatinib study in treatment-naive chronic myeloid leukemia patients trial. J Clin Oncol 2016;34(20):2333–40.
6. Futosi K, Nemeth T, Pick R, et al. Dasatinib inhibits proinflammatory functions of mature human neutrophils. Blood 2012;119(21):4981–91.
7. Saglio G, Kim DW, Issaragrisil S, et al. Nilotinib versus imatinib for newly diagnosed chronic myeloid leukemia. N Engl J Med 2010;362(24):2251–9.
8. Cortes JE, Kim DW, Kantarjian HM, et al. Bosutinib versus imatinib in newly diagnosed chronic-phase chronic myeloid leukemia: results from the BELA trial. J Clin Oncol 2012;30(28):3486–92.

9. Cortes JE, Gambacorti-Passerini C, Deininger MW, et al. Bosutinib versus imatinib for newly diagnosed chronic myeloid leukemia: results from the randomized BFORE trial. J Clin Oncol 2018;36(3):231–7.

10. Cortes JE, Kim DW, Pinilla-Ibarz J, et al. Ponatinib efficacy and safety in Philadelphia chromosome-positive leukemia: final 5-year results of the phase 2 PACE trial. Blood 2018;132(4):393–404.

11. Kim S-H, Kim HJ, Kwak J-Y, et al. Hepatitis B virus reactivation in chronic myeloid leukemia treated with various tyrosine kinase inhibitors: multicenter, retrospective study. Blood 2012;120(21):3738.

12. Benjamini O, Zlotnick M, Ribakovsky E, et al. Evaluation of the risk of hepatitis b reactivation among patients with chronic myeloid leukemia treated with tyrosine kinase inhibitors. Blood 2016;128(22):5429.

13. Byrd JC, Brown JR, O'Brien S, et al. Ibrutinib versus ofatumumab in previously treated chronic lymphoid leukemia. N Engl J Med 2014;371(3):213–23.

14. Byrd JC, Hillmen P, O'Brien S, et al. Long-term follow-up of the RESONATE phase 3 trial of ibrutinib vs ofatumumab. Blood 2019;133(19):2031–42.

15. Byrd JC, Furman RR, Coutre SE, et al. Three-year follow-up of treatment-naive and previously treated patients with CLL and SLL receiving single-agent ibrutinib. Blood 2015;125(16):2497–506.

16. Sharman JP, Coutre SE, Furman RR, et al. Final results of a randomized, phase III study of rituximab with or without idelalisib followed by open-label idelalisib in patients with relapsed chronic lymphocytic leukemia. J Clin Oncol 2019;37(16):1391–402.

17. Ahn IE, Jerussi T, Farooqui M, et al. Atypical Pneumocystis jirovecii pneumonia in previously untreated patients with CLL on single-agent ibrutinib. Blood 2016;128(15):1940–3.

18. Raisch DW, Rafi JA, Chen C, et al. Detection of cases of progressive multifocal leukoencephalopathy associated with new biologicals and targeted cancer therapies from the FDA's adverse event reporting system. Expert Opin Drug Saf 2016;15(8):1003–11.

19. Flinn IW, Hillmen P, Montillo M, et al. The phase 3 DUO trial: duvelisib vs ofatumumab in relapsed and refractory CLL/SLL. Blood 2018;132(23):2446–55.

20. Burger JA, Tedeschi A, Barr PM, et al. Ibrutinib as initial therapy for patients with chronic lymphocytic leukemia. N Engl J Med 2015;373(25):2425–37.

21. Woyach JA, Ruppert AS, Heerema NA, et al. Ibrutinib regimens versus chemoimmunotherapy in older patients with untreated CLL. N Engl J Med 2018;379(26):2517–28.

22. Shanafelt TD, Wang XV, Kay NE, et al. Ibrutinib-rituximab or chemoimmunotherapy for chronic lymphocytic leukemia. N Engl J Med 2019;381(5):432–43.

23. Wang ML, Blum KA, Martin P, et al. Long-term follow-up of MCL patients treated with single-agent ibrutinib: updated safety and efficacy results. Blood 2015;126(6):739–45.

24. Treon SP, Tripsas CK, Meid K, et al. Ibrutinib in previously treated Waldenstrom's macroglobulinemia. N Engl J Med 2015;372(15):1430–40.

25. Dimopoulos MA, Tedeschi A, Trotman J, et al. Phase 3 trial of ibrutinib plus rituximab in waldenstrom's macroglobulinemia. N Engl J Med 2018;378(25):2399–410.

26. Lionakis MS, Dunleavy K, Roschewski M, et al. Inhibition of B cell receptor signaling by ibrutinib in primary CNS lymphoma. Cancer Cell 2017;31(6):833–43.e5.

27. Ruchlemer R, Ben Ami R, Bar-Meir M, et al. Ibrutinib: a risk factor for invasive fungal infections? Blood 2017;130(Suppl 1):4323.
28. Varughese T, Taur Y, Cohen N, et al. Serious infections in patients receiving ibrutinib for treatment of lymphoid cancer. Clin Infect Dis 2018;67(5):687–92.
29. Grommes C, Tang SS, Wolfe J, et al. Phase 1b trial of an ibrutinib-based combination therapy in recurrent/refractory CNS lymphoma. Blood 2019;133(5):436–45.
30. Grommes C, Wolfe J, Gavrilovic I, et al. Phase II of Single-Agent Ibrutinib in Recurrent/Refractory Primary (PCNSL) and Secondary CNS Lymphoma (SCNSL). Blood 2018;132(Supplement 1):2965.
31. Sun C, Gao J, Couzens L, et al. Seasonal influenza vaccination in patients with chronic lymphocytic leukemia treated with ibrutinib. JAMA Oncol 2016;2(12): 1656–7.
32. Byrd JC, Harrington B, O'Brien S, et al. Acalabrutinib (ACP-196) in relapsed chronic lymphocytic leukemia. N Engl J Med 2016;374(4):323–32.
33. Wang M, Rule S, Zinzani PL, et al. Acalabrutinib in relapsed or refractory mantle cell lymphoma (ACE-LY-004): a single-arm, multicentre, phase 2 trial. Lancet 2018;391(10121):659–67.
34. Byrd JC, Owen R, O'Brien S, et al. Pooled analysis of safety data from clinical trials evaluating acalabrutinib monotherapy in hematologic malignancies. Blood 2017;130(Suppl 1):4326.

Epidermal Growth Factor Receptor Inhibitors and Other Tyrosine Kinase Inhibitors for Solid Tumors

Isabel Ruiz-Camps, MD, PhD[a], Juan Aguilar-Company, MD[a,b],*

KEYWORDS

- Kinase inhibitor • Targeted therapy • Immunosuppression • EGFR inhibitors
- ALK inhibitors • mTOR inhibitors • BRAF/MEK inhibitors • VEGFR inhibitors

KEY POINTS

- Kinase inhibitors are small molecules, generally orally administered, that target molecular mechanisms involved in oncogenesis.
- ErbB receptor–targeted kinase inhibitors, including epidermal growth factor receptor inhibitors, are not associated with a significant increase in the risk of infection. Rash is a frequent adverse event, sometimes requiring antibiotics.
- Anaplastic lymphoma kinase and vascular endothelial growth factor receptor inhibitors are not associated with an increase in the risk of infections.
- BRAF and MEK inhibitors are not associated with an increase in risk of infections. Therapy-induced pyrexia and chills are frequent adverse events of these drugs.
- Mammalian target of rapamycin inhibitors are associated with an increase in the number of infections. Screening for latent infections and individualized prophylaxis may be advisable.

INTRODUCTION

This article analyzes, from an infectious diseases perspective, the safety profile of small molecule kinase inhibitors (KIs) used to treat solid organ malignancies, and establishes specific recommendations. This group of drugs is the focus of intense research, and thus is constantly evolving as new agents earn approval or new indications for existing agents are established. Drugs currently approved by the US Food

[a] Infectious Diseases Department, Vall d'Hebron University Hospital, Passeig de la Vall d'Hebron, 119-129, Barcelona 08035, Spain; [b] Oncology Department, Vall d'Hebron University Hospital, Passeig de la Vall d'Hebron, 119-129, Barcelona 08035, Spain
* Corresponding author. Infectious Diseases Department, Vall d'Hebron University Hospital, Passeig de la Vall d'Hebron, 119-129, Barcelona 08035, Spain.
E-mail address: juanaguilarcompany@gmail.com

Infect Dis Clin N Am 34 (2020) 257–270
https://doi.org/10.1016/j.idc.2020.02.005
0891-5520/20/© 2020 Elsevier Inc. All rights reserved.

id.theclinics.com

and Drug Administration, as well as their indications, are listed in **Table 1**. Almost all drugs in this class are administered orally, because of their high oral bioavailability.

Kinases are implicated in cell signaling and frequently promote cell proliferation, survival, and migration. Deregulations in kinases have been found to play a crucial role in the carcinogenesis and metastasization of various types of cancer. Thus, inhibition of distinct kinase pathways has proved to achieve favorable outcomes in certain tumors, and also to be less harmful for noncancerous cells, compared with cytotoxic chemotherapy. Note that KIs may act on 1 or more kinases, also present in normal, healthy cells, thus exerting their effect on multiple pathways.[1] Therefore, susceptibility to infections may be affected in heterogeneous ways. In addition, on individual patients, underlying diseases and previously received treatments also influence the risk of infection. In view of the limited data available so far for many of these agents, clinical reviews, expert recommendations, and scientific society guidelines become the most valuable sources of information.[2–5]

The provided recommendations are open for modification from ongoing and future clinical observations. Increased awareness by clinicians and constant reporting are required to identify infections related to the use of these agents.

This article focuses on 5 groups: KIs targeting ErbB proteins, anaplastic lymphoma kinase (ALK), mammalian target of rapamycin (mTOR), B-type Raf kinase (BRAF) and MAPK (mitogen-activated protein kinase)/ERK (extracellular signal-related kinase) kinases (MEK), and vascular endothelial growth factor receptor (VEGFR). These groups contain the most extensively used agents, for which a greater amount of clinical data is available.

ErbB RECEPTOR TYROSINE KINASE–TARGETED AGENTS: ERLOTINIB (TARCEVA), GEFITINIB (IRESSA), AFATINIB (GIOTRIF), OSIMERTINIB (TAGRISSO), LAPATINIB (TYVERB), AND NERATINIB (NERLYNX)
Mechanism of Action

The epidermal growth factor receptor (EGFR), also known as ErbB1 or human epidermal growth factor receptor 1 (HER1), is a transmembrane glycoprotein comprising a cytoplasmic domain with TK activity. EGFR is one of the 4 proteins in the ErbB (or HER) family of receptor TKs, also including ErbB2/HER2, ErbB3/HER3, and ErbB4/HER4. These receptors are able to initiate intracellular signaling pathways including Ras/MAPK and Ras/phosphatidylinositol 3 kinase (PI3K)/Akt/mTOR, which are linked to cell proliferation, differentiation, and survival. Therefore, its deregulation plays a crucial role in many types of cancer. Several agents are available for targeting ErbB family receptors, as monoclonal antibodies (mAbs) or as KIs.

First-generation EGFR KIs include gefitinib and erlotinib. Afatinib is a second-generation KI that binds irreversibly to all members of the ErbB family.[6–8] The newer generation of KIs includes lapatinib, neratinib, and osimertinib. Osimertinib is active in T790M *EGFR* resistance mutations.

Expected Impact on the Infection Risk

ErbB receptor KIs show a good safety profile. Adverse events consist mainly of rash; diarrhea; hepatotoxicity; and, less frequently, interstitial lung disease. The effects of EGFR blockade on the immune system are not fully understood. Basic research suggests that heparin-binding EGF-like growth factors (HB-EGFs), which act through EGFR, play an important role in regulating the proliferation of hematopoietic maturing cells.[9,10] EGF is also involved in tumor necrosis factor alpha–induced respiratory burst and phagocytic activity through the EGFR TK pathway. Toll-like receptors (TLRs) constitute an important component of the innate immune system. TLR-3 function

Table 1
List of food and drug administration–approved kinase inhibitors for the treatment of solid tumors

Targeted Molecule	Drugs	Currently Approved Indications
ALK	Crizotinib, ceritinib, alectinib, brigatinib, lorlatinib	ALK-positive, ROS1-positive non–small cell lung cancer
B-Raf	Vemurafenib, dabrafenib, encorafenib	BRAF-mutated melanoma Dabrafenib, trametinib: *BRAF*-mutated thyroid cancer and non–small cell lung cancer
CDK family	Palbociclib, ribociclib, abemaciclib	Estrogen receptor–positive breast cancer
c-Kit, PDGF-R, ABL	Imatinib	Gastrointestinal stromal tumors Hematologic malignancies: Ph+ chronic myeloid leukemia and acute lymphoblastic leukemia
c-Met	Crizotinib, cabozantinib	Crizotinib: ALK-positive, ROS1-positive non-small cell lung cancer Cabozantinib: medullary thyroid cancer, hepatocellular carcinoma, renal cell carcinoma
EGFR/HER1, ErbB2/HER2 and other ErbB family members	Erlotinib, gefitinib, afatinib, neratinib, lapatinib, osimertinib, dacomitinib	Neratinib, lapatinib: HER2-positive breast cancer Remaining agents: EGFR-positive lung cancer
mTOR	Temsirolimus, everolimus	Temsirolimus: kidney cancer Everolimus: kidney cancer, neuroendocrine tumors, breast cancer
FGFR	Erdafitinib	Urothelial carcinoma
MEK1/2	Trametinib, cobimetinib, binimetinib	BRAF-mutated melanoma
RET	Vandetanib	Medullary thyroid cancer
TRK, ALK, ROS1	Entrectinib, larotrectinib	NTRK-positive tumors Entrectinib: ROS1-positive non–small cell lung cancer
VEGFR	Axitinib, cabozantinib, lenvatinib, pazopanib, regorafenib, sorafenib, sunitinib, vandetanib	Axitinib: renal cell carcinoma Cabozantinib: renal cell carcinoma, hepatocellular carcinoma Pazopanib: renal cell carcinoma, soft tissue sarcoma Regorafenib: hepatocellular carcinoma, gastrointestinal stromal tumors, colorectal cancer Sunitinib: gastrointestinal stromal tumors, neuroendocrine pancreatic cancer, renal cell carcinoma Lenvatinib, sorafenib: differentiated thyroid cancer, renal cell carcinoma, hepatocellular carcinoma Vandetanib: medullary thyroid cancer

Abbreviations: ABL, Abelson murine leukemia; ALK, anaplastic lymphoma kinase; B-Raf, B-type Raf kinase; CDK, cyclin-dependent kinases; EGFR, epidermal growth factor receptor; FGFR, fibroblast growth factor receptor; MEK, MAPK (mitogen-activated protein kinase)/ERK (extracellular signal-related kinase) kinase; mTOR, mammalian target of rapamycin; PDGF-R, platelet-derived growth factor receptor; Ph+, Philadelphia-positive; RET, rearranged during transfection; TRK and NTRK, neurotrophic tyrosine kinase receptor type 1; VEGFR, vascular endothelial growth factor receptor.

has been found to depend on the activation of 2 TKs, EGFR and Scr.[11] In addition, the EGFR pathway is also responsible for specific protective responses in the airway epithelium, leading to mucin production and secretion, neutrophil recruitment via interleukin-8, and epithelial wound healing; dysregulated EGFR function may contribute to the risk of infection.[12]

Patients treated with EGFR-targeted agents frequently experience dermatologic toxicity, most notably in the form of papulopustular rash, xerosis, and paronychia.[13] EGFR is key in maintaining epidermal homeostasis through regulation of keratinocyte proliferation, differentiation, migration, and survival; its inhibition leads to strong dysregulation in the keratinocyte cycle and inflammatory responses. The occurrence of severe rash is more frequent with mAbs (10%–17%) than with small molecule KIs (5%–9%). Microorganisms do not seem to contribute to the pathogenesis of EGFR-targeted agent–induced rash in the earlier phases, because the initial pustule is sterile, although secondary infection may follow.

Available Clinical Data

In the pivotal phase 3 randomized controlled trials (RCTs) comparing erlotinib with chemotherapy in patients with non–small cell lung cancer (NSCLC) with EGFR mutations, neutropenia was nonexistent in the erlotinib group in contrast with the chemotherapy-based therapy group.[8,14] In a pivotal RCT comparing erlotinib versus placebo as second-line or third-line therapy for advanced NSCLC, infection was reported in 24% of patients receiving erlotinib compared with 15% of those receiving placebo; nevertheless, the grade 3 to 5 infection rate was only 2%, and it has been suggested that this result may reflect prolonged follow-up because of longer survival. Episodes of serious infections included pneumonia, sepsis, and cellulitis.[15]

In a meta-analysis of 4 RCTs comparing gefitinib with chemotherapy, neutropenia was also less frequent in the gefitinib group (all-grade and grade 3–4 neutropenia rates were 7% vs 84% and 3% vs 69%, respectively).[16] As an irreversible pan-ErbB blocker, afatinib is supposed to exert the most potent inhibitory activity. However, rates of infection do not seem to be higher. Cystitis was reported in 13% of patients receiving afatinib compared with 5% of those receiving chemotherapy in an RCT, but the frequency and severity of all-cause adverse events were similar across both study groups. Of note, 2 afatinib-related deaths were caused by infectious complications (pneumonia), whereas 1 patient in the gefitinib group died because of lung infection.[17] A recently published phase 3 RCT comparing osimertinib versus conventional chemotherapy showed a neutropenia rate of 8% (grade 3, 1%).[18] Taken together, these data reflect that neutropenia and infection are infrequent with these drugs.

Skin and soft tissue infections complicating papulopustular rash have been reported in the literature as case reports and retrospective case series. Of note, some of them included serious *Staphylococcus aureus* infections, such as skin abscesses requiring surgical management, or bacteremic infections.[19–22] Two meta-analyses evaluating the efficacy of oral tetracyclines (doxycycline of minocycline) for the prevention of papulopustular rash showed significant benefit in terms of reduced incidence of moderate to severe forms.[23,24] Topical corticosteroids and antibiotics (eg, clindamycin) have been also used as prophylaxis or treatment, although their efficacy has not been adequately evaluated.[23] The use of systemic antibiotic therapy is recommended in cases of severe rash or superinfection.

As for HER2 blockade, data are scarce. A 2015 meta-analysis of 10,094 patients from 13 RCTs treated with trastuzumab (an anti-HER2 mAb) showed a modest but statistically significant increase in the risk of high-grade infection (relative risk [RR], 1.2; 95% confidence interval [CI], 1.07–1.37) and febrile neutropenia (RR, 1.28; 95% CI, 1.08–

1.52). However, this association was mainly driven by studies in which trastuzumab was used in combination with conventional chemotherapy. The investigators concluded that the underlying mechanism remains unclear.[25] Infection or neutropenia were also not reported in RCTs using anti-HER2 KIs without concomitant chemotherapy.[26,27]

Conclusions and Suggested Prevention Strategies

- Therapy with ErbB receptor KIs is not associated with a significant increase in the risk of infection.
- No benefit is expected from the use of anti-infective prophylaxis for patients receiving such therapy.
- Treatment-induced papulopustular rash can lead in some cases to skin infection; patients with severe rash must be closely followed and the need for topical or systemic antibiotic should be evaluated.

ANAPLASTIC LYMPHOMA KINASE INHIBITORS: CRIZOTINIB (XALKORI), CERITINIB (ZYKADIA), ALECTINIB (ALECENSA), BRIGATINIB (ALUNBRIG), LORLATINIB (LORBRENA)
Mechanism of Action

Rearrangements in the gene encoding ALK are found in 3% to 5% of patients with NSCLC They are also present in anaplastic large-cell lymphomas and, rarely, in other solid tumor types. The resultant oncogene promotes cell survival, cell cycle progression, and proliferation. Thus, ALK inhibitors have been developed for its use in patients with ALK-positive tumors, with dramatic improvements in prognosis. Since the introduction of the first-generation ALK TKI crizotinib, more selective and higher central nervous system–penetrant second-generation (ceritinib, alectinib, and brigatinib) and third-generation (lorlatinib) ALK TKIs have been approved, and others are in development.[28]

Expected Impact on the Infection Risk

Few data are available on the implication of ALK in the homeostasis of the immune system. Basic research suggests that ALK plays a role in the innate immune system, upregulating inflammatory response in animal models of sepsis.[29] Nevertheless, it is unclear how this may affect the immune status of patients treated with ALK inhibitors.

Available Clinical Data

For patients treated with crizotinib, data on risk of infection are scarce. In the first-line trials comparing crizotinib with chemotherapy, a higher rate of grade 1 to 2 upper respiratory infections was observed, but grade 3 to 4 infections were only present in the chemotherapy arm.[30,31] For ceritinib, available published data do not describe infections as typically occurring adverse events, and neutropenia was less frequent than in the chemotherapy control arm.[32] Similarly, lorlatinib has not been linked to infectious events.[33] One case of rectal perforation has been reported in possible relation to crizotinib.[34] In summary, the (limited) data suggest infectious complications are infrequent.

Conclusions and Suggested Prevention Strategies

- Therapy with ALK inhibitors is not associated with a significant increase in the risk of infection.
- No benefit is expected from the use of anti-infective prophylaxis.

MAMMALIAN TARGET OF RAPAMYCIN INHIBITORS: RAPAMYCIN/SIROLIMUS (RAPAMUNE), TEMSIROLIMUS (TORISEL), EVEROLIMUS (AFINITOR, VOTUBIA)
Mechanism of Action

The Ras/PI3K/Akt/mTOR pathway plays a crucial role in cell survival, growth, and proliferation. mTOR is a serine/threonine kinase and a member of the PI3K-related kinase superfamily. Two distinct mTOR complexes have been identified: mTORC1 and mTORC2. The effects of mTOR on growth, division, and metabolism are largely attributable to mTORC1, which is regulated by growth factors and cytokine receptors (such as HER2, c-Kit, vascular endothelial growth factor [VEGF] and platelet-derived growth factor [PDGF]) and by changes in intracellular ATP content. mTOR inhibitors comprise a unique drug class in possessing both immunosuppressive and anticancer activity. Rapamycin (also known as sirolimus) and its analogues, the macrolides everolimus and temsirolimus, act by forming an allosteric inhibitory complex with an intracellular receptor (FKBP12) that binds a region in mTORC1, inhibiting its kinase activity. In addition, rapamycin also inhibits angiogenesis and endothelial cell proliferation.

Expected Impact on the Infection Risk

Basic research shows that mTORC1-mediated functions result in both immunosuppressive and immune-activating effects. Although the underlying mechanism is not fully understood, it has been implicated in the normal function of the innate immune system and T and B lymphocyte regulation.[35] Note that patients receiving mTOR inhibitors may have a hampered immune status that is not caused by selective neutropenia or lymphopenia but by an altered immune response. The defects on innate immunity may be further compromised by the effect of mTOR inhibition on stromal cells, which leads to impaired wound healing and stomatitis.

Available Clinical Data

Most common adverse effects attributed to mTOR inhibitors include anemia, thrombocytopenia and increased triglyceride and/or cholesterol levels. Tolerability of these agents has posed a challenge, because discontinuation rates because of adverse events are high. A retrospective analysis of patients treated with PI3K-AKT-mTOR pathway inhibitors showed a higher risk of infections compared with patients treated with other targeted therapies in phase I trials.[36] A systematic review of treatment-related mortality including 12 RCTs reported an increased risk of death from infectious causes (pneumonia and sepsis) in the placebo-controlled subgroup analysis.[37] Of note, noninfectious pneumonitis is a frequent adverse event of mTOR inhibitors, with a reported incidence of 2% to 9.9% and should be included in the differential diagnosis of patients under treatment with these agents who develop pulmonary infiltrates.[38] A recent meta-analysis using data from 12 phase 2 and 3 trials comparing everolimus or temsirolimus versus placebo in patients with cancer also reported a significantly higher risk of infection with mTOR inhibitors, with incidences for all-grade and severe mTOR inhibitor–attributable infection of 9.3% and 2.3%, respectively.[39] The risk substantially varied across different tumor types, being higher for renal cell carcinoma (RCC), lymphoma, and neuroendocrine tumors. Upper respiratory tract infection, urinary tract infection, and pneumonia were the predominant forms, with some examples of opportunistic infection (ie, tuberculosis and herpes zoster) and hepatitis B virus (HBV) reactivation, which has been highlighted in case reports.[40,41] Cases of *Pneumocystis jirovecii* pneumonia in patients with solid cancer treated with everolimus have also been reported, in 1 of them without lymphopenia, reflecting the lymphocyte dysfunction associated with these therapies.[42,43]

Conclusions and Suggested Prevention Strategies

- Therapy with mTOR inhibitors in patients with cancer is associated with an increased risk of infection, especially in those patients with additional risk factors.
- Screening for chronic (latent) infections, including HBV and latent tuberculosis infection, may be advisable before initiating treatment with mTOR inhibitors, followed by appropriate therapy if needed.
- No benefit is expected from the universal use of antimicrobial prophylaxis for patients receiving mTOR inhibitors. Infection risk should be individualized because some patients benefit from targeted prophylaxis (eg, prophylaxis against *P jirovecii* in patients with lymphopenia and/or concomitant treatment with corticosteroids).

BRAF AND MEK KINASE INHIBITORS: VEMURAFENIB (ZELBORAF), DABRAFENIB (TAFINLAR), ENCORAFENIB (BRAFTOVI), TRAMETINIB (MEKINIST), COBIMETINIB (COTELLIC), AND BINIMETINIB (MEKTOVI)
Mechanism of Action

In the MAPK-activating pathway, Ras oncoproteins activate Raf, MEK, and ERKs to direct key cell proliferative and survival signals. Activating mutations of BRAF lead to constitutive activation of the MAPK pathway. Nearly half of the patients with advanced melanoma harbor the activating V600E mutation in the BRAF gene. The introduction of BRAF-directed treatment, often in combination with MEK inhibitors, has dramatically changed the outcome of patients with BRAF-mutated melanoma. Further indications and approved drugs are shown in **Table 1**. The potential use of BRAF inhibitors in BRAF-mutated colorectal carcinoma is also under investigation.

Expected Impact on Susceptibility to Infection

Although some of the antitumor effect of BRAF and MEK KIs is thought to be mediated via the immune response, targeting these pathways does not result in any apparent immunosuppression. Therefore, infection susceptibility is not expected to be directly increased. In a study, vemurafenib and dabrafenib were compared for the effect on lymphocyte counts. Vemurafenib therapy decreased lymphocyte counts and altered CD4+ T-cell phenotype and function compared with dabrafenib. This lymphopenia was found to be more profound when corticosteroids were also administered.[44,45]

As for MEK inhibitors, basic research suggests they may even positively influence the patient's immune status. The MEK pathway is involved in the regulation of FoxP3, a crucial transcription factor that controls function and suppressive activity of regulatory T cells. Ex vivo MEK inhibition with trametinib in blood samples obtained from patients infected with human immunodeficiency virus with tuberculosis downregulated resting and activated regulatory T cells and reduced the production of proinflammatory cytokines in stimulated T cells, resulting in a net improvement of the host's immune response.[46] Trametinib suppresses lipopolysaccharide-induced tumor necrosis factor alpha production and endotoxin shock.[47] Further studies suggest that trametinib may have a potential antimicrobial effect against influenza virus, polyomavirus, or *Schistosoma mansoni*.[48–50]

Available Clinical Data

The most common adverse effects of these drugs are arthralgia, rash, fatigue, nausea, diarrhea, and cutaneous squamous cell carcinoma or keratoacanthoma. Different combinations of BRAF and MEK inhibitors have distinctive profiles of adverse events.[51] Of interest, with the combination of dabrafenib and trametinib, the occurrence of fever and chills has been reported to be as high as 51%, with a median time of onset of 11 days after starting treatment and a median duration of 3 days. For some patients, intermittent fever becomes a pattern of their chronic therapy. Patients under treatment with these drugs should be evaluated in case of fever, but, once infection has been excluded, treatment can be performed on an outpatient basis and symptoms managed with acetaminophen, steroids, and/or temporary drug dose interruption.[52]

In the aforementioned study focusing on lymphopenia in patients treated with vemurafenib, 9 of 102 patients developed an infection; however, the number of events was too small to draw any statistical conclusions. Clinical experience is more limited with cobimetinib, encorafenib, and binimetinib. In a meta-analysis comparing safety and security of BRAF inhibitors alone or in combination with MEK inhibitors, there was no report of an increased risk of infection; nevertheless, the rates of fever and chills were shown to increase 2-fold and 3-fold, respectively, compared with monotherapy.[53]

Conclusions and Suggested Prevention Strategies

- Therapy with BRAF and MEK KIs does not increase the risk of infection.
- Clinicians must be aware of the mimicry of an ongoing infectious complication by some of the most common drug-related adverse effects observed with this therapy (ie, pyrexia, chills, fatigue, arthralgia, and rash).
- No specific prevention strategies are recommended for patients receiving BRAF and MEK inhibitors.

AGENTS TARGETING VASCULAR ENDOTHELIAL GROWTH FACTOR RECEPTOR FAMILY TYROSINE KINASE AND OTHER ANGIOGENIC PATHWAYS: AXITINIB (INLYTA), CABOZANTINIB (COMETRIQ, CABOMETYX), LENVATINIB (LENVIMA), PAZOPANIB (VOTRIENT), REGORAFENIB (STIVARGA), SORAFENIB (NEXAVAR), SUNITINIB (SUTENT)
Mechanism of Action

Angiogenesis constitutes a key process in tumor progression. A complex network of multiple proangiogenic signaling molecules, such as VEGF, PDGF, fibroblast growth factor (FGF), or placental growth factor (PIGF) families and their respective receptors, stimulate intracellular signaling pathways that trigger formation of new blood vessels, tumor growth, and metastatic spread.[54] Inhibition of VEGF family members and their corresponding receptors and downstream signaling pathways has become an attractive therapeutic target, leading to improved outcomes across several tumor types. mAbs targeted against VEGF and PIGF (bevacizumab and aflibercept) have been extensively used, generally in combination with chemotherapy.[55] More recently, KIs targeting VEGFR as well as other angiogenic pathways have been developed. Sorafenib, sunitinib, axitinib, and pazopanib are small molecule multi-KIs that target the VEGF pathway, either alone or in combination with several other pathways, such as PDGF, c-Kit, BRAF, or *fms*-like TK-3. Regorafenib, vandetanib, and cabozantinib are potent KIs targeted not only against VEGFR and previously mentioned pathways but also against Rearranged during Transfection (RET) receptor and angiopoietin-1 receptor.

Expected Impact on Susceptibility to Infection

Neutropenia has been found to occur more frequently during the course of therapy with bevacizumab and aflibercept.[56] Bevacizumab may also modulate intracellular

T-cell immunity within the tumor microenvironment and, eventually, T-cell proliferation, migration, and activation.[57] In addition, the occurrence of gastrointestinal perforation, potentially leading to secondary peritonitis or bacteremia, is a well-established complication of VEGF-targeted agents, with a pooled incidence of 0.9% (and a related mortality of 21.7%).[58] The physiologic proangiogenic role of VEGF in normal tissues also explains the increased risk of delayed postoperative wound healing and postoperative complications (including surgical site infection). Fewer data are available on the effect of KIs in this group. Although these agents may also modulate T-cell functionality within the tumor microenvironment, it is unlikely that such effect exerts a negative impact on the host's immunity. In patients with RCC, sunitinib induced decreases in total leukocyte and neutrophil counts, and also regulated the function of certain peripheral blood lymphocyte subpopulations. The net effects of these changes on host immunity are of unknown significance.[59]

Available Clinical Data

In general terms, KIs in this group show a heterogeneous safety profile, with multitargeted KIs carrying higher toxicity rates. However, the most common adverse events with sorafenib and sunitinib include hand-foot syndrome, hypertension, diarrhea, fatigue, and skin rash, but not infectious events.[60] Although the pooled incidence of all-grade neutropenia with sorafenib therapy was reported to reach 18.0% in a meta-analysis with more than 3000 patients, high-grade neutropenia was rare (5.1%).[61] Infectious complications related to sorafenib have been only rarely reported in clinical trials. Likely because of its more selective action on the VEGFR family, the incidence of cutaneous toxicity and neutropenia seems to be lower with axitinib than with sorafenib.[62] A meta-analysis of fatal adverse events in clinical trials evaluating sorafenib, sunitinib, and pazopanib published before 2011 identified only 3 episodes of fatal sepsis among more than 4000 patients.[63] Recent RCTs assessing the efficacy and safety of cabozantinib or sorafenib versus an mTOR inhibitor for advanced RCC, or regorafenib versus placebo for hepatocellular carcinoma after failure of sorafenib, have not revealed a significant risk of infection.[64–66] Of note, 5 cases of invasive fungal infection (aspergillus pulmonary infection) have been reported in patients treated with sorafenib. Some of the patients had additional risk factors; downregulation of the ERK pathway has been proposed as a possible underlying mechanism.[67] Overall, published results support that the use of KIs related to angiogenic pathways is not associated with a meaningful increase in the risk of infection.

Conclusions and Suggested Prevention Strategies

- Therapy with VEGFR KIs does not increase the risk of infection.
- No benefit is expected from the use of anti-infective prophylaxis for patients receiving this therapy.

SUMMARY

The advent of targeted therapies has changed the landscape of many hematological and solid organ malignancies. Treatment with KIs has resulted in significant changes in prognosis, and precluded the toxic effects of conventional chemotherapy. Although the extent of adverse events is not yet known, risk of infection does not seem to be a major problem associated with the use of these drugs.

ErbB receptor–targeted KIs, including EGFR inhibitors, are not associated with a significant increase in the risk of infection. Rash is a frequent adverse event, sometimes requiring antibiotics. ALK, BRAF/MEK, and VEGFR inhibitors are not associated with an increase in the risk of infections. Therapy-induced pyrexia and chills are frequent with the combination of BRAF and MEK inhibitors. mTOR inhibitors are associated with an increase in the number of infections; screening for latent infections and individualized prophylaxis may be advisable. Because of the limited clinical experience available, recommendations may evolve in the near future.

DISCLOSURE

The authors have no conflicts of interest related to this study. There was no pharmaceutical grant support for the study or the study concept, data analysis, or preparation of the article.

REFERENCES

1. Bhullar KS, Lagarón NO, McGowan EM, et al. Kinase-targeted cancer therapies: progress, challenges and future directions. Mol Cancer 2018;17(1):48.
2. Reinwald M, Silva JT, Mueller NJ, et al. ESCMID Study Group for Infections in Compromised Hosts (ESGICH) Consensus Document on the safety of targeted and biological therapies: an infectious diseases perspective (Intracellular signaling pathways: tyrosine kinase and mTOR inhibitors). Clin Microbiol Infect 2018;24:S53–70.
3. Aguilar-Company J, Fernández-Ruiz M, García-Campelo R, et al. ESCMID Study Group for Infections in Compromised Hosts (ESGICH) Consensus Document on the safety of targeted and biological therapies: an infectious diseases perspective (Cell surface receptors and associated signaling pathways). Clin Microbiol Infect 2018;24:S41–52.
4. Reinwald M, Boch T, Hofmann WK, et al. Risk of infectious complications in hemato-oncological patients treated with kinase inhibitors. Biomark Insights 2015;10s3:55–68.
5. Chamilos G, Lionakis MS, Kontoyiannis DP. Call for action: invasive fungal infections associated with ibrutinib and other small molecule kinase inhibitors targeting immune signaling pathways. Clin Infect Dis 2018;66(1):140–8.
6. Mitsudomi T, Morita S, Yatabe Y, et al. Gefitinib versus cisplatin plus docetaxel in patients with non-small-cell lung cancer harbouring mutations of the epidermal growth factor receptor (WJTOG3405): an open label, randomised phase 3 trial. Lancet Oncol 2010;11(2):121–8.
7. Maemondo M, Inoue A, Kobayashi K, et al. Gefitinib or chemotherapy for non-small-cell lung cancer with mutated EGFR. N Engl J Med 2010;362(25):2380–8.
8. Zhou C, Wu Y-L, Chen G, et al. Erlotinib versus chemotherapy as first-line treatment for patients with advanced EGFR mutation-positive non-small-cell lung cancer (OPTIMAL, CTONG-0802): a multicentre, open-label, randomised, phase 3 study. Lancet Oncol 2011;12(8):735–42.
9. Krampera M, Pasini A, Rigo A, et al. HB-EGF/HER-1 signaling in bone marrow mesenchymal stem cells: Inducing cell expansion and reversibly preventing multilineage differentiation. Blood 2005;106(1):59–66.
10. Vinante F, Rigo A. Heparin-binding epidermal growth factor-like growth factor/diphtheria toxin receptor in normal and neoplastic hematopoiesis. Toxins (Basel) 2013;5(6):1180–201.
11. Yamashita M, Chattopadhyay S, Fensterl V, et al. Epidermal growth factor receptor is essential for toll-like receptor 3 signaling. Sci Signal 2012;5(233):ra50.

12. Burgel P-R, Nadel JA. Epidermal growth factor receptor-mediated innate immune responses and their roles in airway diseases. Eur Respir J 2008;32(4):1068–81.
13. Macdonald JB, Macdonald B, Golitz LE, et al. Cutaneous adverse effects of targeted therapies: part I: inhibitors of the cellular membrane. J Am Acad Dermatol 2015;72(2):203–18 [quiz: 219–20].
14. Rosell R, Carcereny E, Gervais R, et al. Erlotinib versus standard chemotherapy as first-line treatment for European patients with advanced EGFR mutation-positive non-small-cell lung cancer (EURTAC): a multicentre, open-label, randomised phase 3 trial. Lancet Oncol 2012;13(3):239–46.
15. Shepherd FA, Rodrigues Pereira J, Ciuleanu T, et al. Erlotinib in previously treated non–small-cell lung cancer. N Engl J Med 2005;353(2):123–32.
16. Ku GY, Haaland BA, de Lima Lopes G. Gefitinib vs. chemotherapy as first-line therapy in advanced non-small cell lung cancer: meta-analysis of phase III trials. Lung Cancer 2011;74(3):469–73.
17. Soria J-C, Felip E, Cobo M, et al. Afatinib versus erlotinib as second-line treatment of patients with advanced squamous cell carcinoma of the lung (LUX-Lung 8): an open-label randomised controlled phase 3 trial. Lancet Oncol 2015;16(8):897–907.
18. Mok TS, Wu Y-L, Ahn M-J, et al. Osimertinib or platinum–pemetrexed in EGFR T790M–positive lung cancer. N Engl J Med 2017;376(7):629 40.
19. Eilers RE, Gandhi M, Patel JD, et al. Dermatologic infections in cancer patients treated with epidermal growth factor receptor inhibitor therapy. J Natl Cancer Inst 2010;102(1):47–53.
20. Guerriero C, Ricci F, Paradisi A, et al. Subcutaneous abscess as a side-effect of cetuximab therapy. Eur J Dermatol 2011;21(2):277–8.
21. Grenader T, Gipps M, Goldberg A. Staphylococcus aureus bacteremia secondary to severe erlotinib skin toxicity. Clin Lung Cancer 2008;9(1):59–60.
22. Li J, Peccerillo J, Kaley K, et al. Staphylococcus aureus bacteremia related with erlotinib skin toxicity in a patient with pancreatic cancer. JOP 2009;10(3):338–40.
23. Bachet J-B, Peuvrel L, Bachmeyer C, et al. Folliculitis induced by EGFR inhibitors, preventive and curative efficacy of tetracyclines in the management and incidence rates according to the type of EGFR inhibitor administered: a systematic literature review. Oncologist 2012;17(4):555 68.
24. Petrelli F, Borgonovo K, Cabiddu M, et al. Antibiotic prophylaxis for skin toxicity induced by antiepidermal growth factor receptor agents: a systematic review and meta-analysis. Br J Dermatol 2016;175(6):1166–74.
25. Funakoshi T, Suzuki M, Muss HB. Infection risk in breast cancer patients treated with trastuzumab: a systematic review and meta-analysis. Breast Cancer Res Treat 2015;149(2):321–30.
26. Johnston S, Pippen J, Pivot X, et al. Lapatinib combined with letrozole versus letrozole and placebo as first-line therapy for postmenopausal hormone receptor–positive metastatic breast cancer. J Clin Oncol 2009;27(33):5538–46.
27. Martin M, Holmes FA, Ejlertsen B, et al. Neratinib after trastuzumab-based adjuvant therapy in HER2-positive breast cancer (ExteNET): 5-year analysis of a randomised, double-blind, placebo-controlled, phase 3 trial. Lancet Oncol 2017; 18(12):1688–700.
28. McCusker MG, Russo A, Scilla KA, et al. How I treat ALK-positive non-small cell lung cancer. ESMO Open 2019;4(Suppl 2):e000524.
29. Zeng L, Kang R, Zhu S, et al. ALK is a therapeutic target for lethal sepsis. Sci Transl Med 2017;9(412). https://doi.org/10.1126/scitranslmed.aan5689.

30. Shaw AT, Kim D-W, Nakagawa K, et al. Crizotinib versus chemotherapy in advanced ALK -positive lung cancer. N Engl J Med 2013;368(25):2385–94.

31. Solomon BJ, Mok T, Kim D-W, et al. First-line crizotinib versus chemotherapy in ALK-positive lung cancer. N Engl J Med 2014;371(23):2167–77.

32. Soria J-C, Tan DSW, Chiari R, et al. First-line ceritinib versus platinum-based chemotherapy in advanced ALK -rearranged non-small-cell lung cancer (ASCEND-4): a randomised, open-label, phase 3 study. Lancet 2017; 389(10072):917–29.

33. Solomon BJ, Besse B, Bauer TM, et al. Lorlatinib in patients with ALK-positive non-small-cell lung cancer: results from a global phase 2 study. Lancet Oncol 2018;19(12):1654–67.

34. Yanagisawa A, Hayama N, Amano H, et al. Crizotinib-induced rectal perforation with abscess. Intern Med 2017;56(23):3211–3.

35. Limon JJ, Fruman DA. Akt and mTOR in B cell activation and differentiation. Front Immunol 2012;3. https://doi.org/10.3389/fimmu.2012.00228.

36. Rafii S, Roda D, Geuna E, et al. Higher risk of infections with PI3K-AKT-mTOR pathway inhibitors in patients with advanced solid tumors on phase i clinical trials. Clin Cancer Res 2015;21(8):1869–76.

37. Qi W-X, Huang Y-J, Yao Y, et al. Incidence and risk of treatment-related mortality with mTOR inhibitors everolimus and temsirolimus in cancer patients: a meta-analysis. PLoS One 2013;8(6):e65166.

38. Albiges L, Chamming's F, Duclos B, et al. Incidence and management of mTOR inhibitor-associated pneumonitis in patients with metastatic renal cell carcinoma. Ann Oncol 2012;23(8):1943–53.

39. Garcia CA, Wu S. Attributable risk of infection to mTOR inhibitors everolimus and temsirolimus in the treatment of cancer. Cancer Invest 2016;34(10):521–30.

40. Mizuno S, Yamagishi Y, Ebinuma H, et al. Progressive liver failure induced by everolimus for renal cell carcinoma in a 58-year-old male hepatitis B virus carrier. Clin J Gastroenterol 2013;6(2):188–92.

41. Göksu SS. Hepatitis B reactivation related to everolimus. World J Hepatol 2013; 5(1):43.

42. Carbonnaux M, Molin Y, Souquet P-J, et al. Pneumocystis jirovecii pneumonia under everolimus in two patients with metastatic pancreatic neuroendocrine tumors. Invest New Drugs 2014;32(6):1308–10.

43. Saito Y, Nagayama M, Miura Y, et al. A case of pneumocystis pneumonia associated with everolimus therapy for renal cell carcinoma. Jpn J Clin Oncol 2013; 43(5):559–62.

44. Schilling B, Sondermann W, Zhao F, et al. Differential influence of vemurafenib and dabrafenib on patients' lymphocytes despite similar clinical efficacy in melanoma. Ann Oncol 2014;25(3):747–53.

45. Sondermann W, Griewank KG, Schilling B, et al. Corticosteroids augment BRAF inhibitor vemurafenib induced lymphopenia and risk of infection. PLoS One 2015; 10(4):e0124590.

46. Lieske NV, Tonby K, Kvale D, et al. Targeting tuberculosis and HIV infection-specific regulatory T cells with MEK/ERK signaling pathway inhibitors. PLoS One 2015;10(11):e0141903.

47. Shi-lin D, Yuan X, Zhan S, et al. Trametinib, a novel MEK kinase inhibitor, suppresses lipopolysaccharide-induced tumor necrosis factor (TNF)-α production and endotoxin shock. Biochem Biophys Res Commun 2015;458(3):667–73.

48. Haasbach E, Hartmayer C, Planz O. Combination of MEK inhibitors and oseltamivir leads to synergistic antiviral effects after influenza A virus infection in vitro. Antiviral Res 2013;98(2):319–24.

49. Cowan N, Keiser J. Repurposing of anticancer drugs: in vitro and in vivo activities against Schistosoma mansoni. Parasit Vectors 2015;8(1):417.

50. Liu W, Yang R, Payne AS, et al. Identifying the target cells and mechanisms of merkel cell polyomavirus infection. Cell Host Microbe 2016;19(6):775–87.

51. Heinzerling L, Eigentler TK, Fluck M, et al. Tolerability of BRAF/MEK inhibitor combinations: adverse event evaluation and management. ESMO Open 2019;4(3). https://doi.org/10.1136/esmoopen-2019-000491.

52. Welsh SJ, Corrie PG. Management of BRAF and MEK inhibitor toxicities in patients with metastatic melanoma. Ther Adv Med Oncol 2015;7(2):122–36.

53. Liu M, Yang X, Liu J, et al. Efficacy and safety of BRAF inhibition alone versus combined BRAF and MEK inhibition in melanoma: a meta-analysis of randomized controlled trials. Oncotarget 2017;8(19). https://doi.org/10.18632/oncotarget.15632.

54. Hicklin DJ, Ellis LM. Role of the vascular endothelial growth factor pathway in tumor growth and angiogenesis. J Clin Oncol 2005;23(5):1011–27.

55. Hurwitz HI, Tebbutt NC, Kabbinavar F, et al. Efficacy and safety of bevacizumab in metastatic colorectal cancer: pooled analysis from seven randomized controlled trials. Oncologist 2013;18(9):1004–12.

56. Novitskiy SV, Csiki I, Huang Y, et al. Anti-vascular endothelial growth factor treatment in combination with chemotherapy delays hematopoietic recovery due to decreased proliferation of bone marrow hematopoietic progenitor cells. J Thorac Oncol 2010;5(9):1410–5.

57. Kaur S, Chang T, Singh SP, et al. CD47 signaling regulates the immunosuppressive activity of VEGF in T cells. J Immunol 2014;193(8):3914–24.

58. Hapani S, Chu D, Wu S. Risk of gastrointestinal perforation in patients with cancer treated with bevacizumab: a meta-analysis. Lancet Oncol 2009;10(6):559–68.

59. Powles T, Chowdhury S, Bower M, et al. The effect of sunitinib on immune subsets in metastatic clear cell renal cancer. Urol Int 2011;86(1):53–9.

60. Randrup Hansen C, Grimm D, Bauer J, et al. Effects and side effects of using sorafenib and sunitinib in the treatment of metastatic renal cell carcinoma. Int J Mol Sci 2017;18(2):461.

61. Schutz FAB, Je Y, Choueiri TK. Hematologic toxicities in cancer patients treated with the multi-tyrosine kinase sorafenib: A meta-analysis of clinical trials. Crit Rev Oncol Hematol 2011;80(2):291–300.

62. Gunnarsson O, Pfanzelter N, Cohen R, et al. Evaluating the safety and efficacy of axitinib in the treatment of advanced renal cell carcinoma. Cancer Manag Res 2015;7:65.

63. Schutz FAB, Je Y, Richards CJ, et al. Meta-analysis of randomized controlled trials for the incidence and risk of treatment-related mortality in patients with cancer treated with vascular endothelial growth factor tyrosine kinase inhibitors. J Clin Oncol 2012;30(8):871–7.

64. Choueiri TK, Escudier B, Powles T, et al. Cabozantinib versus everolimus in advanced renal cell carcinoma (METEOR): final results from a randomised, open-label, phase 3 trial. Lancet Oncol 2016;17(7):917–27.

65. Hutson TE, Escudier B, Esteban E, et al. Randomized phase iii trial of temsirolimus versus sorafenib as second-line therapy after sunitinib in patients with metastatic renal cell carcinoma. J Clin Oncol 2014;32(8):760–7.

66. Bruix J, Qin S, Merle P, et al. Regorafenib for patients with hepatocellular carcinoma who progressed on sorafenib treatment (RESORCE): a randomised, double-blind, placebo-controlled, phase 3 trial. Lancet 2017;389(10064): 56–66.
67. Chamilos G, Lionakis MS, Kontoyiannis DP. Reply to bazaz and denning. Clin Infect Dis 2018;67(1):157–9.

Infectious Risks Associated with Biologics Targeting Janus Kinase-Signal Transducer and Activator of Transcription Signaling and Complement Pathway for Inflammatory Diseases

Esther Benamu, MD

KEYWORDS

- JAK inhibitor • C5 inhibitor • Infection • Inflammatory disorders
- Autoimmune diseases

KEY POINTS

- C5 inhibitors increase the risk of infections with encapsulated organisms, notably with *Neisseria* spp.
- A combination of vaccination and chemoprophylaxis is needed to mitigate the risk of invasive meningococcal disease in patients receiving C5 inhibitors.
- Janus kinase (JAK) inhibitors directly suppress critical components of the innate and adaptive immune system, increasing the overall risk of infection and of opportunistic diseases such as tuberculosis, *Pneumocystis jirovecii* pneumonia, hepatitis B reactivation, cytomegalovirus, and invasive fungal infections.
- JAK inhibitors (JAKinib) are associated with a markedly increased risk of herpes zoster and efforts should be made to vaccinate patients before therapy, with consideration of prophylaxis in patients at additional risk.
- For JAKinib-treated patients, prophylaxis of opportunistic infections should be individualized based on the net state of immunosuppression and additional risk factors of infection.

INTRODUCTION

Over the last few decades, the medical field has witnessed the breakthrough of biologic targeted therapies for the treatment of a rapidly growing number of conditions across specialties.

University of Colorado Anschutz Campus, RC2 Building -11013, PO Box B-168, Aurora, CO 80045, USA
E-mail address: esther.benamu@cuanschutz.edu

Infect Dis Clin N Am 34 (2020) 271–310
https://doi.org/10.1016/j.idc.2020.02.014
0891-5520/20/© 2020 Elsevier Inc. All rights reserved.

An increasing body of evidence supports the role of complement activation in the pathogenesis of a myriad of inflammatory and autoimmune disorders. The 3 main pathways (classic, lectin, and alternative) of the complement cascade converge at the point of C5 activation, and, thus, C5 inhibition has emerged as an attractive option for the treatment of these diseases.[1]

Similarly, the Janus kinase (JAK)/signal transducer and activator of transcription (STAT) pathway is one of the major channels of cytokine signaling and is increasingly being recognized as playing a critical role in the pathogenesis of inflammatory and immune-mediated diseases.[2] More than 20 JAK inhibitors (JAKinibs) blocking 1 or more JAKs (JAK1, JAk2, JAK3, TyK-2) are at different stages of development for the treatment of multiple cytokine-mediated disorders.

However, because they block specific immune pathways, these agents carry the risk of associated infections. Their rapid development has raised awareness of the need to define these risks and build evidence-based guidelines.

This article reviews the mechanism of action of C5 and JAK-STAT inhibitors; their expected impact on immune responses; and their approved, off-label, and potential indications for the treatment of inflammatory diseases; with special focus on examining the infectious risk deriving from their clinical use, to propose screening, prevention, and risk mitigation strategies.

Complement C5 Inhibitors

Mechanism of action

Eculizumab (Soliris; Alexion) and ravulizumab (Ultomiris; Alexion) are recombinant humanized monoclonal immunoglobulin (Ig) G2/4 antibodies targeting complement protein C5. They block the formation of C5 convertase and its subsequent cleavage into the anaphylatoxin C5a (highly prothrombotic and proinflammatory) and C5b, preventing the formation of the terminal membrane attack complex (MAC) C5b-C9 (**Fig. 1**). This complex plays a key effector role in complement-mediated hemolysis and extracellular killing in pyogenic infections, especially of *Neisseria* spp.[3] Because all 3 arms of the complement cascade converge at the point of C5 activation, C5-targeted therapies have opened horizons for the treatment of disorders resulting from complement overactivation.[1,4]

Indications of C5 inhibitors

Eculizumab was first approved for the treatment of paroxysmal nocturnal hemoglobinuria (PNH) and atypical hemolytic uremic syndrome (aHUS)–associated thrombotic microangiopathy (TMA) in 2007 and 2011 respectively (**Table 1**). Most recently, it was approved for the treatment of refractory acetylcholine receptor antibody (AChRAb)–positive generalized myasthenia gravis (gMG) (2017) and aquaporin-4 antibody-positive neuromyelitis optica spectrum disorder (AQP4NMOsd) (2019).[5]

Paroxysmal nocturnal hemoglobinuria Intravascular hemolysis in PNH results from a deficiency in glycosylphosphatidylinositol (GPI)-anchored proteins CD55 and CD59, which protect cells from complement-mediated destruction.[1] Eculizumab dramatically revolutionized the management of PNH, and its success paved the way for its extended application in inflammation-mediated disorders.

Hemolytic uremic syndrome and thrombotic microangiopathies TMA in aHUS results from hyperactivation of complement's alternative pathway, predisposed by mutations in regulatory genes[6] (see **Fig. 1**). Treatment with eculizumab improves plasma requirements, renal function, and quality of life (QoL), achieving sustained TMA-free status.[7]

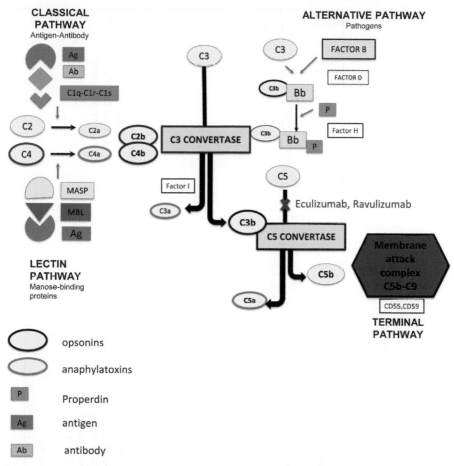

Fig. 1. The complement pathway: mechanism of action of C5 inhibitors.

Using aHUS as an archetypal disease model of complement dysregulation, eculizumab is used in other clinical entities, classified as complement-mediated hemolytic uremic syndrome (HUS), resulting from genetic alterations and/or functional derailment of the complement system leading to inflammatory damage of the glomerular endothelium. Other applications include infection-associated HUS and TMA secondary to malignant hypertension, pregnancy,[8] infection,[9] medications, or autoimmune diseases such as lupus nephritis, antiphospholipid antibody syndrome, scleroderma, or ulcerative colitis (UC).[6,10]

Of particular interest is its application in transplant-associated TMA (TA-TMA) in both hematopoietic stem cell transplant[11] (HSCT) and solid organ transplant (SOT) recipients.[12] Thus far, only case reports/series and small prospective trials have shown a potential benefit, with favorable outcomes in a small cohort of 24 SOT and HSCT recipients.[13] Larger prospective trials are underway to confirm the value of this treatment modality (NCT03518203).

Neurologic disorders In anti-AChR–positive myasthenia gravis, complement inhibition prevents MAC deposition and subsequent destruction of the neuromuscular junction mediated by anti-AChR antibodies.[14] In the REGAIN trial, eculizumab improved

Table 1
Targeted agents, approved indications, and expected infection risks

Drug Class	Drug	Half-Life	Approved Indications	Dosage	Infection Risk	Comments
C5 inhibitors	Eculizumab	11–15 d	PNH	600 mg weekly ×4 wk, then 900 mg every 14 d indefinitely	Neisseria spp. Encapsulated organisms	—
			aHUS	900 mg weekly ×4 wk, then 1200 mg every 14 d		—
			Myasthenia gravis	900 mg weekly ×4 wk, then 1200 mg every 14 d × 26 wk		—
			AQP-4 antibody-positive NMOSD	900 mg weekly ×4 wk, then 1200 mg every 14 d		—
	Ravulizumab	30–50 d	PNH	Weight-based day 1: 40 kg to <60 kg, 2400 mg ; 60 kg to <100 kg, 2700 mg; ≥100 kg, 3000 mg followed by maintenance doses on day 15 and every 8 wk thereafter: 40 kg to <60 kg, 3000 mg; 60 kg to <100 kg, 3300 mg; ≥100 kg, 3600 mg		Noninferior to eculizumab in comparative trials A weekly subcutaneous form is under development

				Overall infection	
JAK inhibitors	Tofacitinib	3 h	Rheumatoid arthritis, Ulcerative colitis	• 5 mg BID • XR 11 mg daily or 22 mg daily	HZ HBV reactivation OIs: PJP, HZ, tuberculosis, CMV, EBV, PML, >IFI	Used in UC at 10 mg BID
	Ruxolitinib	3 h	Myelofibrosis, Polycythemia vera, Acute GVHD	• Myelofibrosis PLT 50–100 × 10^9/L: 5 mg BID PLT 100–200 × 10^9/L: 15 mg BID PLT >200 × 10^9/L: 20 mg BID • PV: 10 mg BID • aGVHD: 5–10 mg BID		Available in 5, 10 mg, 20 mg and 25 mg tabs
	Baricitinib	12.5 h	Rheumatoid arthritis	2 mg daily		—

Abbreviations: aGVHD, acute GVHD; AQP, aquaporin; BID, twice a day; CMV, cytomegalovirus; EBV, Epstein-Barr virus; GVHD, graft-versus-host disease; HBV, hepatitis B virus; HZ, herpes zoster; IFI, invasive fungal infection; IV, intravenous; NMOSD, neuromyelitis optica disorder; OI, opportunistic infection; PJP, *Pneumocystis jirovecii* pneumonia; PLT, platelets; PML, progressive multifocal leukoencephalopathy; PV, polycythemia vera; UC, ulcerative colitis; wk, week; XR, extended release.

muscle strength and QoL, and reduced the rate of exacerbations in patients who had failed immunosuppressants, alone or in combination with immunoglobulin.[15,16]

In AQP4NMOsd, eculizumab reduces MAC-mediated astrocyte and neuronal injury, and reduces the risk of clinical relapse.[16]

Experimental studies suggested a pivotal role of complement in the process of nerve damage in antiganglioside antibody–associated Guillain-Barré syndrome, but a preliminary study failed to show any benefit of eculizumab.[17]

Autoimmune acute hemolytic anemia Warm acute autoimmune hemolytic anemia (AIHA) (75% of AIHA) is typically caused by polyclonal autoantibodies activating complement-mediated hemolysis. Eculizumab showed success treating this disorder in isolated reports, but clinical trials are lacking. In cold agglutinin disease, eculizumab reduced hemolysis and transfusion dependence in a small nonrandomized phase II trial.[18] Targeting higher components of the complement cascade seems more promising and evaluating trials are ongoing[1] (see **Table 1**).

In other conditions, such as catastrophic antiphospholipid syndrome, anecdotal experience suggests a benefit of eculizumab.[1]

C3 glomerulopathies In C3 glomerulopathies (C3Gs), dysregulation of C3 convertase secondary to genetic mutations or autoantibodies leads to glomerular deposition of C3. High soluble levels of C5-C9 are found in C3G patients, but its precise pathogenetic role is incompletely understood. Although evidence of success is limited to isolated reports, experts recommend using eculizumab, especially in patients with short disease duration and high C5-C9 levels.[19] Various clinical trials are underway, mostly evaluating inhibitors of proximal complement.

Eculizumab in transplantation Eculizumab applications have expanded to the prevention and treatment of several deleterious conditions to the transplanted graft, including aHUS, TA-TMA, and also ischemia-reperfusion injury (IRI), delayed graft function (DGF), and antibody-mediated rejection (AMR).

Ischemia-reperfusion injury and delayed graft function C3a and particularly C5a play a pivotal role in IRI leading to DGF.[20] In 2014, eculizumab was granted orphan drug designation for the prevention of DGF in kidney transplantation. However, registration and pilot randomized-controlled trials (RCTs)[21] failed to show any benefit of eculizumab. Results of a European trial (NCT01756508) are pending publication.

Desensitization and antibody-mediated rejection Complement classic pathway plays a key role in the complex pathogenesis of donor-specific antibody-mediated graft injury,[22] and MAC deposition is a poor prognostic factor. Nevertheless, the evidence supporting eculizumab for AMR prevention and treatment is heterogeneous and conflicting. Despite successful reports of AMR reversal, failures have occurred in kidney transplants.[22,23] An open-label trial comparing eculizumab with standard-of-care (SOC) therapy was terminated because of lack of efficacy (NCT01895127).

In a small uncontrolled trial,[24] eculizumab reduced the incidence of AMR by 33% in presensitized cross-match living donor kidney transplant recipients,[25] but a larger phase 2 study failed to show any benefit of prophylactic eculizumab (NCT01399593). Meanwhile, a trial in presensitized deceased-donor kidney transplant recipients showed eculizumab significantly prevented AMR.[26] Application of adjuvant C5 blockade to the prevention of AMR necessitates further investigation. Ongoing trials, including one in heart transplant recipients (NCT02013037), are currently addressing this gap.

Other applications Inhibition of MAC has been explored in the treatment of a diverse array of clinical disorders such as inflammatory ocular diseases[27,28] and asthma.[29]

Indications of ravulizumab Ravulizumab was engineered substituting 4 eculizumab amino acids. It has a longer half-life, allowing a more convenient and effective dosing schedule.[30] In 2 recently published phase III trials, ravulizumab was noninferior to eculizumab both in efficacy and safety for the treatment of PNH,[31,32] and it is now approved for this indication. Moving forward, ravulizumab will likely have expanded indications. Two phase III trials in complement inhibitor–naive patients with HUS are underway (NCT02949128; NCT03131219). In addition, it is being tested for the treatment of gMG (NCT03920293) and IgA nephropathy.[33]

Other targets of the complement pathway A plethora of novel molecules targeting the complement pathway at different levels are under various stages of development for the treatment of multiple inflammatory conditions. **Table 2** summarizes the most relevant agents, trials, and indications investigated.

Infections associated with C5 inhibitors
MAC inhibition results in defective bactericidal activity, particularly against encapsulated organisms. C5b-C9 deficiency is specifically associated with an increased risk of *Neisseria* spp infections (see **Table 1**).[34] Invasive infections with *Streptococcus pneumoniae* or *Haemophilus influenzae* type b are less common with C5 blockage, owing to effective upstream complement function and opsonization. However, the use of C5 inhibitors in patients requiring additional immunosuppressive therapy will present a different risk profile compared with those on targeted blockade alone.

Meningococcal disease Eculizumab-treated patients have 1000-fold to 2000-fold increased risk of meningococcal infection.[35] In the decade following its approval, 158 cases of invasive meningococcal disease (IMD) were reported to the US Food and Drug Administration (FDA) and/or in literature.[36] The estimated crude incidence is 0.25 per 100 patient-years (100PY).[37] Eculizumab is FDA restricted through a Risk Evaluation and Mitigation Strategy (REMS), designed to educate health care providers and patients about this risk and to improve early recognition of IMD. A key element of this program is ensuring patients are immunized before therapy against the most common meningococcal serogroups (in the United States, serogroup B, followed by C and Y) with quadrivalent meningococcal conjugate vaccines (MEN-ACWY), which are more immunogenic than their polysaccharide counterpart, and the recently approved meningococcal B (MEN-B) vaccine. However, breakthrough cases despite vaccination occur. Moreover, IMD with nongroupable *Neisseria meningitidis*, considered a nonpathogenic nasopharyngeal commensal in healthy individuals, is increasingly reported in eculizumab-treated patients. In a recent review of 16 eculizumab-associated cases of IMD (all with meningococcemia; 6 with meningitis), 14 occurred following at least 1 dose of meningococcal vaccine, and 69% of meningococcal strains were nontypable.[38] A summary of meningococcal cases in the literature following eculizumab or ravulizumab is provided in **Table 3**. Many occurred despite vaccination or in the setting of nonprotective specific antibody titers, with varying meningococcal serotypes.[32,38–55]

Meningococcal vaccine response Serum bactericidal antibody (SBA) titers against meningococcal antigens, using human or rabbit complement (hSBA or rSBA, respectively), are the gold standard surrogate of protection against IMD, but these assays are not commercially available. rSBA greater than or equal to 1:8 for MEN-ACWY vaccines; hSBA titers of greater than or equal to 1:4 for MenB vaccines; or 4-fold

Table 2
Novel complement therapeutics, indications and ongoing trials

Complement Target	Drug Name (Company)	Route of Administration	Molecular Category	Disease Indication	Clinical Trials (clinicaltrial.gov)
C1s	BIVV009, sutimlimab (Bioverativ)	IV	mAb	wAIHA, CAD, BP aHUS	NCT02502903; NCT03347396 NCT03347422
MASP-2	OMS721, narsoplimab (Omeros)	IV	mAb	aHUS, TA-TMA C3G, MN, IgAN, LN	NCT03205995; NCT02222545; NCT02682407; NCT02355782; NCT03608033
FB	LNP023 (Novartis)	PO	SM	PNH C3G	NCT03439839; NCT03955445 NCT03832114
FD	ACH_4471, danicopan (Achillion)	PO	SM	PNH C3G	NCT03500549; NCT03369236, NCT03459443
	Lampalizumab (Roche)	IVT	Fab	GA	NCT00973011 NCT01229215 NCT02247479, NCT02247531 NCT02288559
Properdin	CLG561 (Novartis)	IV	mAb	GA	NCT02515942
C3	APL-2, pegcetacoplan (Apellis)	SC IVT	Peptides	wAIHA, CAD C3G, LN, IgAN, LN PNH nAMD GA	NCT03226678 NCT03453619 NCT03500549 NCT02461771 NCT02503332 NCT03525613
	AMY-101, compstatin (Amyndas)	SC	Peptide	PNH	NCT03316521
—	POT4/AL78898A (Potentia/Alcon)	IV	Peptide	nAMD	NCT01157065
C5aR	CCX168, avacopan (Chemocentryx)	PO	SM	C3G ANCA vasculitis	NCT03301467 NCT02994927

Target	Drug	Route	Type	Indication	NCT numbers
C5	ALXN1210, ravulizumab (Alexion)	IV, SC	mAb	PNH, gMG	NCT02946463, NCT03406507; NCT03056040; NCT03920293
	Eculizumab, Soliris (Alexion)	IV	mAb	TA-TMA GA PNH aHUS	NCT03518203 NCT00935883 NCT02352493 NCT03999840
	ALN-CC5, cemdisiran (Alnylam)	SC	RNAi		
	RA101495, zilucoplan (Ra Pharma)	SC	Peptide	PNH, gMG	NCT03030183 NCT03078582 NCT03225287 NCT03315130
	RO7112689, SKY59 (Hoffmann-La Roche)	IV, SC	mAb	PNH	NCT03157635
	REGN3918, pozelimab (Regeneron)	IV, SC	mAb	PNH	NCT03946748
	rVA576, nomacopan (Akari)	SC	Protein	PNH	NCT03427060, NCT03588026 NCT03829449
	ABP-959 (Amgen)	IV	mAb	PNH	NCT03818607
—	LFG316 (Novartis)	IVT	mAb	GA, nAMD GA nAMD	NCT01255462 NCT01527500 NCT01535950
—	ARC1905 (Ophthotech)	IVT	Aptamer	GA nAMD PCV	NCT00950638 NCT02686658 NCT00709527 NCT03362190 NCT03374670
CD59	AAVCAGsCD59 (Hemera)	IVT	Virus	GA	NCT03144999

Abbreviations: ANCA, antineutrophil cytoplasmic antibody; BP, bullous pemphigoid; C3G, C3 glomerulopathies; CAD, cold agglutinin disease; Fab, fragment antibody; FB, factor B; FD, factor D; GA, geographic atrophy; IgAN, IgA nephropathy; IVT, intravitreal; LN, lupus nephritis; mAb, monoclonal antibody; MASP-2, mannose-binding lectin-associated serine protease; MN, membranous nephropathy; nAMD, neovascular age-related macular degeneration; PCV, polypoidal choroidal vasculopathy; PNH, paroxysmal nocturnal hemoglobinuria; PO, by mouth; RNAi, RNA interference; SC, subcutaneous; SM, small molecule; wAIHA, warm autoimmune hemolytic anemia.

Table 3
Case reports and series of meningococcal disease in patients treated with eculizumab, ravulizumab

Report	Age (y), Sex	Underlying Disorder (n)	Vaccine Type	Prophylaxis (Agent)	Meningococcal Serotype	Presentation	Onset Since ECM/RVM or Vaccination	Outcome
Eculizumab								
Hillmen et al,[39] 2013	24, M 54, F	PNH PNH	MEN-ACWY-ps MEN A and C	NA NA	B Y or 135W	Septicemia Septicemia	353 d 14 mo	Recovery Recovery
Vicente et al,[40] 2012	27, M	PNH	MEN-4ps	No	X	Septic shock	16 mo	Death
Rey-Múgica Mde et al,[41] 2013	18, M	PNH	MEN-4ps	Yes, secondary	B	Sepsis	NA	Recovery
Strujik et al,[42] 2013	19, F	aHUS, RT	MEN-4ps	No	W135	Septic shock	18 mo	Recovery
Applegate et al,[43] 2016	41, M	PNH	MEN-4ps	No	NA	Septic shock	3 y	Recovery
Hernando-Real et al,[44] 2017	23, M	PNH	MEN-ACWY, MenB	Yes, secondary (Pen V)	B[a]	Septic shock	4 y after ECM, 10 mo after MenB	Recovery
Friedl et al,[45] 2017	22, M	SLE-TMA	MenB, MenC	Yes, primary/secondary (ciprofloxacin)	W135	WFS, septic shock	11 mo after ECM, 3 mo after MenB/C, 1 mo off prophylaxis	Recovery

Study	Age, Sex	Condition	Vaccine	Prophylaxis	Serogroup	Presentation	Timing	Outcome
Parikh et al,[46] 2017	26, F	aHUS	MenC; MEN-ACWY; MenB	Yes, primary (Pen V)	B	Septicemia, penicillin-resistant strain	4 mo after MenB	Recovery
Polat et al,[47] 2018	11, M	aHUS	MEN-ACWY-D	Yes, primary (Pen V)	Y	Septicemia, shock-isolate with intermediate penicillin susceptibility	18 mo after ECM, 16 mo after MEN-ACWY completed	Death
Cullinan et al,[48] 2015	5, F	aHUS	MEN-ACWY, MenC	Yes, amoxicillin	W	Septicemia; intermediate penicillin susceptibility	30 mo	Recovery
McNamara et al,[38] 2017 (2008-2016, 16 cases)	30 (range: 16-83)	aHUS (n = 10) PNH (n = 5) Other (n = 1)	MEN-ACWY (n = 14), MenB (n = 2)	NA 1 patient: Pen V	Y (n = 4) NT (n = 11) NA (n = 1)	Septicemia (n = 16), meningitis (n = 6)[b]	NA	Death (n = 1) Recovery (n = 15)
Lebel et al,[49] 2018	25, M	PNH	MEN-ACWY-ps	NA	Y	Septicemia	2 wk after MEN-ACWY, 1 wk after ECM	Recovery
Reher et al,[50] 2018	26, F	PNH	MEN-ACWY, MenB	NA	B	Septicemia, shock	6 y after ECM; 2 y after MenB	Recovery
Nolfi-Donegan et al,[51] 2018	16, F	PNH	MEN-ACWY, MenB	NA	NT	Septic shock, WFS	6 mo after vaccination, 24 h after ECM	Death

(continued on next page)

Table 3
(continued)

Report	Age (y), Sex	Underlying Disorder (n)	Vaccine Type	Prophylaxis (Agent)	Meningococcal Serotype	Presentation	Onset Since ECM/RVM or Vaccination	Outcome
Ladhani et al,[52] 2019 9 episodes, 8 patients	22 (range: 20–40)	5 PNH 3 aHUS	MEN-ACWY (n = 7) MenB (n = 3)	Pen V (n = 4) Ciprofloxacin (n = 1) No (n = 1) NA (2)	B (n = 3), NT(B) (n = 3), Y n = 1), W (n = 1), E (n = 1)	IMD, not specified[c]	—	—
Hawkins et al,[53] 2017	18, F	PNH	MEN-ACWY	No primary prophylaxis	NT	Septic shock	2 y	Recovery
Hall et al,[54] 2018	25, M	PNH	MEN-ACWY	Yes, penV	NT	Septic shock	8 mo after vaccination	Recovery
Ravulizumab								
Röth et al,[55] 2018	28, M	PNH	MEN-ACWY, MenB	Yes, Pen V	Y/W135	Septicemia, penicillin intermediate isolate	57 d	Recovery
—	18, M	PNH	MEN-ACWY, MenB	No	Y	Septicemia, penicillin resistant isolate	222 d	Recovery

Abbreviations: ECM, eculizumab; F, female; M, male; MEN, meningococcal vaccine; MEN-4ps, polysaccharide quadrivalent; MEN-ACWY, quadrivalent conjugated; NA, nonavailable; NT, nontypeable; NT(B), nontypeable (interruption of ctrA gene) but genotypically capsular group B; Pen V, penicillin V; PNH, paroxysmal nocturnal hemoglobinuria; RT, renal transplant; RVM, ravulizumab; SLE, systemic lupus erythematous; TMA, thrombotic microangiopathy; WFS, Waterhouse-Friderichsen syndrome.

[a] Molecular analysis showed a strain with the fHbp antigen (variant 2/subfamily A), differing from the variant included in the vaccine (variant 1/subfamily B) and contained the same variant of the Neisseria Heparin Binding Antigen (NHBA) antigen present in the vaccine (allele 1/peptide 2).

[b] Antibiotic susceptibilities for 14 isolates (susceptible, intermediate, resistant); ampicillin (11, 3, 0); ceftriaxone (14, 0, 0); ciprofloxacin (13, 0, 1); penicillin (10, 3, 1); azithromycin (14, 0, 0).

[c] Isolates: 5 penicillin susceptible (2 patients were on penicillin prophylaxis, 1 on ciprofloxacin, 1 on no prophylaxis), 1 penicillin resistant (on penicillin prophylaxis) and 3 NA.

increases in patients with prevaccination titers are considered seroprotective.[56] However, the use of exogenous human complement, which is inactivated by eculizumab, makes hSBA hard to interpret in eculizumab-treated patients. Furthermore, in vitro data suggest that eculizumab interferes with the ability of antimeningococcal antibodies to provide protection despite vaccination, owing to the blockage of C5a-mediated opsonophagocytic and MAC bactericidal effects.[57] Recent studies evaluating the immunogenicity of MEN-ACWY in these patients have shown poor responses (at 35–60 days postvaccination) with rapidly waning immunity after 6 months, and strain-specific disparities.[58,59] The immunogenicity and duration of protection of MenB vaccines is less established. In 85% of healthy adolescents, MenB-4C (Bexsero) induced rapidly waning but protective responses after 18 to 24 months.[60] In a more recent study, responses, albeit lower, were adequate in most children with complement deficiency,[61] suggesting boosters may be beneficial. Durable protection is particularly important in individuals receiving long-standing eculizumab and those under other immunosuppressants that dampen humoral response. With robust vaccine studies lacking in this population, but evidence of unpredictable and individually differing serologic responses as well as waning seroprotection and circulating meningococcal strains that are not covered by administered vaccines, experts are driven to use chemoprophylaxis for the duration of eculizumab therapy and recommend monitoring antibody responses to assess the need for reimmunization.[3,62]

Infections with other *Neisseria* spp Terminal complement inhibition increases the risk of disseminated gonococcal infection (DGI), a rare invasive form of the *Neisseria gonorrhoeae* infection occurring in 0.5% to 3% of patients. DGI can present with skin lesions, tenosynovitis, arthritis, and (rarely) life-threatening gonococcemia, endocarditis, or meningitis. Most patients have evidence of genital, anorectal, or pharyngeal infection.[63] A total of 9 cases of gonorrhea have been reported in patients taking eculizumab, 8 of whom were hospitalized with DGI, 2 in septic shock. One death was attributed to PNH. Eculizumab was discontinued in 1 of the 8 survivors.[64] Crew and colleagues[65] recently reported a case series of invasive infection with typically commensal nonmeningococcal, nongonococcal *Neisseria* spp.. Of note, 4 of the 7 patients had additional immunosuppressive conditions.[65] **Tables 4** and **5** summarize these reports.

Other infections In initial trials, respiratory tract infections were more frequent in eculizumab-treated patients. Urinary tract infections (UTIs) and other viral syndromes were reported in a third of patients.[5] Other reports are anecdotal.

Bacterial infections A handful of cases of severe pseudomonal sepsis during eculizumab therapy have been published.[3] Taking into consideration their coexisting comorbidities, reports of recurrent pseudomonal infections in 2 patients on chronic C5 inhibitor underscore the potentially under-recognized role of terminal complement in the effective killing of these bacteria.[66,67]

Viral infections There is growing evidence suggesting a role of complement in T-cell regulation.[68] Herpes simplex virus (HSV) 1 and respiratory viral syndromes have been reported with eculizumab.[5,69] A kidney-intestine transplant recipient diagnosed with progressive multifocal leukoencephalopathy (PML) improved after discontinuation of C5 blockade and before tapering of other immunosuppression therapy, suggesting a partial role of terminal complement blockade in the development of PML.[70]

Fungal infections A case of aspergillus peritonitis and 1 report of disseminated cryptococcosis in eculizumab-treated patients have shown the theoretic risk of fungal

Table 4

Reported cases of nonmeningococcal, nongonococcal *Neisseria* spp infections in eculizumab-treated patients

Case	*Neisseria* spp	Age (y), Sex	Indication	Catheter, Type	Immunosuppression	Infection Diagnosis, Presentation	Treatment	Outcome
1	*Neisseria sicca* (mucosa)/ subflava	13, M	PNH	CVC	HSCT, neutropenia	Bacteremia	Piperacillin-tazobactam	Recovery
2	*N sicca* (mucosa)/ subflava	6, M	aHUS	SC Port	—	Bacteremia	Ceftriaxone	Recovery
3	*N sicca* (mucosa)	38, F	CAPS	PD catheter, IV port	CVID, lupus, rituximab, steroids	Bacterial peritonitis	Not specified	Recovery
4	*Neisseria cinerea*	17, F	PNH	NA	Lymphoglobulin therapy	Septic shock, bacteremia, possible cholecystitis	Ceftriaxone, metronidazole	Recovery
5	*N cinerea*	38, F	aHUS	HD, AVF	—	Bacteremia	Cefepime	Recovery
6	*Neisseria mucosa*	32, F	PNH	NA	—	Polymicrobial bacteremia, prior gastroenteritis	Ceftriaxone, amoxicillin	Recovery
7	*Neisseria flavescens* (subflava)	4, M	aHUS	NA	HSCT, neutropenia	Neutropenic sepsis	Not specified	Recovery, death from tumor

Abbreviations: AVF, arteriovenous fistula; CAPS, catastrophic antiphospholipid syndrome; CVC, central venous catheter; CVID, common variable immunodeficiency; HD, hemodialysis; HSCT, hematopoietic stem cell transplant; PD, peritoneal dialysis.

Table 5
Reported cases of gonococcal infection in patients receiving eculizumab

Case	Age (y), Sex	Indication	DGI	Culture, Test Positivity	Presentation	Time to Onset (Since ECM)	Treatment	Outcome
1	22, F	PNH	Yes	BC (+)	NR	NR	NR	Resolved
2	28, F	PNH	Yes	BC (+); UG-NAAT (+); LP(−); TTE(−)	Fever, tenosynovitis	16 m	Vancomycin + ceftriaxone, then ceftriaxone + azithromycin (×1)	Resolved
3	23, F	aHUS	Yes	BC (+), UG-NAAT (−)	Fever	46 d	Piperacillin-tazobactam + vancomycin, then ceftriaxone + azithromycin (×1)	Resolved
4	18, F	aHUS	NR	NR	Possible pregnancy	NR	NR	Resolved
5	19, F	PNH	Yes	Cervical culture (+)	Arthralgias Later diagnosed with endocarditis (pathogen NR), thrombotic spleen, CVA	NR	NR	Death ~ 2 mo later, attributed to PNH
6	19, F	PNH	Yes	BC (+); NAAT (−), rectal/genital culture (−)	Fever, RUQ pain and emesis, hypotension	788 d	Vancomycin + ceftriaxone, then meropenem	Resolved
7	42, M	PNH	Yes	BC (+)	Fever, skin lesions	1513 d	Ciprofloxacin	Resolved
8	44, F	PNH	Yes	BC (+)	Fever, arthralgias, body aches	NR	Cefepime, vancomycin, levofloxacin, then ceftriaxone	Resolved
9	28, F	aHUS	Yes	BC (+); LP cultures (−); skin biopsy (−); endocervical GC-PCR (−)	Fever, headache, emesis, maculopapular rash	613 d	Ceftriaxone	Resolved

Abbreviations: BC, blood culture; DGI, disseminated gonococcal infection; GC, gonococcus; LP, lumbar puncture; NAAT, nucleic acid amplification test; NR, not reported; PCR, polymerase chain reaction; RUQ, right upper quadrant; TTE, transthoracic echocardiogram; UG, urogenital.

infection with terminal complement inhibition, previously suggested in experimental data.[71,72] Fungi have a thick cell wall resisting MAC-mediated lysis. However, aspergillus killing relies on C3-dependent opsonization and C5a-mediated inflammatory response leading to efficient phagocytosis.[73] Similarly, *Cryptococcus neoformans* is not affected by MAC (although *Cryptococcus gattii* is), but host defense heavily depends on C5a-mediated chemotaxis and adequate function of phagocytic cells.[72]

Infection prevention and management strategies
Monitoring C5 activity
- The risk of infection during C5-inhibitor therapy can be indirectly assessed via monitoring of complement blockade and eculizumab efficacy (**Table 6**). Soluble C5b-C9, C5 activity, and 50% hemolytic omplement levels have been proposed as surrogate markers of complement inhibition. A complement activity screen assay (Wieslab) showed high sensitivity and specificity detecting C5 activity.[74] However, these biomarkers fail to detect local complement dysregulation, but tissue functional assays are logistically difficult to perform.[75] Test availability and long turnaround time limit routine use of eculizumab drug monitoring. The most promising marker is CH50, which negatively correlates with free eculizumab levels.[76] Appropriate clinical response to Soliris is associated with complete CH50 blockade (CH50<10%), steady eculizumab therapeutic levels (>99 µg/mL), and low sC5-C9 level.[77] Owing to the prolonged half-lives of eculizumab ($\sim$11–15 days) and ravulizumab ($\sim$30–50 days), drug effects can be expected for months (3 or more) after therapy discontinuation.

Meningococcal vaccination
- Eculizumab and ravulizumab carry a black box warning for the risk of IMD and are contraindicated in unvaccinated patients.[5] Prescribers should be familiar with the REMS program and trained to recognize and treat IMD promptly.
- The Advisory Committee on Immunization Practices (ACIP) recommends that patients starting C5 inhibitors be immunized with a quadrivalent vaccine, preferably the more immunogenic conjugated forms (MEN-ACWY), and simultaneously with a recombinant vaccine against serotype B; at least 2 weeks before treatment initiation or as soon as possible if therapy is urgent. Two initial doses of Men-ACWY-D (Menactra, Nimenrix in Europe) or MEN-ACWY-CRM (Menveo) at least 8 to 12 weeks apart are recommended.[78] MEN-B-4C (Bexsero) is indicated as a 2 monthly dose series. MEN-B-FHbp (Trumenba) is licensed in the United States as a 3-dose series administered at 0, 2, and 6 months. A broadly protective promising vaccine against A, B, C, W, and Y serotypes is under investigation.[79]
- rSBA titers should be checked 4 to 6 weeks following completed meningococcal vaccination, then after 6 months and every 1 to 3 years thereafter, with the goal to reimmunize if antibody titers are below protective thresholds.
- The ACIP recommends revaccination with conjugate MEN-ACWY every 5 years, whereas experts recommend boosters every 3 years if C5-inhibitor therapy is continued. According to the ACIP, MEN-B boosters should be given 1 year after initial immunization and every 2 to 3 years while on C5 inhibitors (recommendations yet to be approved by the US Centers for Disease Control and Prevention).[80]

Meningococcal prophylaxis
- During the window period until seroprotection and for at least 2 to 4 weeks following vaccination, meningococcal antibiotic prophylaxis should be administered. However, vaccination cannot ensure sufficient immunoprotection against

Table 6
Recommended infection prevention and management strategies before and during C5-inhibitor therapy (eculizumab, ravulizumab)

Meningococcal Disease			Gonococcal Disease		Other Infections	
Vaccination	Prophylaxis	Monitoring	Screening	Treatment	Prevention	Active Infection
Start at least 2–4 wk before first dose of C5 inhibitor: • MEN-ACWY-D or MEN-ACWY-CRM, 2 doses 8–12 wk apart And[a] • MenB-FHbp: 3 doses at 0, 2, –6 mo Or MenB-4c: 2 doses a month apart Response: SBA titers 4–6 wk after completion Additional doses: • Booster MEN-ACWY every 3–5 y[b] or if rBSA<1:8 • Booster MenB after 1 y and q2-3 y[b] or if hBSA<1:4	• Start with first infusion Penicillin V 250 mg BID; or ciprofloxacin 500 mg/d, or azithromycin 250 mg/d, or cefdinir 300 mg/d, or cefpodoxime 400 mg/d[c] • Minimum duration: 4 wk since last vaccine dose and/or achieved seroprotective titers • Can use SBA to guide continuation of prophylaxis • Consider prophylaxis extension for the duration of C5-inhibitor therapy, especially in immunocompromised hosts	• SBA titers 4–6 wk postvaccination, at 6 mo, 1 y, and yearly while on therapy If titers non-protective: vaccine booster and initiate/resume prophylaxis	Sexually active women younger than 25 y old and patients at high risk of STD Consider yearly screening while on C5 inhibitor and at risk • NAAT for GC/CT	NAAT positive for GC and/or CT: • Ceftriaxone 250 mg IM ×1 And Azithromycin 1 g PO ×1 • During C5-inhibitor therapy: Treat if NAAT positive and evaluate for DGI	Immunize all previously unvaccinated patients for: H influenzae S pneumoniae[d]	• Hold C5-inhibitor if possible, and resume once clinical resolution and/or infection adequately treated • May use CH50 activity (hold C5 inhibitor if <10%) • Consider infectious diseases consultation to guide therapy

(continued on next page)

Table 6
(continued)

	Meningococcal Disease		Gonococcal Disease			Other Infections
Vaccination	Prophylaxis	Monitoring	Screening	Treatment	Prevention	Active Infection
	• C5-inhibitor discontinuation: Continue prophylaxis for at least 5–6 C5-inhibitor elimination half-lives and/or until CH50 normalizes		• Also screen for HIV, HSV, syphilis, hepatitis • Partner evaluation • Counseling	• DGI: ceftriaxone 1–2 g daily + azithromycin 1 g PO ×1 (>7 d; 14 d for meningitis; 4 wk for endocarditis)		• In immunosuppressed host (eg, transplant): reduce immunosuppression if feasible

Abbreviations: CT, *Chlamydia trachomatis*; hBSA, human complement serum bactericidal antibodies; HIV, human immunodeficiency virus; IM, intramuscular; rBSA, rabbit complement serum bactericidal antibodies; STD, sexually transmitted disease.

[a] MEN-ACWY and MenB can be administered simultaneously on different sites.

[b] Evaluate continued seroprotection: enzyme-linked immunosorbent assay serotype-specific antibody titers less than 2 g/mL or SBA titers less than 1:4 (if available) indicate lack of protection and need for revaccination or prophylaxis.

[c] With increasing rates of penicillin resistance or if penicillin allergic, alternatives to penicillin: ciprofloxacin or azithromycin or cephalosporins (if tolerated). Need to consider the adverse effects of these agents when used in the long term.

[d] Thirteen-valent pneumococcal vaccine (Prevnar 13) should not be administered simultaneously with meningococcal vaccines. Administer 4 weeks apart.

IMD in patients receiving C5 inhibitors. Therefore, besides monitoring the vaccine response, chemoprophylaxis for the duration of eculizumab/ravulizumab treatment should be strongly considered.

- Special consideration should be given to immunosuppressed patients, in whom impaired and unpredictable immune responses further compromise humoral protection. Continuation of prophylaxis for the duration of C5-inhibitor therapy is strongly recommended. Monitoring of vaccine titers can direct the need for revaccination and strength of recommendation for continued prophylaxis.
- Long-term penicillin prophylaxis (penicillin VK 250 mg twice daily) is generally considered safe. However, meningococcal penicillin resistance is emerging.[38,51] Alternatives include cefdinir, cefpodoxime, azithromycin, or ciprofloxacin, but long-term toxicities need to be considered. Quality studies evaluating the efficacy or safety of antibiotic prophylaxis in eculizumab recipients are lacking. With the limitations inherent to the data source, Crew and colleagues[36] reviewed 47 cases of IMD reported to the FDA or in the literature over a decade (all previously vaccinated). Compared with non–prophylaxis users, prophylaxed patients (n = 15) had longer median time to onset of first meningococcal episode (835 vs 333 days), although wide ranges were observed in both groups, and higher frequency of reduced penicillin susceptibility (5 of 6 isolates, 83%, vs 2 of 9 isolates, 22%).[36] Prescribers must weigh the potential risks of antibiotic prophylaxis, such as adverse events and antibiotic resistance, against its potential benefits.
- Chemoprophylaxis duration following discontinuation of C5-inhibitor therapy should be guided by the normalization of CH50 levels and (expected) drug clearance.
- Ultimately, neither meningococcal vaccination nor prophylaxis can be expected to fully prevent meningococcal disease in C5-inibitor recipients. Heightened patient awareness of the risks and symptoms of IMD, vaccination of close contacts, early care seeking, and provision of an effective antibiotic to be taken at first signs/symptoms of IMD are additional mitigating strategies.

Prevention of other infections
- Sexually active, high-risk patients and their partners should receive counseling and be screened for gonococcal disease (and other sexually transmitted diseases) before administration of C5 inhibitors and periodically while at risk. Providers should evaluate for signs and symptoms of DGI if *N. gonorrhea* is detected and cases should be reported. Treatment of gonorrhea and DGI should follow guideline recommendations.
- Although the risk of infection is lower for other encapsulated bacteria, unvaccinated patients starting C5 inhibitors should be immunized against *S. pneumoniae* and *H. influenzae* type b, following ACIP guidelines.
- In addition, the role of complement in the prevention and clearance of bacterial, viral, and fungal infections is less well understood. Experimental data suggest an increased risk of fungal infection with complement inhibition. However, the contribution of C5 blockade to these occurrences is insufficiently documented. Therefore, no recommendation can be made on the potential benefit of screening or prophylaxis in these patients. Increased awareness and reporting of infections in the context of C5-inhibitor therapy is encouraged.
- When possible, C5 inhibitors should be held during active infections, until clinically resolved.

Janus Kinase/Signal Transducer and Activator of Transcription Inhibitors

Mechanism of action

The JAK-STAT pathway plays a key role in hematopoiesis, immune-cell signaling and differentiation, and the pathogenesis of many neoplastic and immune-mediated/inflammatory diseases.[2] JAK-STATs mediate cytokine signaling through specific receptors. Type I receptors are used by multiple interleukins (ILs), colony-stimulating factors, and hormones, and type II bind to interferon (IFN) and IL-10-related cytokines. These receptors have various subunits, each associated with specific molecules of the JAK family (JAK1, JAK2, JAK3) and tyrosine-kinase 2 (TyK2), each exerting differential effects. Once activated, JAKs autophosphorylate and transphosphorylate cytokine receptors and STAT molecules. The latter translocate to the cell nucleus, bind DNA, and regulate gene expression (**Fig. 2**).

JAK1 mediates lymphoid development, whereas JAK2 is key to neural development and erythropoiesis. Defects in JAK1 lead to severe combined immunodeficiency (SCID) and impaired immune responses to bacteria and virus. The V617F activating mutation of the JAK2 gene is a hallmark of polycythemia vera (PV), and is present in 50% to 75% of patients with myelofibrosis and essential thrombocythemia. TyK2 deficiency is associated with a suboptimal interferon/IL-12 response, and resistance to arthritis treatment. JAK3 has a key role in the inflammatory cascade and has become a promising target in the treatment of inflammatory diseases and in organ transplantation. Loss-of-function mutations in the JAK3 gene also lead to SCID.[81]

Indications of Janus kinase inhibitors in inflammatory diseases

Three main JAKinibs have been FDA approved (**Tables 1** and **7**). Ruxolitinib (Jakafi, Novartis Pharmaceuticals) targets JAK1 and JAK2 and was approved for the

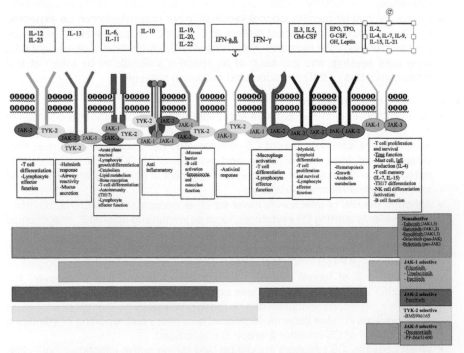

Fig. 2. The JAK-STAT pathway: mechanism of action and effects of JAK-STAT inhibitors. NK, natural killer; TNF, tumor necrosis factor; Treg, T-regulatory cell.

Table 7	
Inflammatory diseases and Janus kinase inhibitors	
Approved Indications	**Investigated Indications and Reported Use**
Rheumatoid arthritis	Psoriasis
Psoriatic arthritis	Ankylosing spondylitis and other spondyloarthropathies
UC	Juvenile idiopathic arthritis and polyarthropathies
aGVHD	Chronic GVHD, GVHD prophylaxis
	Alopecia areata
	Atopic dermatitis
	Dermatomyositis
	Vitiligo
	Lichen sclerosus et atrophicans
	Systemic sclerosis
	Morphea
	Hypereosinophilic syndrome
	Eosinophilic fasciitis
	Contact dermatitis
	SAPHO
	Bullous skin disorders
	Organ transplant rejection
	Posttransplant bronchiolitis obliterans
	Interferonopathies
	SLE
	Sjögren syndrome
	Uveitis (noninfectious)
	Giant cell arteritis and median, large vessel vasculitis
	Atherosclerosis
	Diabetic nephropathy

Abbreviations: SAPHO, synovitis, acne, pustulosis, hyperostosis, and osteitis; SLE, systemic lupus erythematosus.

treatment of myelofibrosis[82] and refractory PV.[83] It recently obtained approval for the treatment of steroid-refractory acute graft-versus-host-disease (aGVHD).[84] Tofacitinib (Xeljanz, Pfizer) blocks JAK1 and JAK3 (and at high concentrations JAK2 and TyK2) and is licensed for the treatment of moderate-to-severe rheumatoid arthritis (RA) and psoriatic arthritis (PsA) in patients unresponsive to or intolerant of disease-modifying antirheumatic drugs (DMARDs),[2] and for the treatment of moderate-severe UC.[85] Baricitinib (Olumiant, Eli Lilly) is a reversible inhibitor of JAK1 and JAK2 approved for refractory RA.[86] Newer generations of more selective JAKinibs are in different stages of development and investigation to treat a wide range of inflammatory diseases, leukemia, and solid malignancies.

Rheumatoid arthritis Clinical trials have shown tofacitinib's efficacy in treating RA, alone or in combination with methotrexate.[87] It has proved to be superior to methotrexate,[88] noninferior to adalimumab,[89] and effective in patients failing multiple biologics.[90] Tofacitinib ameliorates disease activity, functional status, and patient-reported outcomes, preventing disease progression.[2]

Baricitinib was recently approved for the treatment of moderate/severe RA failing 1 or 2 anti–tumor necrosis factor inhibitor (TNFi) agents. Baricitinib significantly improves disease activity, radiographically assessed structural damage, and patient-reported outcomes.[91] It is superior to methotrexate but, contrary to tofacitinib, it outperforms adalimumab.[86]

Peficitinib is a pan-JAK inhibitor with slight JAK3 selectivity that has recently been approved in Japan for treatment of RA. As monotherapy or in combination with methotrexate, it achieves similar results.[2]

Psoriatic arthritis and other arthropathies The role of JAKinibs in other arthritides is incompletely understood, but is thought to be associated with the inhibition of the IL-23/17 axis, which plays a crucial role in the pathogenesis of PsA and spondyloarthropathies, via blockage of IL-22 and IL-23 (which drives IL-17A release), and inhibition of type I IFNs.[92]

Tofacitinib is approved for the treatment of methotrexate-refractory and/or DMARD-refractory or intolerant PsA,[93] and has shown efficacy treating ankylosing spondylitis (AS),[94] which has been associated with polymorphisms of JAK2/STAT2, making JAKinibs a promising alternative to the few available treatment options of seronegative spondyloarthropathies. Following its anecdotal success with treatment-refractory polyarthropathies, tofacitinib is being evaluated for the treatment of juvenile idiopathic arthritis (NCT01500551, NCT02592434).[2] Clinical trials are underway assessing the efficacy and safety of the newer JAK1 inhibitors filgotinib and upadacitinib in PsA and AS.[92]

Graft-versus-host disease Graft-versus-host-disease (GVHD) is caused by donor T-lymphocyte activation by host antigens. Proinflammatory cytokines IL-6 and IFN-γ and T-regulatory cells (Tregs) play a major role in its pathogenesis. Experimental models showed that ruxolitinib and tofacitinib improve and prevent severe GVHD.[95] Favorable results of a retrospective study[84] and phase II trial (response>80%, 55% respectively) led to the approval of ruxolitinib for the treatment of steroid-refractory aGVHD.[96,97] At present, phase III trials are evaluating the efficacy of ruxolitinib and itacitinib for the treatment of aGVHD (NCT02913261, NCT03139604) and chronic GVHD (cGVHD) (NCT03112603, NCT03584516). Itacitinib recently entered 2 phase I studies for prophylactic use.

Inflammatory bowel disease IL-6 is universally implicated in inflammatory bowel disease (IBD) pathogenesis. Other JAK-dependent cytokines, such as IL-9, are thought to play a role in UC but not in Crohn disease (CD), for which IL-12, IL-23, IL-21, IL-22, IL-27, and IFN-γ are key players. Three phase III clinical trials showed that tofacitinib induction (10 mg twice a day) and maintenance (5 or 10 mg twice a day) therapy achieve sustained clinical remission and mucosal healing, improving patient QoL in refractory moderate-severe UC.[85] Results of tofacitinib in CD are less encouraging, but the newer filgotinib and upadacitinib show promise.[92] Variability in clinical response to JAKinibs may be secondary to differential susceptibility of the gastrointestinal mucosa to discrete JAK pathway inhibition (JAK1 vs JAK 2 rather than JAK3) and the detrimental effects of blocking cytokines with antiinflammatory properties (IL-10) or those involved in mucosal barrier integrity (IL-22, IL-9, and indirectly IL-17 via IL-6 and IL-23).

Psoriasis IL-6, IL-22, IL-23, and IFN-γ are implicated in the pathogenesis of psoriasis, suggesting JAKinibs may be powerful treatment options. Although tofacitinib improved disease severity scores in pivotal studies, a recent trial showed that only high dosages of the drug (10 mg twice daily) were noninferior to SOC etanercept.[95,98] Thus, it is not yet FDA approved for this indication, pending additional information on the safety/benefit ratio.

Topical formulations of tofacitinib and ruxolitinib have had less convincing results.[95] Baricitinib (at high doses), the newer peficitinib, and BMS-986165 (Tyk-2 selective) have shown promise in phase 2 studies.[2] Newer JAKinibs (oral and topical) are under investigation in a growing number of trials.

Alopecia areata Alopecia areata results from the upregulation in hair follicles of genes induced by IFN-γ, IL-2, and IL-15, through STAT1, STAT3, and STAT 5.[95] Early-phase clinical trials and large retrospective studies indicate that oral tofacitinib, ruxolitinib, and baricitinib promote hair regrowth, albeit with time-limited effects and recurrences on drug discontinuation.[2,95] Topical ruxolitinib has also shown efficacy.[99] Additional phase II and III trials with oral and topical JAKinibs are underway.

Atopic dermatitis There is growing evidence that atopic dermatitis (AD) is not solely defined by T-helper (Th) 2 cells and related cytokines (IL-4, IL-5, IL-10, IL-13, and IL-31) but also by cytokines linked to other Th responses such as IFN-γ (Th1), IL17, or IL-22 (Th17) and, thus, there is growing interest for JAKinib therapy. Topical formulations, if efficacious and safe, are desirable. The oral and topical JAK1/JAK3-inhibitor tofacitinib, which abrogates IL-4–driven Th2 cell differentiation, showed efficacy in moderate-severe and mild AD, respectively.[100,101] Baricitinib ameliorates AD and spares prolonged topical corticosteroids.[102] Other JAKinibs, such as oclacitinib (JAk1) or the nonselective JTE-052, show promise. Clinical trials further evaluating baricitinib (some with favorable preliminary results), topical ruxolitinib, and newer JAKinibs (PF-04965842, upadacitinib) are underway.[2,92,95]

Other dermatologic conditions The introduction of JAKinibs is enlarging the therapeutic repertoire of a plethora of inflammatory dermatologic disorders.[95] Ruxolitinib and tofacitinib have been successfully used for recalcitrant chronic dermatomyositis. In vitiligo, IFN-γ overexpression results in hypopigmentation. Combined with ultraviolet light, tofacitinib and topical ruxolitinib have shown greater results stimulating repigmentation. A JAK-1 inhibitor (INCB054707) is currently being investigated for the treatment of hidradenitis suppurativa. Therapeutic blockade of IL-17, IL-23, or IFN-γ seems promising in steroid-refractory lichen planus, for which topical ruxolitinib is being investigated (NCT03697460). JAKinibs also have the potential to help in diseases such as lichen sclerosus et atrophicans, systemic sclerosis, morphea, eosinophilic fasciitis, eczema, contact dermatitis, and the syndrome SAPHO (synovitis, acne, pustulosis, hyperostosis, and osteitis); cutaneous manifestations of IBD; and bullous skin disorders.[95]

Organ transplantation JAK-3 blockade is an appealing target for the prevention of T cell–mediated transplant rejection. In phase II studies, tofacitinib showed similar efficacy to tacrolimus or cyclosporine.[103,104] However, it was associated with an unacceptable risk of infection, particularly with cytomegalovirus (CMV) and BK virus, and posttransplant lymphoproliferative disease (PTLD). This finding could be explained by the coadministration of potent immunosuppressants, but also by the high doses of tofacitinib used (10–15 mg twice a day) and high drug levels. Interestingly, therapeutic drug monitoring (TDM) has been proposed as a tool to predict the risk of adverse effects and may allow the reevaluation of JAKinibs as a therapeutic option in transplant rejection.[105]

Itacitinib recently entered a phase I/II study for the treatment of bronchiolitis obliterans following lung transplant (NCT03978637).

Other inflammatory diseases JAKinibs are being investigated for a host of other indications. JAK3-dependent and JAK1-dependent cytokine signaling is critical in chronic inflammation of medium and large arteries. Tofacitinib effectively inhibits core vasculitogenesis.[106] A phase II study testing the efficacy and safety of baricitinib in giant cell arteritis is underway (NCT03026504).

Ruxolitinib and, more recently, baricitinib (through an FDA compassionate program) have been used in the treatment of interferonopathies, with promising results,[92] and in other diseases with interferon signature, namely systemic lupus erythematosus (SLE), dermatomyositis, and Sjögren syndrome. For SLE, a phase II baricitinib study[107] showed consistent clinical improvements. Several clinical trials are ongoing further evaluating the efficacy and safety of this and other JAKinibs for lupus.

Topical JAKinibs may also have a role in treatment of ocular diseases such as dry eye and noninfectious uveitis.[2,92]

The anecdotal success of JAKinibs in treating hypereosinophilic syndrome[108] suggests that JAKinibs might be beneficial in eosinophilic and allergic disorders driven by cytokines IL-4, IL-5, and IL-13.

JAK-STAT pathway inhibition is also being explored for the management of chronic diseases such as diabetic nephropathy, in which it seems to reduce albuminuria by blocking renal inflammation, and atherosclerosis, in which IL-6–driven inflammation plays a key role.[2]

Infections associated with Janus kinase inhibitors

Blockade of JAK-dependent cytokine signaling affects several components of the adaptive and innate immune systems (see **Fig. 2**, **Table 1**). The inhibition of JAK1/3-dependent proinflammatory cytokines result in (1) impaired differentiation and function of dendritic cells; (2) inhibited CD4+ T-cell activation with resulting reduction in Th1, Th17, and Tregs, and cytokine secretion and their mediated responses; and (3) decreased and impaired natural killer (NK) cells, key to the viral immune defense. These effects lead to severe immunodeficiency and increased risk of opportunistic fungal, viral, and parasitic infections (eg, *Toxoplasma*). JAK-1 and TYK-2 inhibition impairs IFN-α/β responses promoting viral infections, whereas inhibition of IL-12 and IFN-γ signaling (JAK1/2) increases the risk of granulomatous infections. In addition, an increased susceptibility to infections can be expected in patients on recent or current immunosuppressive therapy, and those with cytopenias or other comorbidities.

Ruxolitinib

Ruxolitinib is the JAKinib with the longest clinical experience. In a pivotal trial comparing ruxolitinib with best available therapy for myelofibrosis, infections were more frequent in the JAKinib arm, and included UTIs (24.6%), pneumonia (13.1%), herpes zoster (HZ) (11.5%), sepsis/septic shock (7.9%), and tuberculosis (1.0%).[82,109] Infection occurrences decreased over time. However, severe neutropenia was also more frequent, which could have confounded results. In the JUMP expanded-access trial,[110] which included 1144 patients with myelofibrosis, all-grade infections were mainly bacterial and viral, and similar to those described in registry studies. HZ (3.6%), influenza (3%), tuberculosis (n = 3, 0.3%), and legionella pneumonia (n = 1, 0.1%) were reported. Data from a phase III trial in PV showed that, compared with standard therapy, ruxolitinib was associated with an increased rate of HZ (6% vs 0), but there were no significantly higher frequencies of overall (42% vs 37%) or grade 3 or 4 infections (3.6% vs 2.7%).[83] In a retrospective analysis, Polverelli and colleagues[111,112] reported infections twice as often in ruxolitinib-treated patients compared with controls (44% vs 20%, P<.001). Grade 2 or higher infections occurred in 28% of patients, 9% being fatal, and tended to decrease over time. These infections were mostly bacterial (68.9%) (half of the respiratory tract), viral (14.9%) (HZ, HSV), and fungal infections (2.5%). Three cases of tuberculosis (0.7%), 1 aspergillosis, and no case of hepatitis B virus (HBV) (prophylaxis was given to half of patients with reactivation risk) were reported. A previous infectious event and a high international prognostic score system category (stratifying disease severity) were independently associated with infection, whereas improvements in splenomegaly were protective. A recent meta-analysis of a ruxolitinib phase III RCT and phase IV studies linked ruxolitinib with a statistically significant increased risk of HZ compared with control groups (odds ratio [OR], 7.39; 95% confidence interval [CI], 1.33–41).[113]

Opportunistic infections Atypical and opportunistic infections (OIs), albeit rare, are increasingly documented. A recent review identified 32 cases of OIs in literature, occurring at a median of 16 weeks following ruxolitinib initiation[114] and resulting in 5 deaths. The most frequently reported infection was tuberculosis (n = 11, 34%), followed by cryptococcal infection and HBV reactivation (n = 3, 9% each). Cases of *Pneumocystis jirovecii* pneumonia (PJP) (n = 2), CMV and toxoplasma chorioretinitis (1 each), PML,[115,116] *Mycobacterium abscessus*,[117] and disseminated molluscum contagiosum have also been reported.[114] Invasive mold infections,[118] disseminated histoplasmosis[119] and talaromycosis[114] have also occurred.

As for the risk of HBV reactivation, in a series of patients with myelofibrosis with positive anti-hepatitis B core (HBc) antibody but negative hepatitis B surface antigen (HBsAg), and HBV DNA, viral reactivation occurred in 40%, at a median of 10 months of ruxolitinib treatment.[120]

A recent pharmacovigilance study compared FDA-reported cases of mycobacterial infection with ruxolitinib versus all other drugs. Over a 7-year period, 91 cases of tuberculosis and 23 of nontuberculous mycobacteria (NTM) were identified in Jakafi-treated patients. Ruxolitinib was associated with an increased risk of tuberculosis (OR, 9.2%; 95% CI, 7.5–11.4) and NTM infections (OR, 8.3%; 95% CI,5.5–12.6).[121] Based on available data, the incidence of tuberculosis while on ruxolitinib is 0.4 to 0.7/100PY. Of the 14 cases described in literature, 71% were miliary/disseminated, with a mortality of 28.6%.[122]

Opportunistic infections in graft-versus-host disease Data in patients with GVHD derive merely from case series and retrospective reviews, making it difficult to draw conclusions on prevention and prophylaxis strategies. In a small retrospective study of 43 patients, 42% developed greater than or equal to 1 infection (aGVHD 68% vs cGVHD 21%).[123] Uncomplicated viral reactivations (CMV in 21%; HHV6, BK in 11% each) were the most frequent events in patients with aGVHD, followed by bacterial infections, which predominated in the cGVHD group. Only 1 case of invasive fungal infection (IFI) (aspergillosis) occurred in the cGVHD group. Most patients with aGVHD were on antifungal prophylaxis and additional immunosuppressants. The risk of infection was significantly higher with aGVHD, with more frequent CMV reactivations.

Tofacitinib
A pooled analysis of safety data from RA trials and long-term extension studies (LTESs) covering 4789 patients found an incidence of serious infections (SIs) (3.1/100PY) and infection-related mortality (58%) with tofacitinib that, albeit significant, was similar to that observed with other biologic agents.[124] The most common infections were pneumonias, UTIs and skin and soft tissue infections. Age, diabetes, prior corticosteroid therapy, lymphopenia, and higher tofacitinib doses were independent risk factors of SI. A meta-analysis evaluating 66 RA RCTs and 22 LTESs showed a higher incidence of infection with tofacitinib compared with placebo, but again the risk was comparable with that observed with other biologic DMARDs.[125] However, in a later meta-analysis, licensed doses of JAKinibs did not significantly increase this risk.[126]

A head-to-head comparison of tofacitinib and etanercept for psoriasis showed similar rates of infection, predominantly nasopharyngitis and upper respiratory tract infections, across study arms.[98] Two recent trials in patients with conventional DMARD and TNFi-refractory PsA found SIs and HZ more frequently with tofacitinib than with placebo[127] or adalimumab.[128]

In initial UC clinical trials, the most common infections reported were nasopharyngitis (4.9%–13.8%) and influenza (3%). A post hoc analysis pooling all patients (n = 1157) receiving any dose of tofacitinib to manage UC showed higher rates of SI in the treatment group compared with placebo (2.9%, vs 1.0%).[85] These SIs included pneumonia, HZ, anal abscess, and *Clostridium difficile* infection. However, the risk of SI or OI was similar to that of other biologics approved for UC.[129]

Herpes zoster Although the associated risk of bacterial infection is similar to that observed with biologic therapies, a very different risk profile has emerged with regard to varicella zoster virus (VZV) reactivation (ie, HZ). The mechanism, albeit unclear, is thought to be the inhibition of IFN responses and VZV-specific memory T cells through JAK-1 blockade.[130] Interestingly, the incidence of other virus does not seem particularly increased. Winthrop and colleagues[131] examined the risk and characteristics of HZ infections reported cumulatively in studies from tofacitinib programs for RA, psoriasis, and UC. In a pooled analysis of RA studies, the incidence of HZ in tofacitinib-treated patients (4.4/100PY) was 1.5 to 2 times higher than that of adalimumab-treated or placebo groups[131] and twice that of patients taking any biologic DMARD.[132] In psoriatic patients, the crude incidence of HZ was similar in the tofacitinib and etanercept groups (3.4 vs 2.55/100PY). Tofacitinib-associated rates were similar in UC and RA. Overall, in all tofacitinib groups, HZ was more frequent than in placebo groups. Despite this, HZ manifestations were largely limited to cutaneous, uncomplicated disease, with low rates of multidermatomal involvement (0.4%–16.9%), dissemination, visceral or fatal infection. Most patients were able to continue or resume tofacitinib without complications. Across these studies, Asian descent, older age, concomitant use of steroids or methotrexate, and higher tofacitinib (10 mg twice a day) and steroid dose; and in UC and psoriatic patients, prior use of TNFi, were associated with increased HZ risk.[131–134] Newer JAKinibs seem to have similar effects. However, further research is needed to determine whether and how JAK selectivity translates into a differential risk.[131]

Other opportunistic infections With regard to other OIs, estimations of risk are difficult to make because of the heterogeneity in methods and OI definitions across studies. A pooled analysis of phase I/II RCTs and LTESs in RA identified 60 episodes among 5671 subjects (incidence 0.46/100PY) that occurred at a median of 40 weeks (range, 6–179 weeks) following tofacitinib.[135] Tuberculosis was the most common event, with an incidence of 0.2/100PY, similar to that observed with TNFi and nonbiologic DMARDs (5–10 times higher than in the general population). Infection was extrapulmonary in 58% of patients, occurred mostly in high-endemicity areas and in patients receiving higher tofacitinib dose. Importantly, treatment of latent tuberculosis with isoniazid (with at least 1 of 9 months completed before JAKinib initiation) seemed to be protective.[131,135] The incidence of other OIs was 0.25/100PY. These OIs included esophageal candidiasis (n = 9), PJP (n = 4), CMV (n = 6), pulmonary NTM (n = 2), *Cryptococcus* (pneumonia, n = 2; meningitis, n = 1), BK virus encephalopathy (n = 1), and toxoplasmosis (n = 1). Of note, 8 cases of disseminated/multidermatomal HZ were included. In postmarketing studies, at least 1 case of histoplasmosis has been reported. Reactivation of JC and Epstein-Barr virus (EBV) were not documented.[135] Most patients discontinued tofacitinib (69%) and 1 OI-related death occurred (PJP). In studies evaluating tofacitinib application to kidney transplant rejection,[103,104] SIs (including CMV disease, BK nephropathy, and EBV-associated PTLD) were significantly more common among tofacitinib-treated patients compared with the cyclosporine group. Infection susceptibility was associated with high tofacitinib drug levels.[105]

Baricitinib Fewer data are available with baricitinib. In an initial RA study comparing different baricitinib doses with placebo, infection was more frequent among baricitinib-treated patients, although SI rates were comparable across all groups (∼3%).[136] Meta-analysis of RA-specific and combined studies for inflammatory diseases (RA, PsA, IBD, AS) have shown similar incidences of SI, also comparable among baricitinib-treated and placebo groups.[137,138] Across all published studies, baricitinib is associated with an increased and dose-dependent risk of HZ. Although OIs have been reported, no serious case of fungal or CMV infection has been published to date. Tuberculosis cases (n = 10, incidence 0.15/100PY) have mainly occurred in countries with higher background prevalence, but not in Europe, Japan, or North America.

Infection prevention and management strategies
Available data support the need for a thorough assessment of infectious risks before JAKinib therapy. Suggested screening and prevention strategies are summarized in **Table 8**.

- Screening for viral infections, notably Herpesviridae, can prove useful for risk stratification and patient counseling. Interventions such as monitoring of CMV reactivation or universal prophylaxis for CMV/HSV/VZV need further investigation for future guidance. Prophylaxis can be considered in high-risk patients.
- The recognition that HZ disproportionately affects JAKinib-treated patients should prompt efforts to improve vaccination strategies. Patients should be immunized before JAKinib initiation.Owing to the risk of dissemination, the live attenuated vaccine (zoster vaccine live [ZVL], Zostavax, Merck) is contraindicated in immunocompromised hosts. In addition, it has limited efficacy (∼51%) in healthy adults greater than or equal to 60-years old and patients with RA,[139] and protection significantly wanes after 5 years.[140,141] The new recombinant nonlive adjuvanted vaccine (recombinant zoster vaccine [RZV], Shingrix, GlaxoSmithKline) has shown greater efficacy even in older patients (>90%).[142] Its immunogenicity and safety have been shown in patients infected with human immunodeficiency virus, patients with solid tumors receiving chemotherapy, auto-HSCT, and renal transplant recipients.[143–146] Studies in the allo-HSCT population are underway. However, the safety (and efficacy) of RZV in patients with autoimmune diseases has not been evaluated, and there is concern that its highly reactogenic adjuvant component may lead to disease flares. For patients receiving low-dose immunosuppression, ZVL is considered safe,[147] but some experts still favor using RZV.[148,149] However, in highly immunosuppressed patients (high-dose steroids, biologics, JAKinibs), ZVL should be avoided, whereas RZV, although not contraindicated, is not routinely recommended.
- In immunocompetent patients, RZV is preferred to the live ZVL. Shingrix is administered in 2 doses 2 to 6 months apart, and 2 weeks before initiation of JAKinib, whereas Zostavax should be administered once, 4 weeks before commencing treatment.

Table 8				
Prevention strategies for patients with planned initiation of Janus kinase inhibitors				
Infection	Screening, Intervention	Prophylaxis	Monitoring	Other/Comments
Urogenital and bronchopulmonary bacterial infections	None	Prolonged/anticipated neutropenia	Clinical monitoring	Immunize against pneumococcus before treatment[a]
HSV	HSV IgG	HSV IgG (+), consider acyclovir 400 mg BID if additional immunosuppression, risk factors[b]	Clinical monitoring	—
VZV	VZV IgG	VZV IgG (+), consider acyclovir 400 mg BID if additional immunosuppression or risk factors, ±unvaccinated[b]	Clinical monitoring	Immunize with RZV or ZVL before treatment[c,d] ZVL contraindicated in immunosuppressed. RZV lacks safety data in autoimmune diseases
CMV	CMV IgG	CMV IgG (+): not routinely, can consider in higher risk patients (eg, GVHD, additional high-risk immunosuppression)	CMV PCR monitoring in HSCT/GVHD/at risk SOT	—
EBV	EBV IgG	None	EBV PCR monitoring in HSCT/GVHD	—
HBV	HBV sAg, HBV sAb (IgG), HBVcAb (IgG) ± HBV DNA	HBV sAg (+): yes, entecavir 0.5 mg daily or tenofovir 300 mg daily HBV sAg (−), HBc Ab (+): not routine, consider in selected high-risk cases	HBV sAg(+): HBV DNA monthly, LFTs HBV DNA monthly LFTs	Immunize against hepatitis A and B before treatment[a] Consider hepatology consult
HCV	HCV IgG	HCV IgG (+)- no prophylaxis	HCV IgG (+) HCV NAAT	—
PML	± JC virus IgG	None	Clinical monitoring	Screening may help weigh risks and benefits of JAKinib therapy

PJP	None	Strongly consider TMP-SMX or alternative agent in patients with additional immunosuppression/risk factors	Clinical monitoring	—
Fungal infections (eg, Candida, molds)	None	• In selected patients (eg, prolonged neutropenia, high-risk hematologic malignancies, AML/MDS, HSCT, GVHD) • Individualize based on risk factors • anti-mold prophylaxis with echinocandin or triazole: in selected patients^d, eg, expected/prolonged neutropenia, history of IFI, myeloablative allo-HSCT, GVHD on high-dose steroids	Clinical monitoring	DDI of azoles and ruxolitinib>tofacitinib, increase in JAKinib toxicity
Endemic mycosis (Coccidioides, Paracoccidioides, Histoplasma, Blastomyces, Talaromyces, Sporothrix)	Patients at risk: • Coccidioides EIA, ID, CF • Paracoccidioides IgG Poor performance of screening tests for other endemic fungi	Coccidioides serologies positive (but no active infection)/history of infection: consider fluconazole 200–400 mg daily	Serologic monitoring in those with positive screening (coccidioidomycosis), or history of infection (coccidioidomycosis, histoplasmosis)	Insufficient data to recommend prophylaxis in patients with negative serologies living in Coccidioides-endemic area
Cryptococcus	Not recommended	No	Clinical monitoring	—
Toxoplasmosis	Toxoplasma IgG	Toxoplasma IgG (+): consider TMP-SMX or atovaquone if additional immunosuppression or risk factors	Clinical monitoring	—

(continued on next page)

Table 8
(continued)

Infection	Screening, Intervention	Prophylaxis	Monitoring	Other/Comments
Tuberculosis	Quantiferon	Quantiferon (+): isoniazid 300 mg daily ×9 mo	Clinical monitoring	Avoid rifampicin with tofacitinib>ruxolitinib because of drug-drug interactions

Abbreviations: Ab, antibodies; Ag, antigen; AML, acute myeloid leukemia; CF, complement fixation; DDI, drug-drug interactions; EIA, enzyme immunoassay; HCV, hepatitis C virus; ID, immunodiffusion; LFT, liver function test; MDS, myelodysplastic syndrome; RZV, recombinant zoster vaccine, Shingrix; TMP-SMX, trimetho-prim-sulfamethoxazole ZVL, zoster vaccine live, Zostavax.

[a] Recommended: seasonal yearly influenza vaccine; 13-valent pneumococcal vaccine followed by 23-valent vaccine 8 weeks later and hepatitis A/B vaccination. HBV immunization: 1-month postvaccination HBs antibody titers should be checked (>10 IU/mL) to assess need for a booster; annual booster doses for sustained immunity are recommended in immunocompromised hosts.

[b] Additional risk factors: neutropenia, lymphopenia, glucocorticoids, Asian descent, age greater than 65 years, high JAKinib dose, prior use of biologics, concomitant immunosuppression, patients with hematological malignancies, HSCT or SOT recipients.

- RZV: 2 doses at 2 to 6 months apart. Complete shchedule 2 weeks before JAKinib initiation. ZVL: once, 4 weeks before JAKinib.

[c] Immunocompetent patients: either, but RZV preferred.[149]

- Low-dose immunosuppression (prednisone <20 mg/d (or equivalents), methotrexate less than or equal to 0.4 mg/kg/wk, azathioprine less than or equal to 3.0 mg/kg/d, 6-mercaptopurine less than or equal to 1.5 mg/kg/d, hydroxychloroquine, leflunomide, sulfasalazine): can consider ZVL; caution with RZV in auto-immune diseases (no safety data).

- High-dose immunosuppression (prednisone greater than or equal to 20 mg/d or equivalent, biologics, JAK inhibitors, chemotherapy, antirejection medication): ZVL contraindicated. No safety data in autoimmune diseases.

[d] Following guidelines in patients with cancer-related immunosuppression.[150]

- In most immunosuppressed patients, RZV seems safe and immunogenic. Lacking data in allo-HSCT recipients and patients with autoimmune diseases, recommendations cannot be made. Risks and benefits of its administration should be carefully weighed.
- With active HZ, antiviral therapy should be started and tofacitinib temporarily stopped until infection resolves. Secondary prophylaxis can be considered upon resumption of JAKinibs.
- Other recommended immunizations include yearly seasonal influenza, pneumococcal (13 and 23-valent), and hepatitis A/B vaccines. Preferably, these should be completed at least 2 weeks before the first JAKinib dose.
- Live vaccines are contraindicated during JAKinib therapy (and with preexisting immunosuppression). In VZV-naive immunocompetent patients, varicella vaccine (VAR; Varivax, Merck) (2 doses, 4–8 weeks apart) should be administered at least 4 weeks before initiation of JAKinib.
- Clinicians should be aware of the increased risk of OIs (eg, tuberculosis, PJP, HZ, IFI), notably in patients with additional risk factors, and have a low threshold to investigate these.
- Pretreatment screening for latent tuberculosis (and treatment if appropriate) should be pursued based on epidemiologic risk factors, preferably using IFN-γ release assay (ie, Quantiferon).
- Pretreatment screening for chronic HBV infection should be performed in all patients before JAKinib is initiated. It should include Hepatitis B surface antigen (HBs Ag), anti-HBs, and anti-HBc (and HBV DNA if anti-HBc was positive). Patients with anti-HBs titers less than 10 IU/mL should be given an HBV vaccine booster before treatment starts. To prevent reactivation, HBsAg-positive patients should be offered prophylaxis with entecavir or tenofovir while on JAKinib. Serial monitoring of HBV load among HBsAg and anti-HBc–positive/HBsAg-negative patients is warranted.
- Appropriate screening of endemic and geographically restricted infections should be considered (eg, coccidiomycosis).
- During active OIs, dose reduction or discontinuation of JAKinibs (and/or other immunosuppressants) should, if feasible, be pursued.
- In view of (limited) data, the administration of antiviral, anti-*Pneumocystis*, and antifungal prophylaxis should be individualized, but should be favored in patients with additional risk factors or immunosuppression. Guidelines and local protocols for prophylaxis in patients with HSCT, SOT, and GVHD should be followed.
- Given the dose-dependent association of JAKinibs with infection, TDM (eg, tofacitinib) has been proposed as a surrogate marker of infectious risk. This approach needs further investigation.

SUMMARY

Terminal complement and JAK inhibitors have revolutionized the treatment of hematological and inflammatory disorders characterized by complement and JAK pathway activation, improving the understanding of a plethora of conditions potentially benefiting from these agents. C5 inhibitors increase the risk of infection with encapsulated organisms, mainly *Neisseria* spp, whereas other risks are yet to be defined. Therapy with JAKinibs increases the overall risk of infection and OIs, notably HZ. Optimized screening, immunizations, and prophylaxis should mitigate these risks. Reporting of emerging infections occurring in patients receiving C5 or JAK inhibitors is encouraged. Systematic data collection is needed to define and stratify the risk of infectious complications associated with these agents and to standardize prevention and well-defined, solid evidence–based prophylactic strategies.

DISCLOSURE

None.

REFERENCES

1. Patriquin CJ, Kuo KHM. Eculizumab and beyond: the past, present, and future of complement therapeutics. Transfus Med Rev 2019;33(4):256–65.
2. Schwartz DM, Kanno Y, Villarino A, et al. JAK inhibition as a therapeutic strategy for immune and inflammatory diseases. Nat Rev Drug Discov 2017;16(12): 843–62.
3. Benamu E, Montoya JG. Infections associated with the use of eculizumab: recommendations for prevention and prophylaxis. Curr Opin Infect Dis 2016;29(4): 319–29.
4. Reis ES, Mastellos DC, Yancopoulou D, et al. Applying complement therapeutics to rare diseases. Clin Immunol 2015;161(2):225–40.
5. Alexion Pharmaceuticals Inc. Soliris (eculizumab): US prescribing information. 2015. Available at: https://www.accessdata.fda.gov/drugsatfda_ docs/label/2017/125166s422lbl.pdf. Accessed January 30, 2020.
6. Gavriilaki E, Anagnostopoulos A, Mastellos DC. Complement in thrombotic microangiopathies: unraveling Ariadne's thread into the labyrinth of complement therapeutics. Front Immunol 2019;10:337.
7. Licht C, Greenbaum LA, Muus P, et al. Efficacy and safety of eculizumab in atypical hemolytic uremic syndrome from 2-year extensions of phase 2 studies. Kidney Int 2015;87(5):1061–73.
8. Chua J, Paizis K, He SZ, et al. Suspected atypical haemolytic uraemic syndrome in two post-partum patients with foetal-death in utero responding to eculizumab. Nephrology (Carlton) 2017;22(Suppl 1):18–22.
9. Abe T, Sasaki A, Ueda T, et al. Complement-mediated thrombotic microangiopathy secondary to sepsis-induced disseminated intravascular coagulation successfully treated with eculizumab: a case report. Medicine 2017;96(6):e6056.
10. Asif A, Nayer A, Haas CS. Atypical hemolytic uremic syndrome in the setting of complement-amplifying conditions: case reports and a review of the evidence for treatment with eculizumab. J Nephrol 2017;30(3):347–62.
11. Jodele S. Complement in pathophysiology and treatment of transplant-associated thrombotic microangiopathies. Semin Hematol 2018;55(3):159–66.
12. Shochet L, Kanellis J, Simpson I, et al. De novo thrombotic microangiopathy following simultaneous pancreas and kidney transplantation managed with eculizumab. Nephrology (Carlton) 2017;22(Suppl 1):23–7.
13. de Fontbrune FS, Galambrun C, Sirvent A, et al. Use of eculizumab in patients with allogeneic stem cell transplant-associated thrombotic microangiopathy: a study from the SFGM-TC. Transplantation 2015;99(9):1953–9.
14. Dhillon S. Eculizumab: a review in generalized myasthenia gravis. Drugs 2018; 78(3):367–76.
15. Howard JF Jr, Utsugisawa K, Benatar M, et al. Safety and efficacy of eculizumab in anti-acetylcholine receptor antibody-positive refractory generalised myasthenia gravis (REGAIN): a phase 3, randomised, double-blind, placebo-controlled, multicentre study. Lancet Neurol 2017;16(12):976–86.

16. Pittock SJ, Berthele A, Fujihara K, et al. Eculizumab in aquaporin-4-positive neuromyelitis optica spectrum disorder. N Engl J Med 2019;381(7):614–25.

17. Misawa S, Kuwabara S, Sato Y, et al. Safety and efficacy of eculizumab in Guillain-Barré syndrome: a multicentre, double-blind, randomised phase 2 trial. Lancet Neurol 2018;17(6):519–29.

18. Röth A, Bommer M, Hüttmann A, et al. Eculizumab in cold agglutinin disease (DECADE): an open-label, prospective, bicentric, nonrandomized phase 2 trial. Blood Adv 2018;2(19):2543–9.

19. Riedl M, Thorner P, Licht C. C3 glomerulopathy. Pediatr Nephrol 2017;32(1): 43–57.

20. Schröppel B, Legendre C. Delayed kidney graft function: from mechanism to translation. Kidney Int 2014;86(2):251–8.

21. Schröppel B, Akalin E, Baweja M, et al. Peritransplant eculizumab does not prevent delayed graft function in deceased donor kidney transplant recipients: results of two randomized controlled pilot trials. Am J Transplant 2020;20(2): 564–72.

22. Eskandary F, Wahrmann M, Mühlbacher J, et al. Complement inhibition as potential new therapy for antibody-mediated rejection. Transpl Int 2016;29(4): 392–402.

23. Bentall A, Tyan DB, Sequeira F, et al. Antibody-mediated rejection despite inhibition of terminal complement. Transpl Int 2014;27(12):1235–43.

24. Stegall MD, Diwan T, Raghavaiah S, et al. Terminal complement inhibition decreases antibody-mediated rejection in sensitized renal transplant recipients. Am J Transplant 2011;11(11):2405–13.

25. Cornell LD, Schinstock CA, Gandhi MJ, et al. Positive crossmatch kidney transplant recipients treated with eculizumab: outcomes beyond 1 year. Am J Transplant 2015;15(5):1293–302.

26. Glotz D, Russ G, Rostaing L, et al. Safety and efficacy of eculizumab for the prevention of antibody-mediated rejection after deceased-donor kidney transplantation in patients with preformed donor-specific antibodies. Am J Transplant 2019;19(10):2865–75.

27. Park DH, Connor KM, Lambris JD. The challenges and promise of complement therapeutics for ocular diseases. Front Immunol 2019;10:1007.

28. Xu H, Chen M. Targeting the complement system for the management of retinal inflammatory and degenerative diseases. Eur J Pharmacol 2016;787:94–104.

29. Smith SG, Watson B, Clark G, et al. Eculizumab for treatment of asthma. Expert Opin Biol Ther 2012;12(4):529–37.

30. Stern RM, Connell NT. Ravulizumab: a novel C5 inhibitor for the treatment of paroxysmal nocturnal hemoglobinuria. Ther Adv Hematol 2019;10. 2040620719874728.

31. Lee JW, Sicre de Fontbrune F, Wong Lee L, et al. Ravulizumab (ALXN1210) vs eculizumab in adult patients with PNH naive to complement inhibitors: the 301 study. Blood 2019;133(6):530–9.

32. Kulasekararaj AG, Hill A, Rottinghaus ST, et al. Ravulizumab (ALXN1210) vs eculizumab in C5-inhibitor-experienced adult patients with PNH: the 302 study. Blood 2019;133(6):540–9.

33. McKeage K. Ravulizumab: first global approval. Drugs 2019;79(3):347–52.

34. Pettigrew HD, Teuber SS, Gershwin ME. Clinical significance of complement deficiencies. Ann N Y Acad Sci 2009;1173:108–23.

35. Alexion Pharmaceuticals Inc. Soliris (eculizumab): US prescribing information. 2015. Available at: https://www.accessdata.fda.gov/drugsatfda_ docs/label/2017/125166s422lbl.pdf. Accessed December 26, 2019.

36. Crew PE, McNamara L, Waldron PE, et al. Antibiotic prophylaxis in vaccinated eculizumab recipients who developed meningococcal disease: antibiotic prophylaxis and eculizumab. J Infect 2020;80(3):350–71.

37. Socié G, Caby-Tosi M-P, Marantz JL, et al. Eculizumab in paroxysmal nocturnal haemoglobinuria and atypical haemolytic uraemic syndrome: 10-year pharmacovigilance analysis. Br J Haematol 2019;185(2):297–310.

38. McNamara LA, Topaz N, Wang X, et al. High risk for invasive meningococcal disease among patients receiving eculizumab (Soliris) despite receipt of meningococcal vaccine. Am J Transplant 2017;17(9):2481–4.

39. Hillmen P, Muus P, Röth A, et al. Long-term safety and efficacy of sustained eculizumab treatment in patients with paroxysmal nocturnal haemoglobinuria. Br J Haematol 2013;162(1):62–73.

40. Vicente D, Esnal O, Pérez-Trallero E. Fatal Neisseria meningitidis serogroup X sepsis in immunocompromised patients in Spain. Virulence of clinical isolates. J Infect 2012;64(2):184–7.

41. Rey-Múgica Mde L, Hernando-Real S, Carrero-González P, et al. Meningococcemia during eculizumab treatment. Enferm Infecc Microbiol Clin 2013;31(1):62 [in Spanish].

42. Struijk GH, Bouts AHM, Rijkers GT, et al. Meningococcal sepsis complicating eculizumab treatment despite prior vaccination. Am J Transplant 2013;13(3):819–20.

43. Applegate AO, Fong VC, Tardivel K, et al. Notes from the field: meningococcal disease in an international traveler on eculizumab therapy - United States, 2015. MMWR Morb Mortal Wkly Rep 2016;65(27):696–7.

44. Hernando Real S, Vega Castaño S, Pajares García R. Meningococcemia in vaccinated patient under treatment with eculizumab. Enferm Infecc Microbiol Clin 2017;35(3):200–1.

45. Friedl C, Hackl G, Schilcher G, et al. Waterhouse-Friderichsen syndrome due to Neisseria meningitidis infection in a young adult with thrombotic microangiopathy and eculizumab treatment: case report and review of management. Ann Hematol 2017;96(5):879–80.

46. Parikh SR, Lucidarme J, Bingham C, et al. Meningococcal B vaccine failure with a penicillin-resistant strain in a young adult on long-term eculizumab. Pediatrics 2017;140(3) [pii:e20162452].

47. Polat M, Yüksel S, Şahin NÜ. Fatal meningococcemia due to Neisseria meningitidis serogroup Y in a vaccinated child receiving eculizumab. Hum Vaccin Immunother 2018;14(11):2802.

48. Cullinan N, Gorman KM, Riordan M, et al. Case report: benefits and challenges of long-term eculizumab in atypical hemolytic uremic syndrome. Pediatrics 2015;135(6):e1506–9.

49. Lebel E, Trahtemberg U, Block C, et al. Post-eculizumab meningococcaemia in vaccinated patients. Clin Microbiol Infect 2018;24(1):89–90.

50. Reher D, Fuhrmann V, Kluge S, et al. A rare case of septic shock due to Neisseria meningitidis serogroup B infection despite prior vaccination in a young adult with paroxysmal nocturnal haemoglobinuria receiving eculizumab. Vaccine 2018;36(19):2507–9.

51. Nolfi-Donegan D, Konar M, Vianzon V, et al. Fatal nongroupable neisseria meningitidis disease in vaccinated patient receiving eculizumab. Emerg Infect Dis 2018;24(8):1561–4.
52. Ladhani SN, Campbell H, Lucidarme J, et al. Invasive meningococcal disease in patients with complement deficiencies: a case series (2008-2017). BMC Infect Dis 2019;19(1):522.
53. Hawkins KL, Hoffman M, Okuyama S, et al. A case of fulminant meningococcemia: it is all in the complement. Case Rep Infect Dis 2017;2017:6093695.
54. Hall V, Pai Mangalore R, He S, et al. Fulminant meningococcal sepsis due to non-groupable Neisseria meningitidis in a patient receiving eculizumab. Med J Aust 2018;208(11):478–9.
55. Röth A, Rottinghaus ST, Hill A, et al. Ravulizumab (ALXN1210) in patients with paroxysmal nocturnal hemoglobinuria: results of 2 phase 1b/2 studies. Blood Adv 2018;2(17):2176–85.
56. Findlow J, Balmer P, Borrow R. A review of complement sources used in serum bactericidal assays for evaluating immune responses to meningococcal ACWY conjugate vaccines. Hum Vaccin Immunother 2019;15(10):2491–500.
57. Konar M, Granoff DM. Eculizumab treatment and impaired opsonophagocytic killing of meningococci by whole blood from immunized adults. Blood 2017; 130(7):891–9.
58. Alashkar F, Vance C, Herich-Terhürne D, et al. Serologic response to meningococcal vaccination in patients with paroxysmal nocturnal hemoglobinuria (PNH) chronically treated with the terminal complement inhibitor eculizumab. Ann Hematol 2017;96(4):589–96.
59. Alashkar F, Vance C, Herich-Terhürne D, et al. Serologic response to meningococcal vaccination in patients with cold agglutinin disease (CAD) in the novel era of complement inhibition. Vaccine 2019;37(44):6682–7.
60. Santolaya ME, O'Ryan M, Valenzuela MT, et al. Persistence of antibodies in adolescents 18-24 months after immunization with one, two, or three doses of 4CMenB meningococcal serogroup B vaccine. Hum Vaccin Immunother 2013; 9(11):2304–10.
61. Martinón-Torres F, Bernatowska E, Shcherbina A, et al. Meningococcal B vaccine immunogenicity in children with defects in complement and splenic function. Pediatrics 2018;142(3) [pii:e20174250].
62. Winthrop KL, Mariette X, Silva JT, et al. ESCMID Study Group for Infections in Compromised Hosts (ESGICH) Consensus Document on the safety of targeted and biological therapies: an Infectious Diseases perspective (Soluble immune effector molecules [II]: agents targeting interleukins, immunoglobulins and complement factors). Clin Microbiol Infect 2018;24(Suppl 2):S21–40.
63. Workowski KA, Bolan GA, Centers for Disease Control and Prevention. Sexually transmitted diseases treatment guidelines, 2015. MMWR Recomm Rep 2015; 64(RR-03):1–137.
64. Crew PE, Abara WE, McCulley L, et al. Disseminated gonococcal infections in patients receiving eculizumab: a case series. Clin Infect Dis 2019;69(4): 596–600.
65. Crew PE, McNamara L, Waldron PE, et al. Unusual Neisseria species as a cause of infection in patients taking eculizumab. J Infect 2019;78(2):113–8.
66. Webb BJ, Healy R, Child B, et al. Recurrent infection with Pseudomonas aeruginosa during eculizumab therapy in an allogeneic hematopoietic stem cell transplant recipient. Transpl Infect Dis 2016;18(2):312–4.

67. Kawakami T, Nakazawa H, Kurasawa Y, et al. Severe infection of pseudomonas aeruginosa during eculizumab therapy for paroxysmal nocturnal hemoglobinuria. Intern Med 2018;57(1):127–30.
68. Stoermer KA, Morrison TE. Complement and viral pathogenesis. Virology 2011; 411(2):362–73.
69. Borhan WM, Dababo MA, Thompson LDR, et al. Acute necrotizing herpetic tonsillitis: a report of two cases. Head Neck Pathol 2015;9(1):119–22.
70. Gómez-Cibeira E, Ivanovic-Barbeito Y, Gutiérrez-Martínez E, et al. Eculizumab-related progressive multifocal leukoencephalopathy. Neurology 2016;86(4): 399–400.
71. Vellanki VS, Bargman JM. Aspergillus Niger peritonitis in a peritoneal dialysis patient treated with eculizumab. Ren Fail 2014;36(4):631–3.
72. Clancy M, McGhan R, Gitomer J, et al. Disseminated cryptococcosis associated with administration of eculizumab. Am J Health Syst Pharm 2018;75(14): 1018–22.
73. Speth C, Rambach G, Würzner R, et al. Complement and fungal pathogens: an update. Mycoses 2008;51(6):477–96.
74. Volokhina EB, van de Kar NCAJ, Bergseth G, et al. Sensitive, reliable and easy-performed laboratory monitoring of eculizumab therapy in atypical hemolytic uremic syndrome. Clin Immunol 2015;160(2):237–43.
75. Noris M, Galbusera M, Gastoldi S, et al. Dynamics of complement activation in aHUS and how to monitor eculizumab therapy. Blood 2014;124(11):1715–26.
76. Peffault de Latour R, Fremeaux-Bacchi V, Porcher R, et al. Assessing complement blockade in patients with paroxysmal nocturnal hemoglobinuria receiving eculizumab. Blood 2015;125(5):775–83.
77. Jodele S, Fukuda T, Mizuno K, et al. Variable eculizumab clearance requires pharmacodynamic monitoring to optimize therapy for thrombotic microangiopathy after hematopoietic stem cell transplantation. Biol Blood Marrow Transplant 2016;22(2):307–15.
78. Cohn AC, MacNeil JR, Clark TA, et al. Prevention and control of meningococcal disease: recommendations of the Advisory Committee on Immunization Practices (ACIP). MMWR Recomm Rep 2013;62(RR-2):1–28.
79. Welsch JA, Senders S, Essink B, et al. Breadth of coverage against a panel of 110 invasive disease isolates, immunogenicity and safety for 2 and 3 doses of an investigational MenABCWY vaccine in US adolescents - Results from a randomized, controlled, observer-blind phase II study. Vaccine 2018;36(35): 5309–17.
80. Bozio C, Epidemiologist MPH. Evidence to Recommendations Framework (EtR) and Grading of Recommendations, Assessment, Development, and Evaluation (GRADE): Serogroup B Meningococcal (MenB) Vaccine Booster Doses for Persons at increased risk for Serogroup B Meningococcal Disease.
81. Reinwald M, Silva JT, Mueller NJ, et al. ESCMID Study Group for Infections in Compromised Hosts (ESGICH) Consensus Document on the safety of targeted and biological therapies: an infectious diseases perspective (Intracellular signaling pathways: tyrosine kinase and mTOR inhibitors). Clin Microbiol Infect 2018;24(Suppl 2):S53–70.
82. Harrison C, Kiladjian J-J, Al-Ali HK, et al. JAK inhibition with ruxolitinib versus best available therapy for myelofibrosis. N Engl J Med 2012;366(9):787–98.
83. Vannucchi AM, Kiladjian JJ, Griesshammer M, et al. Ruxolitinib versus standard therapy for the treatment of polycythemia vera. N Engl J Med 2015;372(5): 426–35.

84. Zeiser R, Burchert A, Lengerke C, et al. Ruxolitinib in corticosteroid-refractory graft-versus-host disease after allogeneic stem cell transplantation: a multicenter survey. Leukemia 2015;29(10):2062–8.

85. D'Amico F, Parigi TL, Fiorino G, et al. Tofacitinib in the treatment of ulcerative colitis: efficacy and safety from clinical trials to real-world experience. Therap Adv Gastroenterol 2019;12. 1756284819848631.

86. Taylor PC, Keystone EC, van der Heijde D, et al. Baricitinib versus placebo or adalimumab in rheumatoid arthritis. N Engl J Med 2017;376(7):652–62.

87. Burmester GR, Blanco R, Charles-Schoeman C, et al. Tofacitinib (CP-690,550) in combination with methotrexate in patients with active rheumatoid arthritis with an inadequate response to tumour necrosis factor inhibitors: a randomised phase 3 trial. Lancet 2013;381(9865):451–60.

88. Conaghan PG, Østergaard M, Bowes MA, et al. Comparing the effects of tofacitinib, methotrexate and the combination, on bone marrow oedema, synovitis and bone erosion in methotrexate-naive, early active rheumatoid arthritis: results of an exploratory randomised MRI study incorporating semiquantitative and quantitative techniques. Ann Rheum Dis 2016;75(6):1024–33.

89. van Vollenhoven RF, Fleischmann R, Cohen S, et al. Tofacitinib or adalimumab versus placebo in rheumatoid arthritis. N Engl J Med 2012;367(6):508–19.

90. Strand V, Kremer JM, Gruben D, et al. Tofacitinib in combination with conventional disease-modifying antirheumatic drugs in patients with active rheumatoid arthritis: patient-reported outcomes from a phase III randomized controlled trial. Arthritis Care Res 2017;69(4):592–8.

91. Dougados M, van der Heijde D, Chen Y-C, et al. Baricitinib in patients with inadequate response or intolerance to conventional synthetic DMARDs: results from the RA-BUILD study. Ann Rheum Dis 2017;76(1):88–95.

92. Fragoulis GE, McInnes IB, Siebert S. JAK-inhibitors. New players in the field of immune-mediated diseases, beyond rheumatoid arthritis. Rheumatology (Oxford) 2019;58(Supplement_1):i43–54.

93. Pfizer Inc. Xeljanz prescribing information. Available at: http://labeling.pfizer.com/ShowLabeling.aspx?id=959. Accessed January 30, 2020.

94. van der Heijde D, Deodhar A, Wei JC, et al. Tofacitinib in patients with ankylosing spondylitis: a phase II, 16-week, randomised, placebo-controlled, dose-ranging study. Ann Rheum Dis 2017;76(8):1340–7.

95. Solimani F, Meier K, Ghoreschi K. Emerging topical and systemic JAK inhibitors in dermatology. Front Immunol 2019;10:2847.

96. Escamilla Gómez V, García-Gutiérrez V, López Corral L, et al. Ruxolitinib in refractory acute and chronic graft-versus-host disease: a multicenter survey study. Bone Marrow Transplant 2020;55(3):641–8.

97. Modi B, Hernandez-Henderson M, Yang D, et al. Ruxolitinib as salvage therapy for chronic graft-versus-host disease. Biol Blood Marrow Transplant 2019;25(2):265–9.

98. Bachelez H, van de Kerkhof PCM, Strohal R, et al. Tofacitinib versus etanercept or placebo in moderate-to-severe chronic plaque psoriasis: a phase 3 randomised non-inferiority trial. Lancet 2015;386(9993):552–61.

99. Craiglow BG, Tavares D, King BA. Topical ruxolitinib for the treatment of alopecia universalis. JAMA Dermatol 2016;152(4):490–1.

100. Levy LL, Urban J, King BA. Treatment of recalcitrant atopic dermatitis with the oral Janus kinase inhibitor tofacitinib citrate. J Am Acad Dermatol 2015;73(3):395–9.

101. Bissonnette R, Papp KA, Poulin Y, et al. Topical tofacitinib for atopic dermatitis: a phase IIa randomized trial. Br J Dermatol 2016;175(5):902–11.

102. Guttman-Yassky E, Silverberg JI, Nemoto O, et al. Baricitinib in adult patients with moderate-to-severe atopic dermatitis: a phase 2 parallel, double-blinded, randomized placebo-controlled multiple-dose study. J Am Acad Dermatol 2019;80(4):913–21.e9.

103. Vincenti F, Silva HT, Busque S, et al. Evaluation of the effect of tofacitinib exposure on outcomes in kidney transplant patients. Am J Transplant 2015;15(6):1644–53.

104. Busque S, Vincenti FG, Tedesco Silva H, et al. Efficacy and safety of a tofacitinib-based immunosuppressive regimen after kidney transplantation: results from a long-term extension trial. Transplant Direct 2018;4(9):e380.

105. Moore CA, Iasella CJ, Venkataramanan R, et al. Janus kinase inhibition for immunosuppression in solid organ transplantation: is there a role in complex immunologic challenges? Hum Immunol 2017;78(2):64–71.

106. Zhang H, Watanabe R, Berry GJ, et al. Inhibition of JAK-STAT signaling suppresses pathogenic immune responses in medium and large vessel vasculitis. Circulation 2018;137(18):1934–48.

107. Wallace DJ, Furie RA, Tanaka Y, et al. Baricitinib for systemic lupus erythematosus: a double-blind, randomised, placebo-controlled, phase 2 trial. Lancet 2018;392(10143):222–31.

108. King B, Lee AI, Choi J. Treatment of hypereosinophilic syndrome with cutaneous involvement with the JAK inhibitors tofacitinib and ruxolitinib. J Invest Dermatol 2017;137(4):951–4.

109. Cervantes F, Vannucchi AM, Kiladjian J-J, et al. Three-year efficacy, safety, and survival findings from COMFORT-II, a phase 3 study comparing ruxolitinib with best available therapy for myelofibrosis. Blood 2013;122(25):4047–53.

110. Al-Ali HK, Griesshammer M, le Coutre P, et al. Safety and efficacy of ruxolitinib in an open-label, multicenter, single-arm phase 3b expanded-access study in patients with myelofibrosis: a snapshot of 1144 patients in the JUMP trial. Haematologica 2016;101(9):1065–73.

111. Polverelli N, Palumbo GA, Binotto G, et al. Epidemiology, outcome, and risk factors for infectious complications in myelofibrosis patients receiving ruxolitinib: a multicenter study on 446 patients. Hematol Oncol 2018;36:561–9.

112. Polverelli N, Breccia M, Benevolo G, et al. Risk factors for infections in myelofibrosis: role of disease status and treatment. A multicenter study of 507 patients. Am J Hematol 2017;92(1):37–41.

113. Lussana F, Cattaneo M, Rambaldi A, et al. Ruxolitinib-associated infections: a systematic review and meta-analysis. Am J Hematol 2018;93(3):339–47.

114. Dioverti MV, Abu Saleh OM, Tande AJ. Infectious complications in patients on treatment with Ruxolitinib: case report and review of the literature. Infect Dis 2018;50(5):381–7.

115. Wathes R, Moule S, Milojkovic D. Progressive multifocal leukoencephalopathy associated with ruxolitinib. N Engl J Med 2013;369(2):197–8.

116. Reoma LB, Trindade CJ, Monaco MC, et al. Fatal encephalopathy with wild-type JC virus and ruxolitinib therapy. Ann Neurol 2019;86(6):878–84.

117. Salvator H, Berti E, Catherinot E, et al. Pulmonary alveolar proteinosis and Mycobacterium abscessus lung infection related to ruxolitinib after allogeneic stem cell transplantation. Eur Respir J 2018;51 [pii:1701960].

118. Moruno-Rodríguez A, Sánchez-Vicente JL, Rueda-Rueda T, et al. Invasive aspergillosis manifesting as retinal necrosis in a patient treated with ruxolitinib. Arch Soc Esp Oftalmol 2019;94(5):237–41.

119. Prakash K, Richman D. A case report of disseminated histoplasmosis and concurrent cryptococcal meningitis in a patient treated with ruxolitinib. BMC Infect Dis 2019;19(1):287.

120. Gill H, Leung GMK, Seto W-K, et al. Risk of viral reactivation in patients with occult hepatitis B virus infection during ruxolitinib treatment. Ann Hematol 2019;98(1):215–8.

121. Anand K, Burns EA, Ensor J, et al. Mycobacterial infections with ruxolitinib: a retrospective pharmacovigilance review. Clin Lymphoma Myeloma Leuk 2020; 20(1):18–23.

122. Tsukamoto Y, Kiyasu J, Tsuda M, et al. Fatal disseminated tuberculosis during treatment with ruxolitinib plus prednisolone in a patient with primary myelofibrosis: a case report and review of the literature. Intern Med 2018;57(9): 1297–300.

123. Abedin S, McKenna E, Chhabra S, et al. Efficacy, toxicity, and infectious complications in ruxolitinib-treated patients with corticosteroid-refractory graft-versus-host disease after hematopoietic cell transplantation. Biol Blood Marrow Transplant 2019;25(8):1689–94.

124. Cohen S, Radominski SC, Gomez-Reino JJ, et al. Analysis of infections and all-cause mortality in phase II, phase III, and long-term extension studies of tofacitinib in patients with rheumatoid arthritis. Arthritis Rheumatol 2014;66(11): 2924–37.

125. Strand V, Ahadieh S, French J, et al. Systematic review and meta-analysis of serious infections with tofacitinib and biologic disease-modifying antirheumatic drug treatment in rheumatoid arthritis clinical trials. Arthritis Res Ther 2015; 17:362.

126. Bechman K, Subesinghe S, Norton S, et al. A systematic review and meta-analysis of infection risk with small molecule JAK inhibitors in rheumatoid arthritis. Rheumatol 2019;58(10):1755–66.

127. Gladman D, Rigby W, Azevedo VF, et al. Tofacitinib for psoriatic arthritis in patients with an inadequate response to TNF inhibitors. N Engl J Med 2017; 377(16):1525–36.

128. Mease P, Hall S, FitzGerald O, et al. Tofacitinib or adalimumab versus placebo for psoriatic arthritis. N Engl J Med 2017;377(16):1537–50.

129. Trigo-Vicente C, Gimeno-Ballester V, García-López S, et al. Systematic review and network meta-analysis of treatment for moderate-to-severe ulcerative colitis. Int J Clin Pharm 2018;40(6):1411–9.

130. Colombel J-F. Herpes zoster in patients receiving JAK inhibitors for ulcerative colitis: mechanism, epidemiology, management, and prevention. Inflamm Bowel Dis 2018;24(10):2173–82.

131. Winthrop KL. The emerging safety profile of JAK inhibitors in rheumatic disease. Nat Rev Rheumatol 2017;13(4):234–43.

132. Curtis JR, Xie F, Yun H, et al. Real-world comparative risks of herpes virus infections in tofacitinib and biologic-treated patients with rheumatoid arthritis. Ann Rheum Dis 2016;75(10):1843–7.

133. Winthrop KL, Yamanaka H, Valdez H, et al. Herpes zoster and tofacitinib therapy in patients with rheumatoid arthritis. Arthritis Rheumatol 2014;66(10):2675–84.

134. Winthrop KL, Melmed GY, Vermeire S, et al. Herpes Zoster infection in patients with ulcerative colitis receiving tofacitinib. Inflamm Bowel Dis 2018;24(10): 2258–65.
135. Winthrop KL, Park S-H, Gul A, et al. Tuberculosis and other opportunistic infections in tofacitinib-treated patients with rheumatoid arthritis. Ann Rheum Dis 2016;75(6):1133–8.
136. Genovese MC, Kremer J, Zamani O, et al. Baricitinib in patients with refractory rheumatoid arthritis. N Engl J Med 2016;374(13):1243–52.
137. Smolen JS, Genovese MC, Takeuchi T, et al. Safety profile of baricitinib in patients with active rheumatoid arthritis with over 2 years median time in treatment. J Rheumatol 2019;46(1):7–18.
138. Olivera P, Lasa J, Bonovas S, et al. Safety of janus kinase inhibitors in patients with inflammatory bowel diseases or other immune-mediated diseases: a systematic review and meta-analysis. Gastroenterology 2020. Epub ahead of print.
139. Winthrop KL, Wouters AG, Choy EH, et al. The safety and immunogenicity of live zoster vaccination in patients with rheumatoid arthritis before starting tofacitinib: a randomized phase II trial. Arthritis Rheumatol 2017;69(10):1969–77.
140. Baxter R, Bartlett J, Fireman B, et al. Long-term effectiveness of the live zoster vaccine in preventing shingles: a cohort study. Am J Epidemiol 2018;187(1): 161–9.
141. Tseng HF, Harpaz R, Luo Y, et al. Declining effectiveness of herpes zoster vaccine in adults aged ≥60 years. J Infect Dis 2016;213(12):1872–5.
142. Cunningham AL, Lal H, Kovac M, et al. Efficacy of the Herpes Zoster subunit vaccine in adults 70 years of age or older. N Engl J Med 2016;375(11):1019–32.
143. Berkowitz EM, Moyle G, Stellbrink H-J, et al. Safety and immunogenicity of an adjuvanted herpes zoster subunit candidate vaccine in HIV-infected adults: a phase 1/2a randomized, placebo-controlled study. J Infect Dis 2015;211(8): 1279–87.
144. Vink P, Delgado Mingorance I, Maximiano Alonso C, et al. Immunogenicity and safety of the adjuvanted recombinant zoster vaccine in patients with solid tumors, vaccinated before or during chemotherapy: a randomized trial. Cancer 2019;125(8):1301–12.
145. Vink P, Ramon Torrell JM, Sanchez Fructuoso A, et al. Immunogenicity and safety of the adjuvanted recombinant zoster vaccine in chronically immunosuppressed adults following renal transplant: a phase 3, randomized clinical trial. Clin Infect Dis 2020;70(2):181–90.
146. Bastidas A, de la Serna J, El Idrissi M, et al. Effect of recombinant zoster vaccine on incidence of Herpes Zoster after autologous stem cell transplantation: a randomized clinical trial. JAMA 2019;322(2):123–33.
147. Khan N, Shah Y, Trivedi C, et al. Safety of Herpes Zoster vaccination among inflammatory bowel disease patients being treated with anti-TNF medications. Aliment Pharmacol Ther 2017;46(7):668–72.
148. Singh JA, Saag KG, Bridges SL Jr, et al. 2015 American College of Rheumatology Guideline for the Treatment of Rheumatoid Arthritis. Arthritis Rheumatol 2016;68(1):1–26.
149. Dooling KL, Guo A, Patel M, et al. Recommendations of the Advisory Committee on Immunization practices for use of Herpes Zoster vaccines. MMWR Morb Mortal Wkly Rep 2018;67(3):103–8.
150. Taplitz RA, Kennedy EB, Bow EJ, et al. Antimicrobial prophylaxis for adult patients with cancer-related immunosuppression: ASCO and IDSA clinical practice guideline update. J Clin Oncol 2018;36(30):3043–54.

Herpesvirus Infections Potentiated by Biologics

Dora Y. Ho, MD, PhD[a],*, Kyle Enriquez, MS[b], Ashrit Multani, MD[c]

KEYWORDS

- Herpesvirus - Herpes simplex - Varicella-zoster - Cytomegalovirus
- Biologic agents

KEY POINTS

- Herpesviruses such as herpes simplex virus (HSV) type 1 and 2, varicella-zoster virus (VZV), and cytomegalovirus (CMV) maintain lifelong latency in the host after primary infection and can reactivate periodically either as asymptomatic viral shedding or as clinical disease.
- Immunosuppression, including biologic therapy, may increase frequency and severity of herpesvirus reactivation and infection.
- Licensed biologics are reviewed regarding their risks of potentiating HSV, VZV, and CMV reactivation and infection.
- Approaches to prophylaxis against HSV, VZV, and CMV infection or reactivation are discussed.

INTRODUCTION

Herpesviruses (members of family Herpesviridae) are enveloped, double-stranded DNA viruses that are ubiquitous in the animal kingdom. Eight of them are known human pathogens, which are grouped into 3 subfamilies based on their genomic and biological characteristics: *Alphaherpesvirinae* (herpes simplex virus [HSV] type 1 and 2 and varicella-zoster virus [VZV]), *Betaherpesvirinae* (cytomegalovirus [CMV], human herpesvirus [HHV] 6 and HHV-7), and *Gammaherpesvirinae* (Epstein-Barr virus and Kaposi sarcoma–associated herpesvirus [also known as HHV-8]). One prominent characteristic of the HHVs is their ability to establish and maintain lifelong latency in infected hosts and reactivate periodically, either as asymptomatic viral shedding or as clinic syndromes or diseases. Reactivation of HHVs is more frequent and has

[a] Division of Infectious Diseases and Geographic Medicine, Department of Medicine, Stanford University School of Medicine, 300 Pasteur Drive, Lane Building L-135, Stanford, CA 94305-5107, USA; [b] Stanford University, 450 Serra Mall, Stanford, CA 94305, USA; [c] Division of Infectious Diseases, Department of Medicine, David Geffen School of Medicine at UCLA, 10833 Le Conte Avenue CHS 37-121, Los Angeles, CA 90095-1688, USA
* Corresponding author.
E-mail address: doraywho@stanford.edu

Infect Dis Clin N Am 34 (2020) 311–339
https://doi.org/10.1016/j.idc.2020.02.006
0891-5520/20/© 2020 Elsevier Inc. All rights reserved.

id.theclinics.com

more severe consequences in immunocompromised hosts. Among the HHVs, HSV, VZV, and CMV are of particular interest, because their reactivation can lead to significant morbidity and mortality, but such harm can be mitigated using prophylactic or preemptive approaches. As discussed in other articles in this issue, biologics can modulate or suppress the immune system via various mechanisms and pathways. This article provides a survey of biologics currently in clinical use regarding their possible risks of potentiating infection or reactivation of HSV, VZV, and CMV, and discusses approaches for antiviral prophylaxis.

BIOLOGY AND PATHOGENESIS OF HERPESVIRUSES

Herpesviruses have developed complex mechanisms to evade the host immune system. A detailed discussion of their pathogenesis and host immune response is beyond the scope of this article.

Herpes Simplex Virus 1 and 2

Primary HSV infection usually occurs after exposure of the oral or anogenital mucosa to the virus and is commonly subclinical. After initial replication of the virus in the epidermis, the virus undergoes retrograde axonal transport to the neuronal cell body, where it can establish a lifelong latency within the trigeminal and/or dorsal root ganglia.[1] Reactivation of the virus may result in asymptomatic viral shedding or symptomatic diseases. Multiple arms of the immune system (including both innate and adoptive immunity) participate in the host defense against HSV.[2,3] In particular, cluster of differentiation (CD) 4 and CD8 T cells, the key components of the cell-mediated immune response, play critical roles in controlling HSV infection. T-cell responses at the ganglion level as well as immune surveillance at the epithelium can influence the frequency and severity of HSV reactivation. While CD4 T cells help orchestrate multiple facets of the immune response (eg, activation of B cells, production of interferon, and recruitment of CD8 T cells), CD8 T cells have the important role of killing virus-infected cells and allowing viral clearance. The role of antibody-mediated protection against HSV pathogenesis is less clear, but neutralizing antibodies might reduce acquisition of the infection as well as the frequency of recurrent lesions and viral shedding.

Although HSV-1 and HSV-2 are well known to cause oral and genital herpes, a wide range of clinical manifestations may develop, depending on the anatomic sites involved and the immune status of the host.[3] In immunocompromised patients, HSV can cause extensive mucocutaneous infection and can disseminate to cause multiorgan involvement (**Table 1**).

Varicella-zoster Virus

Exposure of a susceptible host to VZV results in the primary form of infection termed varicella or chickenpox. Unlike other HHVs, which are in general transmitted by direct contact, VZV is transmitted by the respiratory route. After inoculation of respiratory mucosal sites and replication in regional lymphoid tissue (targeting primarily T lymphocytes), infected T cells transport VZV to the skin via a cell-associated viremia. Infection of the skin then produces the characteristic vesicular rash. The virus can gain access to the sensory nerve cell body from the nerve endings or via cell-associated viremia, to establish lifelong latent infection within the sensory ganglia. Reactivation of the virus leads to anterograde transport of the virions along the neuronal exons back to the skin, resulting in herpes zoster (HZ), which is most commonly manifested as a

Table 1
Genome size, sites of latency, and clinical manifestations of herpes simplex virus, varicella-zoster virus, and cytomegalovirus

Virus	Genome Size (kbp)	Sites of Latency	Primary Infection in Immuno-competent Hosts	Reactivation in Immunocompetent Hosts	Infection in Immunocompromised Hosts
HSV	152	Sensory ganglia	Gingivostomatitis Genital herpes Keratocon-junctivitis Neonatal herpes	Oral or genital mucocutaneous infection Keratoconjunctivitis Aseptic meningitis Encephalitis	Disseminated or visceral infection Severe mucocutaneous infection Meningoencephalitis Pneumonitis Hepatitis Esophagitis
VZV	125	Sensory ganglia	Varicella	Zoster	Disseminated or visceral infection
CMV	236	Myeloid progenitor cells (eg, CD34+ cells)	Mononucleosis Congenital CMV disease	Asymptomatic viral shedding	Asymptomatic viremia CMV syndrome Disseminated or visceral infection Encephalitis Pneumonitis Hepatitis Retinitis Gastroenteritis

Abbreviation: kbp, kilobase pairs.

localized dermatomal rash. In immunocompromised patients, VZV reactivation may result in a multidermatomal rash or dissemination with multiorgan involvement (see **Table 1**).

The maintenance of VZV latency is influenced directly by the host response, as shown from the high incidence of VZV reactivation when VZV-specific immunity is impaired (eg, after hematopoietic stem cell transplant [HSCT]).[4] Similar to HSV, humoral immunity seems to be less important in the host response to VZV than cell-mediated immunity.[5] Preexisting immunoglobulin (Ig) G antibody seropositivity does not prevent VZV reactivation, although it may decrease the viral load. In contrast, diminished VZV-specific T-cell proliferation correlates with increased susceptibility to HZ among immunocompromised hosts.[4]

Cytomegalovirus

Primary infection of CMV in healthy individuals is usually asymptomatic, but the virus can cause severe to life-threatening infections in neonates or immunocompromised patients. Despite a robust response of both the innate and cellular immunities to the primary infection, CMV establishes lifelong latency in infected hosts. CMV maintains latency in myeloprogenitor cells (eg, CD34+ cells), but other cell types, including those of endothelial or epithelial origins, might also harbor the virus in a chronic, "smoldering" form.[6,7] Being the largest virus to infect humans, CMV encodes many gene products that can directly modulate the host immune system. The interplay between CMV and the host immune response to control viral latency, reactivation, as well as the extent of active viral replication and disease is far from clear and is a subject of intense research.[6] Viral reactivation is a frequent phenomenon among HSCT and solid organ transplant (SOT) recipients and can result in asymptomatic viremia or severe end-organ disease (see **Table 1**). For nontransplant settings, the risk and consequence of CMV reactivation is less well studied, but certain forms of immunosuppression, including treatment with biologics, can potentiate CMV reactivation, as discussed later.

HERPESVIRUS INFECTIONS WITH BIOLOGICS

A large number of biologics have been licensed for clinical use and many more are in development. Please refer to other articles in this issue for the mechanism of action of each individual biologic agent. The licensed agents and their risks of herpesvirus infection are summarized in **Table 2**. Only those with increased risk of herpesvirus infection are discussed.

Tumor Necrosis Factor Alpha Inhibitors (Adalimumab, Certolizumab, Etanercept, Golimumab, Infliximab)

Herpesviruses encode genes that target tumor necrosis factor (TNF)–related cytokines and receptors in order to modulate the host immune response.[8] Treatment with TNF-α inhibitors has been associated with severe HSV and VZV disease (including examples of hepatitis, encephalitis, and disseminated disease from HSV[9–12]; and meningitis, pneumonitis, and disseminated disease from VZV[13–17]). Whether anti-TNF therapy increases risk of VZV reactivation has been evaluated in several studies and the results are conflicting. Several European studies showed that anti-TNF treatment is associated with significantly increased risk of HZ,[18–20] but a large multicenter cohort study in the United States that studied patients treated with anti-TNF (n = 33,324) or nonbiologic disease-modifying antirheumatic drugs (DMARDs) (n = 25,742) for rheumatoid arthritis (RA) or other inflammatory diseases did not show any increased HZ risk.[21] It is thought that the discrepancies of these conflicting results might reflect a different practice in the use of corticosteroid therapy between the practitioners in the United States and in Europe.[22]

Cases of CMV reactivation have also been reported with infliximab,[23] from acute CMV syndrome,[24] retinitis,[25] colitis,[26] and hepatitis[27] to disseminated disease.[28]

Conclusion

Severe infections with HSV, VZV, or CMV have been associated with TNF-α inhibition. Routine antiviral prophylaxis may not be indicated, but physicians should be aware of the risk and monitor patients closely.

AGENTS TARGETING B CELLS

Anti–CD20 agents (obinutuzumab, ocrelizumab, ofatumumab, rituximab, ^{90}Y-ibritumomab tiuxetan)

Rituximab is the first licensed CD20-targeted agent. A recent review of 20 years of its clinical experience noted that grade 3/4 infections occurred in approximately 4% of patients treated with rituximab as monotherapy in randomized studies, more common than those of observation groups.[29] Serious or fatal infections with HSV, VZV, and CMV have been reported.[30–32]

Obinutuzumab has been compared with rituximab in a large phase 3 randomized clinical trial (RCT) for previously untreated patients with follicular lymphoma.[33] This study showed a higher rate of infection in the obinutuzumab group (n = 595) than

Table 2
Biologic agents and herpesvirus risk

Pharmacologic Agent	HSV/VZV/CMV Risks	Prophylaxis/Monitoring/Comments
TNF-α Inhibitors		

TNF-α inhibitors
  Adalimumab
  Certolizumab
  Etanercept
  Golimumab
  Infliximab
	Yes, but HZ risk may depend on concomitant use of steroids	No current recommendations for routine antiviral prophylaxis or for monitoring of CMV reactivation

Agents Targeting B Cells		

Anti-CD20 agents
  Obinutuzumab
  Ocrelizumab
  Ofatumumab
  Rituximab
  ^{90}Y-ibritumomab tiuxetan
	Yes; most notable with HZ	Consider antiviral prophylaxis for HZ, depending on other concomitant immunosuppression
		No current recommendations for routine monitoring of CMV reactivation

Anti-CD30 agent Brentuximab vedotin	Yes; most notable with CMV	Consider antiviral prophylaxis CMV-seropositive patients should be monitored for CMV reactivation/infection
Anti-CD38 agent Daratumumab	Yes	Prophylaxis for HZ is recommended

PI3K inhibitors
  Idelalisib
  Buparlisib
  Rigosertib
  Duvelisib
	Yes	Consider acyclovir prophylaxis
		CMV-seropositive patients should be monitored for CMV reactivation/infection

Anti-C19 agents Blinatumomab	No	NA

Anti-CD22 agents
  Epratuzumab
  Inotuzumab ozogamicin
  Moxetumomab pasudotox
	No	NA

Bcl-2 inhibitor Venetoclax	No	NA
B cell–activating factor inhibitor Belimumab	No	NA
Agents Targeting T-cell Activation		

CTLA-4 IgG: CD28-CD80/86 blockade
  Abatacept
  Belatacept
	Possible increase risk	No current recommendations for routine antiviral prophylaxis or for monitoring of CMV reactivation

LFA-3/CD-2 inhibitor Alefacept	No	NA

(continued on next page)

Table 2
(continued)

Pharmacologic Agent	HSV/VZV/CMV Risks	Prophylaxis/Monitoring/ Comments
IL-12/23 p40-targeted agents and IL-23 inhibitors Guselkumab Risankizumab Tildrakizumab Ustekinumab	No	NA
IL-17 inhibitors Brodalumab Ixekizumab Secukinumab	No	NA
Direct T-cell Inhibitors and Agents Targeting T-cell Migration and Chemotaxis		
Anti-CD52 agent Alemtuzumab	Yes	Antiviral prophylaxis for HSV and VZV is recommended CMV-seropositive patients should be monitored for CMV reactivation/infection
Alpha4-integrin inhibitors Natalizumab Vedolizumab	No	NA
IL-2 receptor inhibitors Basiliximab Daclizumab[a]	No	NA
IL-1, IL-4, IL-5, IL-6, and IgE Inhibitors		
IL-4 inhibitor Dupilumab	Possible increased risk of HZ	No current recommendations for routine antiviral prophylaxis
IL-5 inhibitors Benralizumab Mepolizumab Reslizumab	Possible increased risk of HZ	No current recommendations for routine antiviral prophylaxis Package insert of mepolizumab recommends consideration of varicella vaccination before starting therapy
IL-6 inhibitors Sarilumab Tocilizumab	Increased risk of HZ	No current recommendations for routine antiviral prophylaxis
IL-1 inhibitors Anakinra Canakinumab Rilonacept	No	NA
IgE inhibitor Omalizumab	No	NA
Checkpoint Inhibitors		
Atezolizumab Avelumab Cemiplimab Durvalumab	No, but immunosuppression therapy used to treat immune-mediated complications might	NA

(continued on next page)

Table 2
(continued)

Pharmacologic Agent	HSV/VZV/CMV Risks	Prophylaxis/Monitoring/Comments
Ipilimumab Nivolumab Pembrolizumab	increase risks of herpesvirus reactivation	
Tyrosine Kinase Inhibitors for Hematologic Malignancies		

Small molecule BCR-ABL tyrosine kinase inhibitors
    Bafetinib
    Bosutinib
    Dasatinib
    Imatinib
    Nilotinib
    Ponatinib
	Yes	No current recommendations for routine antiviral prophylaxis or for monitoring of CMV reactivation

Bruton tyrosine kinase inhibitors
    Acalabrutinib
    Ibrutinib
	No	NA

EGFR Inhibitors and Other Tyrosine Kinase Inhibitors for Solid Tumors		

EGFR tyrosine kinase inhibitors
    Afatinib
    Erlotinib
    Gefitinib
    Lapatinib
    Neratinib
    Osimertinib
	No	NA

EGFR-inhibiting monoclonal antibodies
    Cetuximab
    Panitumumab
	No	NA

Other tyrosine kinase inhibitors
    Axitinib
    Cabozantinib
    Pazopanib
    Ramucirumab
    Regorafenib
    Sorafenib
    Sunitinib
    Vandetanib
	No	NA

VEGF inhibitors
    Aflibercept
    Bevacizumab
	No	NA

Targeting JAK-STAT Signaling and Complement Pathway for Inflammatory Diseases		

Janus kinase inhibitors
    Baricitinib ruxolitinib
    Tofacitinib
	Increased risk of HZ	Antiviral prophylaxis for HSV and VZV is recommended CMV-seropositive patients should be monitored for CMV reactivation/infection

C5 inhibitors	No	NA

(continued on next page)

Table 2
(continued)

Pharmacologic Agent	HSV/VZV/CMV Risks	Prophylaxis/Monitoring/Comments
Eculizumab Ravulizumab		
Miscellaneous		
S1P receptor modulator Fingolimod	Increased risk of HZ	Routine antiviral prophylaxis has not recommended, but can be considered with concomitant steroid use
Proteasome inhibitors Bortezomib Carfilzomib Ixazomib	Increased risk of HZ	Antiviral prophylaxis should be considered
Anti-SLAMF7 agent Elotuzumab	Increased risk of HZ	Antiviral prophylaxis should be considered
Anti-CCR4 agent Mogamulizumab	Yes	Antiviral prophylaxis is recommended CMV-seropositive patients should be closely monitored for CMV reactivation/disease
Anti-CD33 agent Gemtuzumab	No	NA
BRAF and MEK kinase inhibitors Vemurafenib Dabrafenib Trametinib Cobimetinib Selumetinib Encorafenib (+binimetinib)	No	NA

Abbreviations: CTLA-4, cytotoxic T lymphocyte–associated protein 4; EGFR, epidermal growth factor receptor; IL, interleukin; NA, not applicable; TNF, tumor necrosis factor; VEGF, vascular endothelial growth factor.
 [a] Voluntarily withdrawn from market in the United States in 2018.

the rituximab group (n = 597) (20% vs 16%). Approximately 10% of patients in the obinutuzumab group and 6.7% of patients in the rituximab group developed HZ but no cases of CMV disease were reported. A subgroup analysis for patients enrolled in Japan[34] also showed higher HZ incidence in the obinutuzumab group (n = 65) compared with the rituximab group (n = 58) (13.8% vs 3.4%).

For the other anti-CD20 agents, fewer data regarding herpesvirus reactivation are available. A phase 3 RCT that studied ocrelizumab in primary progressive multiple sclerosis (MS) noted more frequent oral HSV reactivation with ocrelizumab than with placebo.[35] A case of HSV-2 encephalitis was reported in a patient with MS treated with ocrelizumab.[36] A phase 3 RCT that studied ofatumumab in relapsed chronic lymphocytic leukemia (CLL) did not report any cases of CMV; only a few cases of HZ were noted in both ofatumumab and the comparator groups.[37] For ^{90}Y-ibtriumomab, no herpesvirus infection was reported in its pivotal phase 3 RCT for advanced-stage follicular lymphoma.[38]

Conclusion

Risk of herpesvirus reactivation is most notable with VZV among patients treated with rituximab or ofatumumab. At present, there are no recommendations for routine antiviral prophylaxis.

Anti–CD30 agent (brentuximab vedotin)

In a pivotal phase 3 RCT that studied brentuximab vedotin as consolidation therapy after autologous HSCT in patients with Hodgkin lymphoma,[39] no increase in serious herpesvirus reactivation was reported, but a subsequent safety analysis of this RCT reported more cases of HSV and HZ in the brentuximab arm (HSV, 7 out of 167, 4%; HZ, 12 out of 167, 7%) than in the placebo arm (HSV, 1 out of 160, 1%; HZ, 6 out of 160, 3%) despite antiviral prophylaxis per protocol.[40]

A retrospective study on 39 patients that received brentuximab vedotin reported CMV reactivation in 6 patients.[41] This agent was also linked to a case of severe CMV retinitis, which relapsed on rechallenge with the same biologic.[42]

Conclusion

Brentuximab vedotin may increase risk of herpesvirus reactivation. Antiviral prophylaxis can be considered. CMV-seropositive patients should be monitored for CMV reactivation. Secondary anti-CMV prophylaxis should be considered in those who need additional doses of brentuximab vedotin.[43]

Anti–CD38 agent (daratumumab)

From monotherapy studies and RCTs, VZV reactivation rates in the daratumumab arms ranged from 2% to 5%, but it should be noted that these patients also received other immunomodulatory agents, including proteasome inhibitors and corticosteroids.[43] Reported cases of herpesvirus reactivation included HSV encephalitis, CMV syndrome, retinitis, and enterocolitis, as well as VZV reactivation despite acyclovir prophylaxis.[44–46]

Conclusion

Prophylaxis for VZV reactivation was recommended for patients in some clinical trials. Per package insert, antiviral prophylaxis to prevent HZ reactivation should be initiated within 1 week after starting daratumumab and continued for 3 months following treatment.[47]

Phosphatidylinositol 3 kinase (PI3K) inhibitors (idelalisib, buparlisib, rigosertib, duvelisib)

In a pivotal phase 3 RCT[48] that studied idelalisib in combination with ofatumumab for treatment of relapsed CLL, serious opportunistic infections were noted in the idelalisib arm, including 3 cases (2%) of CMV reactivation. Grade 3 reactivations of HSV (n = 1), HZ (n = 2; 1 with dissemination), and oral herpes (n = 1) were also noted in the idelalisib group, whereas no herpesvirus reactivations/infections were noted in the control group. Other investigators have also reported cases of CMV reactivation/disease with idelalisib treatment.[49,50]

For the newer phosphatidylinositol 3 kinase (PI3K) inhibitors, fewer data are available. Buparlisib is licensed for the treatment of advanced or metastatic HR-positive/HER2-negative breast cancer and RCTs did not identify any increased risks for herpesvirus reactivation, but the underlying risk of opportunistic infections for patients with breast cancer is likely less than for patients with CLL. Similar to idelalisib, duvelisib is also marketed for treatment of relapsed or refractory CLL and follicular lymphoma. Per package insert, CMV reactivation occurred in 1% of patients taking duvelisib.[51] In the RCTs of this agent, prophylaxis for HSV/VZV (and for *Pneumocystis jirovecii*) was used.[52,53]

Conclusion

Patients who receive these agents for the treatment of hematologic malignancies should be checked for CMV IgG antibody, and those who are seropositive should have regular clinical and laboratory monitoring for CMV reactivation during treatment.[51,54] Of note, duvelisib's package insert recommends to "consider prophylactic antivirals during duvelisib treatment to prevent CMV infection including CMV reactivation." However, usual doses of acyclovir and valacyclovir for HSV or VZV prophylaxis are unlikely to be effective for CMV, whereas anti-CMV prophylaxis with valganciclovir is not a routine practice among patients with hematologic malignancies because of its potential myelotoxicity.

AGENTS TARGETING T-CELL ACTIVATION
Cytotoxic T lymphocyte–associated protein 4 (CTLA4)- IgG: blockade of CD28–CD80/86 interaction (abatacept, belatacept)

Treatment of RA with abatacept has been associated with serious infections.[55] For herpesvirus infections, a phase 2/3 RCT that studied abatacept in lupus nephritis showed that HZ occurred at higher rates in abatacept-treated groups compared with the placebo group.[56] In a large cohort of patients with RA who used abatacept or TNF-α inhibitors as a first-line or second-line biologic agent, the risks of HZ were similar between abatacept and TNF-α inhibitors.[57]

An initial phase 3 RCT of belatacept in kidney transplant recipients did not show any increased risk of herpesvirus infection.[58] However, more recent studies showed that belatacept treatment might increase herpesvirus reactivation risk. In a study that followed the safety and efficacy outcomes of kidney transplant recipients 3 years after switching from a calcineurin inhibitor to belatacept, more patients in the belatacept group versus the group that continued calcineurin inhibitor had any-grade viral infections (14.6 vs 11.0 per 100 patient-years) including herpes virus infection (1.71 vs 0.84), CMV viremia (1.71 vs 0.00), and HZ (1.29 vs 0.85), although overall incidence remained low.[59] Another phase 3 RCT that studied the long-term outcomes in belatacept-treated versus cyclosporine-treated renal transplant recipients also showed a slightly higher incidence of CMV infection and HZ in the belatacept arms.[60] Other reports of herpesvirus reactivation in renal transplant patients treated with belatacept include a fatal case of HZ[61] and 2 cases of CMV retinitis.[62]

Conclusion

These agents may be associated with an increased risk of herpesvirus reactivation, although antiviral prophylaxis has not been recommended.

DIRECT T-CELL INHIBITORS
Anti–CD52 agent (alemtuzumab)

Alemtuzumab is approved by the US Food and Drug Administration (FDA) for the treatment of B-cell CLL and for relapsing-remitting MS (under different trade names, Campath and Lemtrada, respectively), but it has also been studied extensively for other off-label uses, including treatment of other hematologic malignancies and graft-versus-host disease after HSCT, as well as induction therapy for immunosuppression in SOT.

Regarding risks of infection, CMV reactivation is frequent in patients treated with alemtuzumab for hematologic malignancies, reported in 15% to 66% of patients.[63] In a study that monitored 10 patients prospectively for CMV reactivation after being treated with alemtuzumab, all 10 patients developed CMV reactivation, including pneumonitis and hepatitis.[64] RCTs also showed significantly higher rates of asymptomatic and symptomatic CMV reactivation with the alemtuzumab arms than the comparator arms.[65,66] Thus, frequent monitoring for and early treatment of CMV reactivation should be instituted during alemtuzumab therapy.

For the use of alemtuzumab in MS, multiple studies reported increased risks of HSV and VZV.[67] In a phase 3 RCT that compared alemtuzumab with interferon-β-1a, 62 of 376 (16%) patients treated with alemtuzumab had herpesvirus reactivation (12 cases of HZ and 50 cases of HSV) compared with 3 of 187 (2%) patients treated with interferon-β-1a (all with HSV).[68] Another phase 3 RCT for MS also noted increased herpesvirus reactivation with alemtuzumab (16% of alemtuzumab groups vs 4% in the interferon-β-1a group), even though some patients of the alemtuzumab groups received acyclovir prophylaxis.[69] Although CMV risk was not prominent in RCTs for MS, multiple cases of CMV reactivation with end-organ disease have been reported.[70–72]

For SOT recipients who received alemtuzumab as induction therapy, the risk of herpesvirus reactivation is difficult to assess, because patients frequently received antiviral prophylaxis per transplant protocol.

Conclusion
Given the Increased risk of HSV and VZV infections, the manufacturer recommends antiviral prophylaxis with acyclovir starting on the first day of treatment and continuing for at least 2 months after alemtuzumab therapy or until the CD4+ lymphocyte count is greater than or equal to 200 cells per microliter, whichever occurs later. Patients with positive CMV serostatus should also be monitored closely for signs or symptoms of CMV reactivation.

INTERLEUKIN (IL)-4, IL-5, AND IL-6 INHIBITORS
IL-4 inhibitor (dupilumab)

The infection risk of dupilumab has been analyzed using pooled data from 7 RCTs of dupilumab in adults with moderate-to-severe atopic dermatitis.[73] Herpesvirus reactivation rates overall were slightly higher with dupilumab than placebo (mostly caused by oral HSV), but clinically important herpesvirus reactivations such as eczema herpeticum and HZ were less common with dupilumab (risk ratio, 0.31; $P<.01$). However, recurrent HSV uveitis and VZV meningitis have been linked to dupilumab use.[74]

Conclusion
Possible increased risk of HSV or VZV, but routine prophylaxis is not indicated.

IL-5 inhibitors (benralizumab, mepolizumab, and reslizumab)

Rare cases of HZ were observed in the mepolizumab treatment arm of RCTs for refractory or severe eosinophilic asthma[75,76]; otherwise, no increased risk of herpesvirus reactivation was noted.[77–79] However, the risk of developing HZ is included in its product monograph, with the recommendation of considering VZV vaccination before starting therapy with mepolizumab. Phase 3 RCTs[80,81] and a long-term safety and efficacy study[82] of reslizumab did not report any cases of herpesvirus infection. For benralizumab, a pivotal RCT that randomized more than 1300 patients reported only 1 case of HZ, which occurred in the benralizumab group.[83] A study that analyzed the incidence of adverse events in published RCTs of benralizumab did not identify any increased risk of opportunistic infections. A case of disseminated VZV was reported in a patient after initiation of benralizumab treatment of severe asthma,[84] but causality was unclear.

Conclusion

No significant increase of herpesvirus risk, although few cases of HZ were reported. Routine prophylaxis is not indicated, but package insert of mepolizumab recommends consideration of varicella vaccination before initiating treatment.

IL-6 inhibitors (sarilumab, siltuximab, tocilizumab)

These agents have been linked to increased risk of infectious complications, including that of herpesviruses. In a postmarketing surveillance of 7901 patients in Japan with RA who received tocilizumab,[85] 86 cases of HZ (with 18 rated as serious) were noted with an incidence rate of 1.09% and a rate of 2.24 episodes per 100 patient-years. Using a large population-based study using Medicare data, incidence rate of HZ among older patients with RA treated with tocilizumab was 2.15 episodes per 100 patient-years.[86] Cases of severe CMV disease have also been reported.[87,88]

For sarilumab, phase 3 RCTs[89,90] did not report any cases of herpesvirus reactivation. In a study that[91] assessed its long-term safety among 2887 patients that received sarilumab in combination with conventional synthetic DMARDs and 471 patients that received sarilumab monotherapy, incidence rates of HZ per 100 patient-years were 0.6 and 0.5 respectively; no cases were disseminated.

Fewer data on herpesvirus infection are available for siltuximab. In a phase 2 study for relapsed or refractory multiple myeloma, only 1 case of HZ was reported.[92]

CONCLUSION

Among the interleukin (IL)-6 inhibitors, available data suggest tocilizumab is associated with an increased risk HZ, although there is currently no recommendation for routine prophylaxis with acyclovir.

Checkpoint Inhibitors

Cytotoxic T Lymphocyte–associated protein 4 targetedagents (Ipilimumab and Tremelimumab) and programmed cell death protein1/programmed death-ligand 1 targeted agents (nivolumab, pembrolizumab, andatezolizumab).

Although treatment with checkpoint inhibitors may not directly lead to herpesvirus reactivation, they can cause a constellation of adverse effects that mimic infectious syndromes. The management of their adverse effects frequently involves treatment with corticosteroids and/or other immunosuppressive agents, such as TNF-α inhibitors, which might then increase risk for herpesvirus reactivation. For instance, patients who received corticosteroids and/or infliximab to manage immune-mediated colitis might develop CMV colitis.[93,94] In a retrospective review[95] of 740 patients with melanoma who received ipilimumab and nivolumab, serious infectious complications occurred in 54 patients (7.3%), including 3 cases of disseminated or facial HZ and 1 case of CMV enterocolitis. The main risk factors for infectious complications among these patients were receipt of corticosteroids and/or infliximab, but it was unclear whether those patients with herpesvirus infection had received other immunosuppressive agents.

Conclusion

Checkpoint inhibitors may not directly increase risk of herpesvirus reactivation. However, for those patients who develop new signs or symptoms during management of immune-related adverse events, the possibility of herpesvirus reactivation should be considered.

TYROSINE KINASE (TK) INHIBITORS FOR HEMATOLOGIC MALIGNANCIES
BCR-ABL tyrosine kinase inhibitors (bosutinib, dasatinib, imatinib, nilotinib, ponatinib)

The BCR-ABL tyrosine kinase (TK) inhibitors can interfere with T-cell activation and suppress CMV specific CD8+ T-cell responses.[96,97] Interestingly, in vitro studies showed that TK inhibitors have direct antiviral effects by binding to platelet-derived growth factor receptor-α, which is the critical receptor for CMV cell entry.[98] A recent phase 2 study that repurposed nilotinib as CMV prophylaxis after allogeneic HSCT showed that this approach is safe, and a multicenter RCT is currently ongoing.[99]

Although the anti-CMV effect of TK inhibitors is yet to be shown in clinical settings, CMV reactivation or disease has been linked to dasatinib treatment, including hepatitis,[100] colitis,[101,102] and pneumonitis.[103] In a study of 109 patients who received dasatinib to prevent disease relapse after HSCT for treatment of chronic myelogenic leukemia (CML) or Philadelphia chromosome–positive acute lymphocytic leukemia, dasatinib use was associated with a significantly increased risk of CMV reactivation (adjusted hazard ratio, 7.65; 95% confidence interval, 1.84–31.7).[104]

Occasional cases of oral herpes or HZ have been reported with TK inhibitors in RCTs or case reports.[105,106] In a retrospective analysis of 771 patients treated with imatinib for CML, 16 patients had VZV de novo infection or reactivation (~2% with 5.25 cases per 100 patient-years).[107]

Conclusion
Herpesvirus reactivation is linked with these agents but routine antiviral prophylaxis has not been recommended.

TARGETING JANUS KINASE (JAK)–STAT SIGNALING AND COMPLEMENT PATHWAY FOR INFLAMMATORY DISEASES
JAK inhibitors (baricitinib, ruxolitinib, tofacitinib)

Treatment with JAK inhibitors is associated with markedly increased risk of infectious complications, including HZ. In a phase 3 RCT that compared ruxolitinib with standard therapy for the treatment of polycythemia vera, HZ was noted in 6% of ruxolitinib group compared with 0% in the control group.[108] In a phase 4 postmarketing study for ruxolitinib with 1144 patients, HZ was the most frequent infectious complication, with an incidence of 8%.[109] A recent meta-analysis that evaluated ruxolitinib-associated infectious complications also noted a significant increased risk of HZ with ruxolitinib (odds ratio of 7.39 compared with controls).[110]

Similarly, phase 3 RCTs also showed an increased risk of HZ with tofacitinib treatment of RA, plaque psoriasis, or psoriatic arthritis compared with placebo control.[111–114] In a study that evaluated 3623 patients with psoriasis for HZ incidence, 130 patients (3.6%) developed HZ. Of these, 9 patients (7%) required hospitalization and 8 (6%) had multidermatomal HZ.[115] For patients with inflammatory bowel disease, tofacitinib also confers a higher HZ risk compared with other immunosuppressive regimens.[116,117] For subsequent RCTs with tofacitinib, zoster vaccine was used ~4 weeks in advance of study treatment at investigator discretion.[118]

Baricitinib is mostly studied for treatment of RA, and RCTs also reported increased HZ risk with its use.[119,120]

CMV reactivation has been rarely reported with these agents. In a review of phase 2, phase 3, and long-term extension clinical trial data with a total of 5671 patients that received tofacitinib for RA, 6 cases of CMV reactivation, including hepatitis, retinitis, and gastritis, were identified.[121] In a phase 2b study that compared tofacitinib with cyclosporine A for immunosuppression in kidney transplant recipients, CMV viremia and disease occurred more frequently with tofacitinib, and the incidence of CMV disease was reduced by one-third with the use of antiviral prophylaxis.[122]

Conclusion

JAK inhibitors are associated with a markedly increased risk of infectious complications, including HZ, and antiviral prophylaxis is recommended. Vaccination against VZV can also be considered if it can be administered at least 4 weeks before the start of immunosuppression, although the efficacy of VZV vaccination in this setting has not been studied. The possibility of CMV reactivation, although infrequent, should also be considered, particularly among transplant recipients.

MISCELLANEOUS
Sphingosine-1-phosphate (S1P) receptor modulator (fingolimod)

Fingolimod is used mostly for treatment of MS. It prevents lymphocyte egress from lymph nodes and causes a marked reduction of CD3 T cells. Patients treated with fingolimod have reduced antiviral T-cell response[123] and more frequent VZV reactivation (as measured by VZV polymerase chain reaction [PCR] in saliva or blood).[123,124] Rates of VZV reactivation among patients with relapsing-remitting MS treated with fingolimod were evaluated by Arvin and colleagues.[125] Based on phase 2 and 3 clinical studies and ongoing uncontrolled extension phases, VZV rates were low (7–11 per 1000 patient-years), but higher than placebo in clinical trials. Severe or complicated cases of HZ were uncommon. The investigators recommended establishing each patient's VZV serostatus before initiating fingolimod therapy and immunization for patients susceptible to primary VZV infection. Routine antiviral prophylaxis is not generally needed, but risk-benefit ratio should be assessed if the patient receives concomitant pulsed corticosteroid therapy.[125]

Cases of severe HSV encephalitis have also been reported with fingolimod.[126,127]

Conclusion

Fingolimod therapy can increase risk of HZ. Routine antiviral prophylaxis is not generally needed, but risk-benefit ratio should be assessed if the patient receives concomitant pulsed corticosteroid therapy.[125]

Proteasome inhibitors (bortezomib, carfilzomib, and ixazomib)

Bortezomib treatment significantly reduced VZV-specific cell-mediated immunity[128] and clinical studies have shown a significantly increased risk for HZ with this agent.[128–130] For example, a phase 3 clinical trial that compared bortezomib with high-dose dexamethasone for the treatment of relapsed multiple myeloma showed that incidence of HZ was higher in the bortezomib group than in the dexamethasone group (13% vs 5%, $P<.001$).[129] In subsequent clinical trials using bortezomib, antiviral prophylaxis was made mandatory.[131] Apparently, treatment with bortezomib-based regimens might also confer higher risk of CMV or HHV-6 reactivation after autologous HSCT.[132,133]

Fewer data are available with ixazomib and carfilzomib, but a phase 3 RCT also showed increased HZ risk with ixazomib.[134] For carfilzomib, phase 3 RCTs used antiviral prophylaxis, and no cases of breakthrough HZ were reported.[135,136]

Conclusion

These agents significantly increase risk of HZ. Antiviral prophylaxis should be considered.

Anti-SLAMF7 agent (elotuzumab)

In RCTs that studied elotuzumab for treatment of multiple myeloma, this biologic was associated with an increased risk of infectious complications, particularly caused by HZ. Comparing the elotuzumab group with the control group, incidence of HZ was 4.1 versus 2.2 episodes per 100 patient-years in 1 study[137] and 6.6 versus 2.9 episodes per 100 patient-years in another.[138] Higher rates of HZ were also confirmed in extended 4-year follow-up[139] (7% vs 3%).

Conclusion

Antiviral prophylaxis should be considered for VZV-seropositive patients who receive elotuzumab.

CCR4 inhibitor (mogamulizumab)

In its first single-arm phase 2 study for the treatment of relapsed adult T-cell leukemia-lymphoma, patients received prophylaxis with acyclovir, trimethoprim-sulfamethoxazole, and fluconazole; no data on infectious complications were reported.[140] For its second single-arm study of 37 patients, no prophylaxis was used; 1 case of HSV esophagitis as well as 2 cases of CMV retinitis were reported.[141] A subsequent phase 2 RCT that studied dose-intensified chemotherapy alone or in combination with mogamulizumab in newly diagnosed aggressive adult T-cell leukemia-lymphoma noted 6 cases of CMV (including 2 cases of pneumonia) in the mogamulizumab arm, but none with the control arm.[142] In a postmarketing surveillance study,[143] CMV reactivation constituted the most common infection-related adverse event. Forty cases of CMV disease (including chorioretinitis, enterocolitis, and pneumonia) or CMV viremia were noted among 484 patients (8.3%). Fatal CMV diseases have also been reported.[144,145]

Conclusion

Antiviral prophylaxis is recommended. CMV-seropositive patients should be closely monitored for CMV reactivation.

PREVENTION OF HERPESVIRUS INFECTION

Herpes Simplex Virus and Varicella-zoster Virus

The major antiviral agents used for prophylaxis (and treatment) of HSV and VZV are acyclovir, its valyl-ester valacyclovir, and famciclovir (**Table 3**).[146] Other agents, such as ganciclovir (or its valyl-ester valganciclovir), foscarnet, and cidofovir, are also active against HSV and VZV, but they have significantly more toxicities compared with acyclovir, valacyclovir, or famciclovir. As such, foscarnet and cidofovir are used primarily for the treatment of acyclovir-resistant HSV or VZV (as well as for ganciclovir-resistant CMV).

Acyclovir prophylaxis to prevent VZV reactivation has been studied extensively in the setting of HSCT. There is substantial variability of doses used, ranging from a total daily dose of 200 mg to 2400 mg.[147] Notably, even the low doses (200 mg or 400 mg daily) were efficacious in preventing VZV reactivation. The most commonly used regimens for HSV or VZV prophylaxis include acyclovir 400 mg twice daily to 800 mg twice daily, valacyclovir 500 mg once or twice daily, or famciclovir 250 mg twice daily.[148,149] A new class of antivirals with a novel mechanism against HSV ($\pm$ VZV) by targeting the viral helicase-primase complex is currently in development. These agents are active against thymidine kinase–deficient viral strains that are resistant to acyclovir or famciclovir. Of these agents, pritelivir has been studied in RCTs as suppressive therapy for genital HSV-2 infection,[150,151] and amenamevir has been studied for treatment of HZ.[152]

Table 3
Antiviral agents against herpes simplex virus, varicella-zoster virus, and cytomegalovirus[146]

| | | Activities Against | | | | Licensed Antiviral Agents | |
Drug	Mechanisms	HSV	VZV	CMV	Route	Dosage for Prophylaxis[a,b]	Dosage for Treatment[a,b]
Acyclovir	Activated by viral kinase to become an inhibitor of viral DNA polymerase	+	+	±[c]	PO IV	400 mg BID to 800 mg BID —	400 mg TID to 800 mg 5× daily 5–10 mg/kg Q 8 h
Valacyclovir	Valyl-ester prodrug of acyclovir	+	+	±[c]	PO	500 mg QD to BID, or 1g QD	1g BID to TID
Cidofovir	A nucleotide analog that inhibits viral DNA polymerase	+	+	+	IV	—	5 mg/kg q week for 2 wk, then every other week
Famciclovir	A prodrug of penciclovir; activated by viral kinase to become an inhibitor of viral DNA polymerase	+	+	−	PO	250 mg BID	250 mg TID to 500 mg TID
Foscarnet	An inorganic pyrophosphate analog that inhibits viral DNA polymerase	+	+	+	IV	—	For HSV: 40 mg/kg Q 8 h to Q 12 h For CMV: Induction: 60 mg/kg Q 8 h or 90 mg/kg Q 12 h Maintenance: 90–120 mg/kg IV QD
Ganciclovir	Activated by viral kinase to become an inhibitor of viral DNA polymerase	+	+	+	IV	—	Induction: 5 mg/kg Q 12 h
Valganciclovir	Valyl-ester prodrug of ganciclovir	+	+	+	PO	450 mg QD to 900 mg BID	Induction: 900 mg BID Maintenance: 900 mg QD
Letermovir	An inhibitor of the viral terminase enzyme complex	−	−	+	PO/IV	480 mg QD[d]	—

Novel Antiviral Agents in Development[e]

| Drug | Mechanisms | Activities Against | | | Route | Major Published Clinical Trials | |
		HSV	VZV	CMV		For Prophylaxis	For Treatment
Amenamevir	Inhibits the viral helicase-primase complex	+	+	–	PO	—	Against HZ[152]
Brincidofovir (CMX001)	A lipid-conjugated prodrug of cidofovir	+	+	+	PO	Against CMV in HSCT[165]	Against adenovirus in pediatric HSCT[166]
Maribavir	Inhibits viral protein kinase UL97 to block viral egress	–	–	+	PO	Against CMV in HSCT[163] Against CMV in SCT[164]	Against CMV in HSCT[162]
Pritelivir	Inhibits the viral helicase-primase complex	+	–	–	PO	Against HSV-2[150,151]	—

Abbreviations: BID, twice a day; IV, intravenous; PO, by mouth; Q, every; QD, every day; TID, 3 times a day.

a Dosing for normal renal function only; dose adjustment needed for renal impairment.
b Dosing varies based on indications. A range of the most common dosages is listed.
c High-dose acyclovir or valacyclovir has limited activities against CMV.
d Decrease dose to 240 mg every day if coadministered with cyclosporine.
e Only those agents with published phase 2 or phase 3 clinical trial data are listed.

Vaccination is another well-recognized approach to prevent viral complications. No HSV vaccines have been marketed to date, but several vaccines are available to protect against VZV infection. A live attenuated varicella vaccine (VAR, Varivax) and a live attenuated zoster vaccine (ZVL, Zostavax) have been in use since 1995 and 2006, respectively. However, the use of these live vaccines is contraindicated in highly immunocompromised patients; if used, should be administered 4 weeks or more before initiating immunosuppressive therapy.[153] In October 2017, an inactive recombinant subunit zoster vaccine (RZV; Shingrix) was approved by the FDA for the prevention of HZ in adults 50 years of age and older. RZV is composed of recombinant VZV glycoprotein E reconstituted with a new adjuvant formulation ASO1$_B$. It is now recommended by the Advisory Committee on Immunization Practices as the preferred zoster vaccine given its excellent efficacy (overall efficacy of 97.2% among older adults of $\geq$50 years of age)[154] and prolonged duration of protection (efficacy of $\geq$84.7% in adults aged $\geq$70 years in all 4 years after vaccination).[155] RZV has also been studied in immunocompromised patients, including those with autologous HSCT,[156] human immunodeficiency virus,[157] or renal transplant[158] and was found to be immunogenic and safe.[159] Although RZV has not been studied specifically among those patient populations that undergo biologic therapy, it is a reasonable approach to decrease risk of VZV reactivation if the vaccine can be administered before initiation of immunosuppression.

Cytomegalovirus

CMV prophylaxis with valganciclovir or ganciclovir is commonly used for SOT recipients, but their use in HSCT is limited given their potential myelotoxicity.[160] Letermovir, a novel CMV viral terminase inhibitor, was recently approved for CMV prophylaxis in allogeneic HSCT recipients.[161] Clinical trials studying its use for CMV prophylaxis in SOT and for CMV treatment are currently ongoing. Maribavir is another novel anti-CMV agent that is under development. It blocks nuclear egress of viral capsids through the inhibition of protein kinase UL97 and has been studied in RCTs as prophylaxis or treatment (see **Table 3**).[162–164] Although foscarnet and cidofovir are not useful as prophylactic agents because of their intravenous formulation and nephrotoxicity, an oral lipid-conjugated prodrug brincidofovir (also called CMX001) with an improved safety profile has been studied as CMV prophylaxis in HSCT[165] and is currently being studied for treatment of other DNA viruses.[166]

As discussed earlier, several biologics can potentiate CMV reactivation, but antiviral prophylaxis against CMV is generally not indicated and has not been recommended for patients receiving biologic therapy. In post-HSCT settings, CMV PCR is performed regularly to monitor for CMV reactivation in at-risk patients, and antiviral treatment should be initiated if viremia is detected.[160] Such a preemptive approach is currently not adopted for most patients who undergo biologic therapy. Instead, patients should be closely monitored for any concerning signs or symptoms that might suggest CMV reactivation or disease. Although CMV PCR is useful to detect peripheral viral replication, CMV end-organ disease is not always accompanied by viremia. Therefore, other diagnostic procedures, such as bronchoscopy, endoscopy, and/or tissue biopsy, might be needed to rule out CMV disease.

Several CMV vaccines have been in development,[167,168] but none are currently licensed for use.

SUMMARY

Herpesviruses, including HSV, VZV, and CMV, have developed complex mechanisms to evade host immune responses to maintain latency. Once reactivated, these viruses can cause significant morbidity and mortality among immunocompromised patients. Biologics that are used to treat inflammatory diseases, hematologic malignancies, and solid tumor malignancies modulate the host immune system through different pathways, and some have been shown to potentiate herpesvirus reactivation and disease. Understanding the relationship between these biologics and herpesviruses helps mitigate the risk of infectious complications and also furthers the understanding of the intricate interplay between herpesviruses and the immune system.

REFERENCES

1. Miranda-Saksena M, Denes CE, Diefenbach RJ, et al. Infection and transport of herpes simplex virus type 1 in neurons: role of the cytoskeleton. Viruses 2018;10(2).
2. Truong NR, Smith JB, Sandgren KJ, et al. Mechanisms of immune control of mucosal HSV infection: a guide to rational vaccine design. Front Immunol 2019;10:373.
3. Schiffer JT, Corey L. Herpes simplex virus. In: Bennett JE, Dolin R, Blaser MJ, editors. Principles and practice of infectious diseases, vol. 2, 8th edition. Philadelphia: Elsevier Saunders; 2015. p. 1713–30.
4. Ho DY, Arvin AM. Varicella zoster virus infections. In: Forman SJ, Negrin RS, Antin JH, et al, editors. Thomas' hematopoietic cell transplantation, vol. 2. West Sussex (UK): Wiley; 2016. p. 1085–104.
5. Laing KJ, Ouwendijk WJD, Koelle DM, et al. Immunobiology of varicella-zoster virus infection. J Infect Dis 2018;218(suppl_2):S68–74.
6. Collins-McMillen D, Buehler J, Peppenelli M, et al. Molecular determinants and the regulation of human cytomegalovirus latency and reactivation. Viruses 2018; 10(8) [pii:E444].
7. Dupont L, Reeves MB. Cytomegalovirus latency and reactivation: recent insights into an age old problem. Rev Med Virol 2016;26(2):75–89.
8. Sedy JR, Spear PG, Ware CF. Cross-regulation between herpesviruses and the TNF superfamily members. Nat Rev Immunol 2008;8(11):861–73.
9. Haag LM, Hofmann J, Kredel LI, et al. Herpes simplex virus sepsis in a young woman with crohn's disease. J Crohns Colitis 2015;9(12):1169–73.
10. Justice EA, Khan SY, Logan S, et al. Disseminated cutaneous Herpes Simplex Virus-1 in a woman with rheumatoid arthritis receiving infliximab: a case report. J Med Case Rep 2008;2:282.
11. Crusio RH, Singson SV, Haroun F, et al. Herpes simplex virus encephalitis during treatment with etanercept. Scand J Infect Dis 2014;46(2):152–4.
12. Schepers K, Hernandez A, Andrei G, et al. Acyclovir-resistant herpes simplex encephalitis in a patient treated with anti-tumor necrosis factor-alpha monoclonal antibodies. J Clin Virol 2014;59(1):67–70.
13. Manzano V, Ruiz P, Torres M, et al. Severe pneumonia by aciclovir-resistant varicella-zoster virus during etanercept therapy. Rheumatology (Oxford) 2010; 49(9):1791–3.
14. Skuhala T, Atelj A, Prepolec J, et al. A case report of severe recurrent varicella in an ankylosing spondylitis patient treated with adalimumab - a new side effect after 15 years of usage. BMC Infect Dis 2019;19(1):127.
15. Ma C, Walters B, Fedorak RN. Varicella zoster meningitis complicating combined anti-tumor necrosis factor and corticosteroid therapy in Crohn's disease. World J Gastroenterol 2013;19(21):3347–51.

16. Kunz AN, Rajnik M. Disseminated cutaneous varicella zoster virus infections during infliximab therapy for Crohn's disease: case report of two pediatric patients at one institution. Clin Pediatr (Phila) 2011;50(6):559–61.

17. Tresch S, Trueb RM, Kamarachev J, et al. Disseminated herpes zoster mimicking rheumatoid vasculitis in a rheumatoid arthritis patient on etanercept. Dermatology 2009;219(4):347–9.

18. Galloway JB, Mercer LK, Moseley A, et al. Risk of skin and soft tissue infections (including shingles) in patients exposed to anti-tumour necrosis factor therapy: results from the British Society for Rheumatology Biologics Register. Ann Rheum Dis 2013;72(2):229–34.

19. Garcia-Doval I, Perez-Zafrilla B, Descalzo MA, et al. Incidence and risk of hospitalisation due to shingles and chickenpox in patients with rheumatic diseases treated with TNF antagonists. Ann Rheum Dis 2010;69(10):1751–5.

20. Serac G, Tubach F, Mariette X, et al. Risk of herpes zoster in patients receiving anti-TNF-alpha in the prospective French RATIO registry. J Invest Dermatol 2012;132(3 Pt 1):726–9.

21. Winthrop KL, Baddley JW, Chen L, et al. Association between the initiation of anti-tumor necrosis factor therapy and the risk of herpes zoster. JAMA 2013; 309(9):887–95.

22. Baddley JW, Cantini F, Goletti D, et al. ESCMID Study Group for Infections in Compromised Hosts (ESGICH) Consensus Document on the safety of targeted and biological therapies: an infectious diseases perspective (Soluble immune effector molecules [I]: anti-tumor necrosis factor-alpha agents). Clin Microbiol Infect 2018;24(Suppl 2):S10–20.

23. Ali T, Kaitha S, Mahmood S, et al. Clinical use of anti-TNF therapy and increased risk of infections. Drug Healthc Patient Saf 2013;5:79–99.

24. Shimojima Y, Ishii W, Matsuda M, et al. Cytomegalovirus-induced infectious mononucleosis-like syndrome in a rheumatoid arthritis patient treated with methotrexate and infliximab. Intern Med 2010;49(10):937–40.

25. Haerter G, Manfras BJ, de Jong-Hesse Y, et al. Cytomegalovirus retinitis in a patient treated with anti-tumor necrosis factor alpha antibody therapy for rheumatoid arthritis. Clin Infect Dis 2004;39(9):e88–94.

26. Sari I, Birlik M, Gonen C, et al. Cytomegalovirus colitis in a patient with Behcet's disease receiving tumor necrosis factor alpha inhibitory treatment. World J Gastroenterol 2008;14(18):2912–4.

27. Mizuta M, Schuster MG. Cytomegalovirus hepatitis associated with use of anti-tumor necrosis factor-alpha antibody. Clin Infect Dis 2005;40(7):1071–2.

28. Helbling D, Breitbach TH, Krause M. Disseminated cytomegalovirus infection in Crohn's disease following anti-tumour necrosis factor therapy. Eur J Gastroenterol Hepatol 2002;14(12):1393–5.

29. Salles G, Barrett M, Foa R, et al. Rituximab in B-cell hematologic malignancies: a review of 20 years of clinical experience. Adv Ther 2017;34(10):2232–73.

30. Okamoto A, Abe A, Okamoto M, et al. Severe hepatitis associated with varicella zoster virus infection in a patient with diffuse large B cell lymphoma treated with rituximab-CHOP chemotherapy. Int J Hematol 2012;96(4):516–20.

31. Okamoto A, Abe A, Okamoto M, et al. A varicella outbreak in B-cell lymphoma patients receiving rituximab-containing chemotherapy. J Infect Chemother 2014;20(12):774–7.

32. Aksoy S, Harputluoglu H, Kilickap S, et al. Rituximab-related viral infections in lymphoma patients. Leuk Lymphoma 2007;48(7):1307–12.

33. Marcus R, Davies A, Ando K, et al. Obinutuzumab for the first-line treatment of follicular lymphoma. N Engl J Med 2017;377(14):1331–44.
34. Ohmachi K, Tobinai K, Kinoshita T, et al. Efficacy and safety of obinutuzumab in patients with previously untreated follicular lymphoma: a subgroup analysis of patients enrolled in Japan in the randomized phase III GALLIUM trial. Int J Hematol 2018;108(5):499–509.
35. Montalban X, Hauser SL, Kappos L, et al. Ocrelizumab versus placebo in primary progressive multiple sclerosis. N Engl J Med 2017;376(3):209–20.
36. Dudek MIR, Thies K, Kammenhuber S, et al. HSV-2-encephalitis in a patient with multiple sclerosis treated with ocrelizumab. J Neurol 2019;266(9):2322–3.
37. van Oers MH, Kuliczkowski K, Smolej L, et al. Ofatumumab maintenance versus observation in relapsed chronic lymphocytic leukaemia (PROLONG): an open-label, multicentre, randomised phase 3 study. Lancet Oncol 2015;16(13): 1370–9.
38. Morschhauser F, Radford J, Van Hoof A, et al. Phase III trial of consolidation therapy with yttrium-90-ibritumomab tiuxetan compared with no additional therapy after first remission in advanced follicular lymphoma. J Clin Oncol 2008; 26(32):5156–64.
39. Moskowitz CH, Nademanee A, Masszl T, et al. Brentuximab vedotin as consolidation therapy after autologous stem-cell transplantation in patients with Hodgkin's lymphoma at risk of relapse or progression (AETHERA): a randomised, double-blind, placebo-controlled, phase 3 trial. Lancet 2015;385(9980): 1853–62.
40. Nademanee A, Sureda A, Stiff P, et al. Safety analysis of brentuximab vedotin from the phase III AETHERA trial in hodgkin lymphoma in the post-transplant consolidation setting. Biol Blood Marrow Transplant 2018;24(11):2354–9.
41. Clarivet B, Vincent L, Vergely L, et al. Adverse reactions related to brentuximab vedotin use: a real-life retrospective study. Therapie 2019;74(3):343–6.
42. Tudesq JJ, Vincent L, Lebrun J, et al. Cytomegalovirus infection with retinitis after brentuximab vedotin treatment for CD30(+) lymphoma. Open Forum Infect Dis 2017;4(2):ofx091.
43. Drgona L, Gudiol C, Lanini S, et al. ESCMID Study Group for Infections in Compromised Hosts (ESGICH) Consensus Document on the safety of targeted and biological therapies: an infectious diseases perspective (Agents targeting lymphoid or myeloid cells surface antigens [II]: CD22, CD30, CD33, CD38, CD40, SLAMF-7 and CCR4). Clin Microbiol Infect 2018;24(Suppl 2):S83–94.
44. Frerichs KA, Bosman PWC, Nijhof IS, et al. Cytomegalovirus reactivation in a patient with extensively pretreated multiple myeloma during daratumumab treatment. Clin Lymphoma Myeloma Leuk 2019;19(1):e9–11.
45. Lavi N, Okasha D, Sabo E, et al. Severe cytomegalovirus enterocolitis developing following daratumumab exposure in three patients with multiple myeloma. Eur J Haematol 2018. https://doi.org/10.1111/ejh.13164.
46. Nahi H, Chrobok M, Gran C, et al. Infectious complications and NK cell depletion following daratumumab treatment of Multiple Myeloma. PLoS One 2019; 14(2):e0211927.
47. Available at: https://www.accessdata.fda.gov/drugsatfda_docs/label/2016/761036s004lbl.pdf.
48. Jones JA, Robak T, Brown JR, et al. Efficacy and safety of idelalisib in combination with ofatumumab for previously treated chronic lymphocytic leukaemia: an open-label, randomised phase 3 trial. Lancet Haematol 2017;4(3):e114–26.

49. Goldring L, Kumar B, Gan TE, et al. Idelalisib induced CMV gastrointestinal disease: the need for vigilance with novel therapies. Pathology 2017;49(5):555–7.

50. Lampson BL, Kasar SN, Matos TR, et al. Idelalisib given front-line for treatment of chronic lymphocytic leukemia causes frequent immune-mediated hepatotoxicity. Blood 2016;128(2):195–203.

51. Available at: https://www.accessdata.fda.gov/drugsatfda_docs/label/2018/211155s000lbl.pdf.

52. Flinn IW, Hillmen P, Montillo M, et al. The phase 3 DUO trial: duvelisib vs ofatumumab in relapsed and refractory CLL/SLL. Blood 2018;132(23):2446–55.

53. Flinn IW, Miller CB, Ardeshna KM, et al. DYNAMO: a phase II study of duvelisib (IPI-145) in patients with refractory indolent non-hodgkin lymphoma. J Clin Oncol 2019;37(11):912–22.

54. Reinwald M, Silva JT, Mueller NJ, et al. ESCMID Study Group for Infections in Compromised Hosts (ESGICH) Consensus Document on the safety of targeted and biological therapies: an infectious diseases perspective (Intracellular signaling pathways: tyrosine kinase and mTOR inhibitors). Clin Microbiol Infect 2018;24(Suppl 2):S53–70.

55. Blair HA, Deeks ED. Abatacept: a review in rheumatoid arthritis. Drugs 2017; 77(11):1221–33.

56. Furie R, Nicholls K, Cheng TT, et al. Efficacy and safety of abatacept in lupus nephritis: a twelve-month, randomized, double-blind study. Arthritis Rheumatol 2014;66(2):379–89.

57. Chen SK, Liao KP, Liu J, et al. Risk of hospitalized infection and initiation of abatacept versus TNF inhibitors among patients with rheumatoid arthritis: a propensity score-matched cohort study. Arthritis Care Res (Hoboken) 2020;72(1):9–17.

58. Vincenti F, Rostaing L, Grinyo J, et al. Belatacept and long-term outcomes in kidney transplantation. N Engl J Med 2016;374(4):333–43.

59. Grinyo JM, Del Carmen Rial M, Alberu J, et al. Safety and efficacy outcomes 3 years after switching to belatacept from a calcineurin inhibitor in kidney transplant recipients: results from a phase 2 randomized trial. Am J Kidney Dis 2017;69(5):587–94.

60. Durrbach A, Pestana JM, Florman S, et al. Long-term outcomes in belatacept-versus cyclosporine-treated recipients of extended criteria donor kidneys: final results from BENEFIT-EXT, a phase III randomized study. Am J Transplant 2016; 16(11):3192–201.

61. Helou E, Grant M, Landry M, et al. Fatal case of cutaneous-sparing orolaryngeal zoster in a renal transplant recipient. Transpl Infect Dis 2017;19(4). https://doi.org/10.1111/tid.12704.

62. Fan J, Gong D, Truong C, et al. Cytomegalovirus retinitis with belatacept immunosuppression. Retin Cases Brief Rep 2019. https://doi.org/10.1097/ICB.0000000000000928.

63. Thursky KA, Worth LJ, Seymour JF, et al. Spectrum of infection, risk and recommendations for prophylaxis and screening among patients with lymphoproliferative disorders treated with alemtuzumab*. Br J Haematol 2006;132(1):3–12.

64. Cheung WW, Tse E, Leung AY, et al. Regular virologic surveillance showed very frequent cytomegalovirus reactivation in patients treated with alemtuzumab. Am J Hematol 2007;82(2):108–11.

65. Mikulska M, Lanini S, Gudiol C, et al. ESCMID Study Group for Infections in Compromised Hosts (ESGICH) Consensus Document on the safety of targeted and biological therapies: an infectious diseases perspective (Agents targeting

lymphoid cells surface antigens [I]: CD19, CD20 and CD52). Clin Microbiol Infect 2018;24(Suppl 2):S71–82.

66. Skoetz N, Bauer K, Elter T, et al. Alemtuzumab for patients with chronic lymphocytic leukaemia. Cochrane Database Syst Rev 2012;(2):CD008078.

67. Sorensen PS, Sellebjorg F. Pulsed immune reconstitution therapy in multiple sclerosis. Ther Adv Neurol Disord 2019;12. 1756286419836913.

68. Cohen JA, Coles AJ, Arnold DL, et al. Alemtuzumab versus interferon beta 1a as first-line treatment for patients with relapsing-remitting multiple sclerosis: a randomised controlled phase 3 trial. Lancet 2012;380(9856):1819–28.

69. Coles AJ, Twyman CL, Arnold DL, et al. Alemtuzumab for patients with relapsing multiple sclerosis after disease-modifying therapy: a randomised controlled phase 3 trial. Lancet 2012;380(9856):1829–39.

70. Clerico M, De Mercanti S, Artusi CA, et al. Active CMV infection in two patients with multiple sclerosis treated with alemtuzumab. Mult Scler 2017;23(6):874–6.

71. Barone S, Scannapieco S, Torti C, et al. Hepatic microabscesses during CMV reactivation in a multiple sclerosis patient after alemtuzumab treatment. Mult Scler Relat Disord 2018;20:6–8.

72. Buonomo AR, Sacca F, Zappulo E, et al. Bacterial and CMV pneumonia in a patient treated with alemtuzumab for multiple sclerosis. Mult Scler Relat Disord 2019;27:44–5.

73. Eichenfield LF, Bieber T, Beck LA, et al. Infections in dupilumab clinical trials in atopic dermatitis: a comprehensive pooled analysis. Am J Clin Dermatol 2019; 20(3):443–56.

74. Ivert LU, Wahlgren CF, Ivert L, et al. Eye complications during dupilumab treatment for severe atopic dermatitis. Acta Derm Venereol 2019;99(4):375–8.

75. Haldar P, Brightling CE, Hargadon B, et al. Mepolizumab and exacerbations of refractory eosinophilic asthma. N Engl J Med 2009;360(10):973–84.

76. Shimoda T, Odajima H, Okamasa A, et al. Efficacy and safety of mepolizumab in Japanese patients with severe eosinophilic asthma. Allergol Int 2017;66(3): 445–51.

77. Ortega HG, Liu MC, Pavord ID, et al. Mepolizumab treatment in patients with severe eosinophilic asthma. N Engl J Med 2014;371(13):1198–207.

78. Lugogo N, Domingo C, Chanez P, et al. Long-term efficacy and safety of mepolizumab in patients with severe eosinophilic asthma: a multi-center, open-label, phase IIIb study. Clin Ther 2016;38(9):2058–70.e1.

79. Pavord ID, Chanez P, Criner GJ, et al. Mepolizumab for eosinophilic chronic obstructive pulmonary disease. N Engl J Med 2017;377(17):1613–29.

80. Bjermer L, Lemiere C, Maspero J, et al. Reslizumab for inadequately controlled asthma with elevated blood eosinophil levels: a randomized phase 3 study. Chest 2016;150(4):789–98.

81. Castro M, Zangrilli J, Wechsler ME, et al. Reslizumab for inadequately controlled asthma with elevated blood eosinophil counts: results from two multicentre, parallel, double-blind, randomised, placebo-controlled, phase 3 trials. Lancet Respir Med 2015;3(5):355–66.

82. Murphy K, Jacobs J, Bjermer L, et al. Long-term safety and efficacy of reslizumab in patients with eosinophilic asthma. J Allergy Clin Immunol Pract 2017; 5(6):1572–81.e3.

83. FitzGerald JM, Bleecker ER, Nair P, et al. Benralizumab, an anti-interleukin-5 receptor alpha monoclonal antibody, as add-on treatment for patients with severe, uncontrolled, eosinophilic asthma (CALIMA): a randomised, double-blind, placebo-controlled phase 3 trial. Lancet 2016;388(10056):2128–41.

84. Mishra AK, Sahu KK, James A. Disseminated herpes zoster following treatment with benralizumab. Clin Respir J 2019;13(3):189–91.

85. Koike T, Harigai M, Inokuma S, et al. Effectiveness and safety of tocilizumab: postmarketing surveillance of 7901 patients with rheumatoid arthritis in Japan. J Rheumatol 2014;41(1):15–23.

86. Yun H, Xie F, Delzell E, et al. Risks of herpes zoster in patients with rheumatoid arthritis according to biologic disease-modifying therapy. Arthritis Care Res (Hoboken) 2015;67(5):731–6.

87. Fromhold-Treu S, Erbersdobler A, Turan M, et al. CMV associated acute liver failure in a patient receiving tocilizumab for systemic lupus erythematosus. Z Gastroenterol 2017;55(5):467–72 [in German].

88. Komura T, Ohta H, Nakai R, et al. Cytomegalovirus reactivation induced acute hepatitis and gastric erosions in a patient with rheumatoid arthritis under treatment with an anti-il-6 receptor antibody, tocilizumab. Intern Med 2016;55(14): 1923–7.

89. Genovese MC, van Adelsberg J, Fan C, et al. Two years of sarilumab in patients with rheumatoid arthritis and an inadequate response to MTX: safety, efficacy and radiographic outcomes. Rheumatology (Oxford) 2018;57(8):1423–31.

90. Burmester GR, Lin Y, Patel R, et al. Efficacy and safety of sarilumab monotherapy versus adalimumab monotherapy for the treatment of patients with active rheumatoid arthritis (MONARCH): a randomised, double-blind, parallel-group phase III trial. Ann Rheum Dis 2017;76(5):840–7.

91. Fleischmann R, Genovese MC, Lin Y, et al. Long-term safety of sarilumab in rheumatoid arthritis: an integrated analysis with up to 7 years' follow-up. Rheumatology (Oxford) 2020;59(2):292–302.

92. Voorhees PM, Manges RF, Sonneveld P, et al. A phase 2 multicentre study of siltuximab, an anti-interleukin-6 monoclonal antibody, in patients with relapsed or refractory multiple myeloma. Br J Haematol 2013;161(3):357–66.

93. Franklin C, Rooms I, Fiedler M, et al. Cytomegalovirus reactivation in patients with refractory checkpoint inhibitor-induced colitis. Eur J Cancer 2017;86: 248–56.

94. Uslu U, Agaimy A, Hundorfean G, et al. Autoimmune colitis and subsequent CMV-induced hepatitis after treatment with ipilimumab. J Immunother 2015; 38(5):212–5.

95. Del Castillo M, Romero FA, Arguello E, et al. The spectrum of serious infections among patients receiving immune checkpoint blockade for the treatment of melanoma. Clin Infect Dis 2016;63(11):1490–3.

96. Seggewiss R, Lore K, Greiner E, et al. Imatinib inhibits T-cell receptor-mediated T-cell proliferation and activation in a dose-dependent manner. Blood 2005; 105(6):2473–9.

97. Fei F, Yu Y, Schmitt A, et al. Dasatinib exerts an immunosuppressive effect on CD8+ T cells specific for viral and leukemia antigens. Exp Hematol 2008; 36(10):1297–308.

98. Soroceanu L, Akhavan A, Cobbs CS. Platelet-derived growth factor-alpha receptor activation is required for human cytomegalovirus infection. Nature 2008;455(7211):391–5.

99. Lin CT, Hsueh PR, Wu SJ, et al. Repurposing nilotinib for cytomegalovirus infection prophylaxis after allogeneic hematopoietic stem cell transplantation: a single-arm, phase ii trial. Biol Blood Marrow Transplant 2018;24(11):2310–5.

100. Davalos F, Chaucer B, Zafar W, et al. Dasatinib-induced CMV hepatitis in an immunocompetent patient: a rare complication of a common drug. Transl Oncol 2016;9(3):248–50.

101. Yassin MA, Nashwan AJ, Soliman AT, et al. Cytomegalovirus-induced hemorrhagic colitis in a patient with chronic myelold leukemia (chronic phase) on dasatinib as an upfront therapy. Clin Med Insights Case Rep 2015;8:77–81.

102. Aldoss I, Gaal K, Al Malki MM, et al. Dasatinib-induced colitis after allogeneic stem cell transplantation for philadelphia chromosome-positive acute lymphoblastic leukemia. Biol Blood Marrow Transplant 2016;22(10):1900–3.

103. Knoll BM, Seiter K. Infections in patients on BCR-ABL tyrosine kinase inhibitor therapy: cases and review of the literature. Infection 2018;46(3):409–18.

104. Prestes DP, Arbona E, Nevett-Fernandez A, et al. Dasatinib use and risk of cytomegalovirus reactivation after allogeneic hematopoietic-cell transplantation. Clin Infect Dis 2017;65(3):510–3.

105. Lipton JH, Chuah C, Guerci-Bresler A, et al. Ponatinib versus imatinib for newly diagnosed chronic myeloid leukaemia: an international, randomised, open-label, phase 3 trial. Lancet Oncol 2016;17(5):612–21.

106. Durosinmi MA, Ogbe PO, Salawu L, et al. Herpes zoster complicating imatinib mesylate for gastrointestinal stromal tumour. Singapore Med J 2007;48(1): e16–8.

107. Mattiuzzi GN, Cortes JE, Talpaz M, et al. Development of Varicella-Zoster virus infection in patients with chronic myelogenous leukemia treated with imatinib mesylate. Clin Cancer Res 2003;9(3):976–80.

108. Vannucchi AM, Kiladjian JJ, Griesshammer M, et al. Ruxolitinib versus standard therapy for the treatment of polycythemia vera. N Engl J Med 2015;372(5): 426–35.

109. Al-Ali HK, Griesshammer M, le Coutre P, et al. Safety and efficacy of ruxolitinib in an open-label, multicenter, single-arm phase 3b expanded-access study in patients with myelofibrosis: a snapshot of 1144 patients in the JUMP trial. Haematologica 2016;101(9):1065–73.

110. Lussana F, Cattaneo M, Rambaldi A, et al. Ruxolitinib-associated infections: a systematic review and meta-analysis. Am J Hematol 2018;93(3):339–47.

111. Asahina A, Etoh T, Igarashi A, et al. Oral tofacitinib efficacy, safety and tolerability in Japanese patients with moderate to severe plaque psoriasis and psoriatic arthritis: a randomized, double-blind, phase 3 study. J Dermatol 2016;43(8): 869–80.

112. Cohen SB, Tanaka Y, Mariette X, et al. Long-term safety of tofacitinib for the treatment of rheumatoid arthritis up to 8.5 years: integrated analysis of data from the global clinical trials. Ann Rheum Dis 2017;76(7):1253–62.

113. Gladman D, Rigby W, Azevedo VF, et al. Tofacitinib for psoriatic arthritis in patients with an inadequate response to TNF inhibitors. N Engl J Med 2017; 377(16):1525–36.

114. Mease P, Hall S, FitzGerald O, et al. Tofacitinib or adalimumab versus placebo for psoriatic arthritis. N Engl J Med 2017;377(16):1537–50.

115. Winthrop KL, Lebwohl M, Cohen AD, et al. Herpes zoster in psoriasis patients treated with tofacitinib. J Am Acad Dermatol 2017;77(2):302–9.

116. Winthrop KL, Melmed GY, Vermeire S, et al. Herpes zoster infection in patients with ulcerative colitis receiving tofacitinib. Inflamm Bowel Dis 2018;24(10): 2258–65.

117. Caldera F, Hayney MS, Cross RK. Using number needed to harm to put the risk of herpes zoster from tofacitinib in perspective. Inflamm Bowel Dis 2019;25(6):955–7.
118. Fleischmann R, Mysler E, Hall S, et al. Efficacy and safety of tofacitinib monotherapy, tofacitinib with methotrexate, and adalimumab with methotrexate in patients with rheumatoid arthritis (ORAL Strategy): a phase 3b/4, double-blind, head-to-head, randomised controlled trial. Lancet 2017;390(10093):457–68.
119. Genovese MC, Kremer J, Zamani O, et al. Baricitinib in patients with refractory rheumatoid arthritis. N Engl J Med 2016;374(13):1243–52.
120. Smolen JS, Genovese MC, Takeuchi T, et al. Safety profile of baricitinib in patients with active rheumatoid arthritis with over 2 years median time in treatment. J Rheumatol 2019;46(1):7–18.
121. Winthrop KL, Park SH, Gul A, et al. Tuberculosis and other opportunistic infections in tofacitinib-treated patients with rheumatoid arthritis. Ann Rheum Dis 2016;75(6):1133–8.
122. Vincenti F, Tedesco Silva H, Busque S, et al. Randomized phase 2b trial of tofacitinib (CP-690,550) in de novo kidney transplant patients: efficacy, renal function and safety at 1 year. Am J Transplant 2012;12(9):2446–56.
123. Ricklin ME, Lorscheider J, Waschbisch A, et al. T-cell response against varicella-zoster virus in fingolimod-treated MS patients. Neurology 2013;81(2):174–81.
124. Aramideh Khouy R, Karampoor S, Keyvani H, et al. The frequency of varicella-zoster virus infection in patients with multiple sclerosis receiving fingolimod. J Neuroimmunol 2019;328:94–7.
125. Arvin AM, Wolinsky JS, Kappos L, et al. Varicella-zoster virus infections in patients treated with fingolimod: risk assessment and consensus recommendations for management. JAMA Neurol 2015;72(1):31–9.
126. Pfender N, Jelcic I, Linnebank M, et al. Reactivation of herpesvirus under fingolimod: A case of severe herpes simplex encephalitis. Neurology 2015;84(23):2377–8.
127. Cohen JA, Barkhof F, Comi G, et al. Oral fingolimod or intramuscular interferon for relapsing multiple sclerosis. N Engl J Med 2010;362(5):402–15.
128. Kim JW, Min CK, Mun YC, et al. Varicella-zoster virus-specific cell-mediated immunity and herpes zoster development in multiple myeloma patients receiving bortezomib- or thalidomide-based chemotherapy. J Clin Virol 2015;73:64–9.
129. Richardson PG, Sonneveld P, Schuster MW, et al. Bortezomib or high-dose dexamethasone for relapsed multiple myeloma. N Engl J Med 2005;352(24):2487–98.
130. San Miguel JF, Schlag R, Khuageva NK, et al. Bortezomib plus melphalan and prednisone for initial treatment of multiple myeloma. N Engl J Med 2008;359(9):906–17.
131. Robak T, Huang H, Jin J, et al. Bortezomib-based therapy for newly diagnosed mantle-cell lymphoma. N Engl J Med 2015;372(10):944–53.
132. Marchesi F, Mengarelli A, Giannotti F, et al. High incidence of post-transplant cytomegalovirus reactivations in myeloma patients undergoing autologous stem cell transplantation after treatment with bortezomib-based regimens: a survey from the Rome transplant network. Transpl Infect Dis 2014;16(1):158–64.
133. Horowitz N, Oren I, Lavi N, et al. New rising infection: human herpesvirus 6 is frequent in myeloma patients undergoing autologous stem cell

transplantation after induction therapy with bortezomib. Bone Marrow Res 2012;2012:409765.

134. Hou J, Jin J, Xu Y, et al. Randomized, double-blind, placebo-controlled phase III study of ixazomib plus lenalidomide-dexamethasone in patients with relapsed/ refractory multiple myeloma: China Continuation study. J Hematol Oncol 2017; 10(1):137.

135. Dimopoulos MA, Goldschmidt H, Niesvizky R, et al. Carfilzomib or bortezomib in relapsed or refractory multiple myeloma (ENDEAVOR): an interim overall survival analysis of an open-label, randomised, phase 3 trial. Lancet Oncol 2017; 18(10):1327–37.

136. Stewart AK, Rajkumar SV, Dimopoulos MA, et al. Carfilzomib, lenalidomide, and dexamethasone for relapsed multiple myeloma. N Engl J Med 2015;372(2): 142–52.

137. Lonial S, Dimopoulos M, Palumbo A, et al. Elotuzumab therapy for relapsed or refractory multiple myeloma. N Engl J Med 2015;373(7):621–31.

138. Dimopoulos MA, Dytfeld D, Grosicki S, et al. Elotuzumab plus pomalidomide and dexamethasone for multiple myeloma. N Engl J Med 2018;379(19): 1811–22.

139. Dimopoulos MA, Lonial S, Betts KA, et al. Elotuzumab plus lenalidomide and dexamethasone in relapsed/refractory multiple myeloma: Extended 4-year follow-up and analysis of relative progression-free survival from the randomized ELOQUENT-2 trial. Cancer 2018;124(20):4032–43.

140. Ishida T, Joh T, Uike N, et al. Defucosylated anti-CCR4 monoclonal antibody (KW-0761) for relapsed adult T-cell leukemia-lymphoma: a multicenter phase II study. J Clin Oncol 2012;30(8):837–42.

141. Ogura M, Ishida T, Hatake K, et al. Multicenter phase II study of mogamulizumab (KW-0761), a defucosylated anti-cc chemokine receptor 4 antibody, in patients with relapsed peripheral T-cell lymphoma and cutaneous T-cell lymphoma. J Clin Oncol 2014;32(11):1157–63.

142. Ishida T, Jo T, Takemoto S, et al. Dose-intensified chemotherapy alone or in combination with mogamulizumab in newly diagnosed aggressive adult T-cell leukaemia-lymphoma: a randomized phase II study. Br J Haematol 2015; 169(5):672–82.

143. Ishitsuka K, Yurimoto S, Kawamura K, et al. Safety and efficacy of mogamulizumab in patients with adult T-cell leukemia-lymphoma in Japan: interim results of postmarketing all-case surveillance. Int J Hematol 2017;106(4):522–32.

144. Ishii Y, Itabashi M, Numata A, et al. Cytomegalovirus pneumonia after anti-CC-chemokine receptor 4 monoclonal antibody (mogamulizumab) therapy in an angioimmunoblastic T-cell lymphoma patient. Intern Med 2016;55(6):673–5.

145. Ohyama Y, Kumode T, Eguchi G, et al. Induction of molecular remission by using anti-CC-chemokine receptor 4 (anti-CCR4) antibodies for adult T cell leukemia: a risk of opportunistic infection after treatment with anti-CCR4 antibodies. Ann Hematol 2014;93(1):169–71.

146. Aoki F. Antivirals against Herpes viruses. In: Bennett JE, Dolin R, Blaser MJ, editors. Principles and practice of infectious diseases, vol. 1. Philadelphia: Elsevier Saunders; 2015. p. 546–62.

147. Wada-Shimosato Y, Tanoshima R, Hiratoko K, et al. Effectiveness of acyclovir prophylaxis against varicella zoster virus disease after allogeneic hematopoietic cell transplantation: a systematic review and meta-analysis. Transpl Infect Dis 2019;21(3):e13061.

148. Sandherr M, Hentrich M, von Lilienfeld-Toal M, et al. Antiviral prophylaxis in patients with solid tumours and haematological malignancies–update of the Guidelines of the Infectious Diseases Working Party (AGIHO) of the German Society for Hematology and Medical Oncology (DGHO). Ann Hematol 2015;94(9): 1441–50.

149. Available at: https://www.nccn.org/professionals/physician_gls/pdf/ infections.pdf.

150. Wald A, Corey L, Timmler B, et al. Helicase-primase inhibitor pritelivir for HSV-2 infection. N Engl J Med 2014;370(3):201–10.

151. Wald A, Timmler B, Magaret A, et al. Effect of pritelivir compared with valacyclovir on genital HSV-2 shedding in patients with frequent recurrences: a randomized clinical trial. JAMA 2016;316(23):2495–503.

152. Kawashima M, Nemoto O, Honda M, et al. Amenamevir, a novel helicase-primase inhibitor, for treatment of herpes zoster: A randomized, double-blind, valaciclovir-controlled phase 3 study. J Dermatol 2017;44(11):1219–27.

153. Rubin LG, Levin MJ, Ljungman P, et al. 2013 IDSA clinical practice guideline for vaccination of the immunocompromised host. Clin Infect Dis 2014;58(3): e44–100.

154. Lal H, Cunningham AL, Godeaux O, et al. Efficacy of an adjuvanted herpes zoster subunit vaccine in older adults. N Engl J Med 2015;372(22):2087–96.

155. Cunningham AL, Lal H, Kovac M, et al. Efficacy of the herpes zoster subunit vaccine in adults 70 years of age or older. N Engl J Med 2016;375(11):1019–32.

156. Stadtmauer EA, Sullivan KM, Marty FM, et al. A phase 1/2 study of an adjuvanted varicella-zoster virus subunit vaccine in autologous hematopoietic cell transplant recipients. Blood 2014;124(19):2921–9.

157. Berkowitz EM, Moyle G, Stellbrink HJ, et al. Safety and immunogenicity of an adjuvanted herpes zoster subunit candidate vaccine in HIV-infected adults: a phase 1/2a randomized, placebo-controlled study. J Infect Dis 2015;211(8): 1279–87.

158. Available at: https://idsa.confex.com/idsa/2017/webprogram/Paper65338.html.

159. James SF, Chahine EB, Sucher AJ, et al. Shingrix: the new adjuvanted recombinant herpes zoster vaccine. Ann Pharmacother 2018;52(7):673–80.

160. Zaia JA. Cytomegalovirus infection. In: Forman SJ, Negrin RS, Antin JH, et al, editors. Thomas' hematopoietic cell transplantation, vol. 2. West Sussex (UK): Wiley; 2016. p. 1069–77.

161. Razonable RR. Role of letermovir for prevention of cytomegalovirus infection after allogeneic haematopoietic stem cell transplantation. Curr Opin Infect Dis 2018;31(4):286–91.

162. Maertens J, Cordonnier C, Jaksch P, et al. Maribavir for preemptive treatment of cytomegalovirus reactivation. N Engl J Med 2019;381(12):1136–47.

163. Marty FM, Ljungman P, Papanicolaou GA, et al. Maribavir prophylaxis for prevention of cytomegalovirus disease in recipients of allogeneic stem-cell transplants: a phase 3, double-blind, placebo-controlled, randomised trial. Lancet Infect Dis 2011;11(4):284–92.

164. Winston DJ, Saliba F, Blumberg E, et al. Efficacy and safety of maribavir dosed at 100 mg orally twice daily for the prevention of cytomegalovirus disease in liver transplant recipients: a randomized, double-blind, multicenter controlled trial. Am J Transplant 2012;12(11):3021–30.

165. Marty FM, Winston DJ, Rowley SD, et al. CMX001 to prevent cytomegalovirus disease in hematopoietic-cell transplantation. N Engl J Med 2013;369(13): 1227–36.

166. Hiwarkar P, Amrolia P, Sivaprakasam P, et al. Brincidofovir is highly efficacious in controlling adenoviremia in pediatric recipients of hematopoietic cell transplant. Blood 2017;129(14):2033–7.
167. Anderholm KM, Bierle CJ, Schleiss MR. Cytomegalovirus vaccines: current status and future prospects. Drugs 2016;76(17):1625 45.
168. Diamond DJ, La Rosa C, Chiuppesi F, et al. A fifty-year odyssey: prospects for a cytomegalovirus vaccine in transplant and congenital infection. Expert Rev Vaccines 2018;17(10):889–911.

Hepatitis B Virus Reactivation Potentiated by Biologics

Eiichi Ogawa, MD, PhD[a], Mike T. Wei, MD[b],
Mindie H. Nguyen, MD, MAS[b],*

KEYWORDS

• Hepatitis B virus • Reactivation • Prophylaxis • Nucleos(t)ide analogue

KEY POINTS

• Hepatitis B virus (HBV) reactivation can be a serious complication for patients with chronic (HBsAg+) as well as resolved HBV (HBsAg−/anti-HBc+) infection when treated with biologics. All patients should be screened for HBsAg, anti-HBc, and HBV DNA before starting biologics.

• Patients with chronic HBV infection should generally receive prophylactic treatment with nucleos(t)ide analogues before the initiation of biologics, except in cases of biologics with very low risk of immunosuppression.

• Patients with resolved HBV infection can generally be observed except for high-risk patients such as those receiving anti-CD20 agents who should receive anti-HBV prophylaxis. Moderate-risk patients require a more individualized approach with regard to anti-HBV prophylaxis based on comorbidities, feasibility of monitoring, and the duration of biologics.

• Once anti-HBV prophylaxis is decided and initiated, treatment should be continued during biologic therapy and for at least 6 months after discontinuation of most biologics and for at least 12 months for patients receiving anti-CD20 agents.

INTRODUCTION

Globally, more than 2 billion people are estimated to have been exposed to the hepatitis B virus (HBV),[1] and approximately 292 million are chronically infected,[2] making chronic hepatitis B (CHB) one of the leading causes of cirrhosis, liver decompensation, and hepatocellular carcinoma (HCC).[3] Except for older agents such as lamivudine, adefovir, and telbivudine, newer nucleos(t)ide analogues (NAs) such as entecavir

[a] Department of General Internal Medicine, Kyushu University Hospital, 3-1-1 Maidashi Higashi-ku, Fukuoka 8128582, Japan; [b] Division of Gastroenterology and Hepatology, Department of Medicine, Stanford University Medical Center, 750 Welch Road, Suite 210, Palo Alto, CA 94304, USA
* Corresponding author.
E-mail address: mindiehn@stanford.edu

Infect Dis Clin N Am 34 (2020) 341–358
https://doi.org/10.1016/j.idc.2020.02.009
0891-5520/20/© 2020 Elsevier Inc. All rights reserved.

id.theclinics.com

(ETV), tenofovir disoproxil fumarate (TDF), and tenofovir alafenamide (TAF) are highly effective in inhibiting HBV replication with excellent short-term and long-term safety profiles.[4] Long-term NA treatment also can improve liver histology and reduce HCC incidence.[5,6]

In recent decades, innovation and rapid expansion in the field of biologics have revolutionized the management of many oncologic and nononcologic diseases. As a result, immunosuppression and concern for HBV reactivation are no longer relevant in oncologic practice alone but also in many other disciplines such as rheumatologic, hematologic, dermatologic, and gastrointestinal inflammatory bowel disease, among others.[7–9] Moreover, B-cell depleting biologics such as anti-CD20 agents are associated with even higher risk of HBV reactivation than more traditional cytotoxic chemotherapeutic agents. Therefore, it is important for practitioners in diverse settings to screen all patients being considered for biologics for evidence of ongoing as well as resolved HBV infection. This synopsis will help define HBV reactivation and screening tests, summarize the different classes of biologics associated with HBV reactivation, stratify the various reactivation risk levels by HBV status and biologic agents, and review management strategies on who to monitor, who to treat, how to treat, and for how long.

GENERAL INFORMATION ON HEPATITIS B VIRUS REACTIVATION
Definition and Epidemiology

HBV reactivation is characterized by an abrupt elevation of serum HBV DNA in patients with chronic (hepatitis B surface antigen [HBsAg]- positive) or resolved HBV infection (HBsAg-negative, hepatitis B core antibody [anti-HBc]-positive and undetectable HBV DNA).[10] HBV reactivation in HBsAg-positive patients is defined as a ≥ 2 log rise in HBV DNA from baseline (3 log if baseline is negative, 4 log if baseline unknown).[4] In the case of HBsAg-negative/anti-HBc-positive patients, having detectable HBV DNA or reversion of HBsAg from negative to positive indicates HBV reactivation.[4] HBV reactivation may or may not be associated with hepatitis flares, which is defined with increase in alanine aminotransferase (ALT) to greater than 100 U/L or 3 times the baseline or higher.[4]

It is important to note that CHB is a global disease and is still endemic throughout much of Asia, sub-Saharan Africa, certain areas of South America, and certain areas of Eastern and Southern Europe.[2] In Western Europe and North America, CHB is prevalent among immigrants coming from endemic regions. Besides individuals with CHB, there is an even larger reservoir of individuals with resolved HBV infection in the general population who remain at risk for HBV reactivation from latent infection with covalently closed circular DNA (cccDNA) in the nuclei of hepatocytes (see the Pathophysiology section, later in this article). Therefore, all patients being considered for immunosuppressive therapy including biologics should be screened for active as well as prior exposure to HBV with HBsAg, anti-HBc, and HBV DNA (**Fig. 1**).[4]

Clinical Manifestations

After exposure to immunosuppressive treatments, HBV replication may abruptly increase, although the patient may remain asymptomatic during this stage. The timing of occurrence of HBV reactivation varies depending on the host status, disease status, and type of immunosuppressive treatment(s).[7–9] Reactivation may occur as early as within the first 2 weeks of initiation of immunosuppressive drugs or up to a year after their cessation or even longer.

A rapid rise in serum ALT level can occur within a few weeks or months of HBV DNA elevation. In general, ALT rise often lags behind HBV DNA rise or does not occur at all

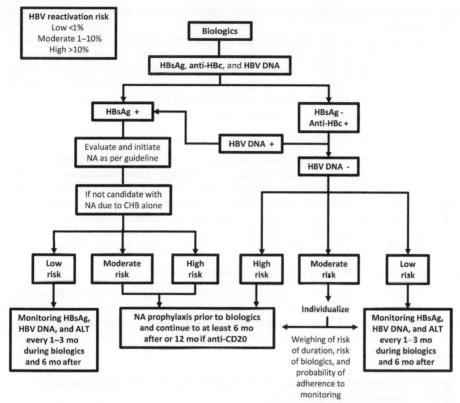

Fig. 1. Algorithm for management of hepatitis B reactivation based on HBV serology and low to moderate to high-risk biologic categories for HBV reactivation.

in mild cases. A small percentage of patients may experience worsening bilirubin level, progression to severe liver failure characterized by jaundice, prolonged prothrombin time, development of ascites, and hepatic encephalopathy.[11] Some of these patients may need a liver transplant if they are candidates, despite initiation of NA. If unrecognized or untreated, these patients have a high risk of death from liver failure. On the other hand, most patients will recover from HBV reactivation after the initiation of NA or with the cessation of immunosuppressive treatment.[10] In general, many patients only develop transient HBV DNA elevation, with or without ALT elevation, whereas some can develop hepatitis flares or even life-threatening liver failure.

Pathophysiology

HBV virions enter hepatocytes by binding to specific receptor sodium-taurocholate cotransporting polypeptide.[12] After entry, the partially double-strand relaxed circular DNA is converted to cccDNA in the nuclei of hepatocytes to serve as the template for transcription of viral RNAs.[13,14] The cccDNA is quite stable structurally and can persist in a latent state and serve as a reservoir for HBV reactivation.[13-15] Resolution of HBV infection is generally contributed by cytotoxic CD8-positive T cells destroying infected hepatocytes and thus contributing to viral clearance.[16,17] However, this is not sufficiently adequate to eradicate the infected hepatocytes harboring HBV cccDNA that escape targeting by the HBV-specific immune cells. HBV cccDNA contained in the hepatocytes by host immune during latent infection provides the source for active

HBV DNA replication once immune control mechanisms are suppressed, leading to HBV reactivation.[11,13–15,17,18]

Liver injury resulting from HBV reactivation goes through 2 patterns during immunosuppressive treatment. First, drug-induced immune suppression may lead to remarkable HBV replication, which can result in infected hepatocytes suffering direct damage. Second, cessation of immunosuppressive drugs may lead to reconstitution of immune function, which can cause severe injury of hepatocytes secondary to immune clearance and destruction of HBV-infected hepatocytes.[11]

Responsible Agents for Hepatitis B Virus Reactivation

HBV reactivation can occur spontaneously but is more often associated with medical treatments affecting host immune function. Historically, immunosuppressive treatments with steroid and other immunosuppressant drugs or with anticancer chemotherapy have been shown to cause HBV reactivation by inhibiting production of interleukin (IL), which is crucial for lymphocyte proliferation.[18] Recently, with its increasingly widespread use, molecularly targeted biologic treatments acting on specific host pathways have been associated increasingly with HBV reactivation.[8]

Risk Categories for Hepatitis B Virus Reactivation

Generally, patients with 10% or higher risk of developing HBV reactivation are considered to be high risk, 1% to 10% as moderate, and less than 1% as low risk.[9] Both HBV status at baseline and the type of biologics used determine the risk for HBV reactivation, which is sometimes difficult to discern due to lack of high-quality data, especially for newer agents.

HEPATITIS B VIRUS REACTIVATION FOR HEPATITIS B SURFACE ANTIGEN–POSITIVE PATIENTS TREATED WITH BIOLOGICS

For HBsAg-positive patients receiving biologics, the risk of HBV reactivation is moderate to high in most cases, particularly if a tumor necrosis factor-alpha (TNF-α) inhibitor or B-cell-depleting agent is used (**Table 1**). Therefore, in the vast majority of cases, HBsAg-positive patients should be considered for antiviral prophylaxis and should be referred to an infectious disease, gastroenterology, or hepatology specialist who is familiar with HBV management.

Tumor Necrosis Factor-α Inhibitors

TNF-α and related cytokines are proinflammatory agents in the host defense mechanism against many intracellular pathogens.[19] By stimulating HBV-specific cytotoxic CD8-positive T-cell response, TNF-α can suppress HBV replication and promote HBV eradication.[20] Recently, TNF-α has been found to activate a specific endogenous antiviral pathway related to degradation of HBV cccDNA in liver cells.[21] TNF-α inhibitors are widely used for treatment of rheumatologic and dermatologic diseases, such as rheumatoid arthritis, ankylosing spondylitis, and psoriasis. HBV reactivation may occur directly due to a lack of TNF-α, or indirectly via diminished T-cell activation, although the precise mechanism remains largely unknown.[22] TNF-α inhibitors, including infliximab, adalimumab, and etanercept have a high risk of promoting HBV reactivation (15.4%) in HBsAg-positive patients.[23]

Agents Targeting B Cells

A representative agent that targets B cells well characterized to associate with HBV reactivation is rituximab, a chimeric anti-CD20 antibody widely used in the treatment

Table 1
Risk of HBV reactivation associated with biologics for hepatitis B surface antigen–positive patients

Biologics, grouped by mechanism of action	Reactivation Risk		
	Low (<1%) or Unknown (Probable Low Risk)	Moderate (1 to <10%)	High (≥10%)
TNF-α inhibitors			Infliximab Adalimumab Certolizumab Etanercept Golimumab

Agents targeting B cells
  Anti-CD20
  Anti-CD38
  Anti-CD30
  Inhibit B-cell activating factor
			Rituximab
			Ofatumumab
			Ocrelizumab
			Obinutuzumab
			Ibritumomab
			Daratumumab
			Brentuximab
			Belimumab

Agents targeting T-cell
  activation
  Anti-CD80/86
  Anti-CD2
  IL-23 inhibitors
  IL-17 inhibitors
			Belatacept
			Abatacept
			Alefacept
			Ustekinumab
			Guselkumab
			Tildrakizumab
			Secukinumab
			Ixekizumab
			Brodalumab

Direct T-cell inhibition and
  agents targeting T-cell
  migration and chemotaxis
  Blocking alpha4-integrin
  Anti-CD52
		Natalizumab
		Vedolizumab
			Alemtuzumab

Interleukin inhibitors
  IL-1 inhibitors
  IL-6 inhibitors
		Anakinra
		Canakinumab
		Rilonacept
		Tocilizumab
		Sarilumab	

Checkpoint inhibitors	Ipilimumab Atezolizumab Durvalumab Nivolumab Pembrolizumab Cemiplimab Avelumab		

Tyrosine kinase inhibitors
  for heme malignancies
  Bruton tyrosine kinase
    inhibitors
  Small-molecule Bcr-Abl
    tyrosine kinase inhibitors
		Ibrutinib
		Acalabrutinib
		Imatinib
		Nilotinib
		Dasatinib
		Bosutinib
		Ponatinib
		Bafetinib	

(continued on next page)

Table 1 (continued)			
	Reactivation Risk		
Biologics, grouped by mechanism of action	**Low (<1%) or Unknown (Probable Low Risk)**	**Moderate (1 to <10%)**	**High (≥10%)**
EGFR inhibitors and other tyrosine kinase inhibitors for solid tumors EGFR tyrosine kinase inhibitors EGFR inhibiting monoclonal antibody Other tyrosine kinase inhibitors VEGF inhibitors VEGF and FGFR inhibitors	Cetuximab Panitumumab Sorafenib Sunitinib Bevacizumab Lenvatinib	Gefitinib Erlotinib Osimertinib Afatinib Dacomitinib	
Targeting JAK-STAT signaling and complement pathway JAK inhibitors C5 inhibitors	Eculizumab Ravulizumab	Ruxolitinib Tofacitinib Baricitinib	

Abbreviations: EGFR, epidermal growth factor receptor; FGFR, fibroblast growth factor receptor; HBV, hepatitis B; IL, interleukin; JAK, janus kinase; STAT, signal transducer and activator of transcription; TNF, tumor necrosis factor; VEGF, vascular endothelial growth factor.

of B-cell non-Hodgkin lymphoma. The pathophysiology of HBV reactivation induced by rituximab remains unclear but is likely more complex than simple B-cell depletion and may be associated with insufficient induction of CD4-positive T-cell activation and proliferation.[24] Among HBsAg-positive patients treated with rituximab for non-Hodgkin lymphoma who did not receive antiviral prophylaxis, HBV reactivation occurred in up to 28.5%.[25] Patients taking other anti-CD20 monoclonal antibodies, such as ofatumumab, ocrelizumab, obinutuzumab, and ibritumomab are also at high risk of HBV reactivation, as in the case of rituximab. Moreover, HBV reactivation has been reported to persist long after discontinuation of anti-CD20 agents; therefore, prophylactic antiviral therapy should be continued for at least 12 months after the end of anti-CD20 therapy,[4] and it may be prudent to treat for even a longer duration in some cases. HBV reactivation beyond 12 months after the last dose of rituximab has been reported, due to delayed immune recovery.[26]

Daratumumab and brentuximab are antibodies against CD38 and CD30, respectively, which are expressed on both B cells and activated T cells.[27] Belimumab is a human immunoglobulin (Ig)G1-λ monoclonal antibody that binds soluble B-cell stimulator and inhibits the survival of B cells, including autoreactive B cells, reducing their differentiation into Ig-producing plasma cells.[28] Although there is a lack of clinical data regarding the association between HBV reactivation and these B-cell targeting agents, given the data for rituximab, prophylaxis for HBV reactivation would be prudent.

Agents Targeting T-Cell Activation

Belatacept and abatacept, which differ by only 2 amino acids, inhibit T-cell activation by blocking a costimulatory signal by binding to CD80/CD86 on antigen-presenting cells.[29,30] Alefacept interrupts CD2-mediated T-cell costimulation and depletes T cells via a natural killer cell–dependent mechanism.[31] In a retrospective case series,

4 HBsAg-positive patients given antiviral prophylaxis remained clinically stable, whereas an additional 4 not given prophylaxis developed HBV reactivation.[32] Given their mechanism of action, these biologics likely have a reactivation rate that is moderate to high.

Ustekinumab is an IL-12/23 p40 monoclonal antibody, and guselkumab and tildrakizumab are anti–IL-23 p19 monoclonal antibodies.[33] Secukinumab, ixekizumab, and brodalumab are anti–IL-17 agents that block the IL-17 pathway of proinflammatory cytokine secreted by a variety of immunologic cells, including T-helper cells.[34] IL-17 is thought to play an important role in suppressing HBV activity.[35] Circulating and intrahepatic T-helper 17 cell numbers are increased in HBV-infected patients with CHB, and IL-17 expression is positively related to the severity of liver injury and inflammation progression.[35] In one small series of anti–HBs-positive patients, 2 (28.6%) of 7 treated with ustekinumab[36] and 6 (24.0%) of 25 treated with secukinumab[37] who did not receive antiviral prophylaxis experienced reactivation. Overall, anti–IL-23/17 agents are considered high risk for HBV reactivation.

Direct T-Cell Inhibition and Agents Targeting T-Cell Migration and Chemotaxis

Natalizumab and vedolizumab are humanized anti-α4 integrin monoclonal antibodies.[38,39] They bind the α4 subunit of α4β1 or α4β7 integrins, which are cell adhesion molecules. Although integrins seem to affect lymphocyte trafficking in the liver, the implication for HBV reactivation is unclear. Only 1 case of potential HBV reactivation has been reported,[40] but further information on HBV-infected patients should become available in the near future.

In contrast, alemtuzumab, an anti-CD52 monoclonal antibody, causes profound B-lymphocyte lymphocytopenia, as it does for T-lymphocytes. As is the case with anti-CD20 antibodies, alemtuzumab is considered to be a high-risk agent for HBV reactivation.[41]

Interleukin Inhibitors

Anakinra, canakinumab, and rilonacept are recombinant interleukin (IL)-1 receptor antagonists. IL-1 is produced in response to various microbial and nonmicrobial stimuli, and is a major mediator of the inflammatory response.[42] Tocilizumab and sarilumab are IL-6 receptor antagonists. IL-6, a pleiotropic proinflammatory cytokine, is referred to as B-cell stimulatory factor-2, and it plays an essential role in the final differentiation of B cells into immunoglobulin secreting cells, which are involved in diverse physiologic processes.[43] Few data have been obtained on HBV reactivation by patients treated with IL inhibitors, but based on the limited clinical studies available,[44,45] interleukin inhibitors should probably be considered moderate risk for HBV reactivation.

Checkpoint Inhibitors

Checkpoint inhibitors have generally shown efficacy in restoring T-cell function of patients with malignancy. PD-1, PD-L1, and CTLA-4 inhibitors disrupt immune checkpoint signaling and restore suppressed effector T cells.[46,47] This mechanism may have the potential to increase specific anti-HBV activity within the liver, unlike other biologics. A recent pilot study by Gane and colleagues[48] provided data on the decline of HBV DNA on nivolumab, a PD-1/PD-L1 inhibitor, likely secondary to the restoration of HBV-specific immune responses. Therefore, the risk of HBV reactivation is unknown, but considered to be probably low. Further studies will be needed to elucidate the influence of checkpoint inhibitors on chronic HBV infection.

Tyrosine Kinase Inhibitors for Hematologic Malignancies

Ibrutinib (first generation) and acalabrutinib (second generation) inhibit Bruton tyrosine kinase (BTK) and thereby interrupt B-cell receptor signaling. These agents are currently used in the treatment of chronic lymphocytic leukemia,[49] mantle cell lymphoma,[50] and Waldenstrom macroglobulinemia.[51] HBV reactivation could be a potential complication from the standpoint of the B-cell signaling inhibitory activity of BTK inhibitors. Although there are few data to date to inform practice of the risk for HBV reactivation associated with these agents, given their mechanism of action, it would be prudent to consider these agents to be of moderate risk until further data are available.

Imatinib, nilotinib, and dasatinib are small-molecule tyrosine kinase inhibitors (TKIs) that block the ATP binding site of BCR/ABL. Although the mechanism of TKI-induced HBV reactivation remains unclear, TKIs can inhibit T-cell activation and proliferation.[52] Therefore, TKIs likely have moderate risk for HBV reactivation, although data are currently sparse, with only a few case reports and small case series to date.[53–55]

Epidermal Growth Factor Receptor Inhibitors and Other Tyrosine Kinase Inhibitors for Solid Tumors

Epidermal growth factor receptor (EGFR) TKIs, including gefitinib, erlotinib, osimertinib, and afatinib, have become first-line therapies for advanced non–small-cell lung cancer. A recent study reported an HBV reactivation rate of 9.36% (16 of 171) among patients treated with EGFR TKIs.[56] Likewise, the TKIs sorafenib and sunitinib have potential to cause HBV reactivation, although there are few clinical data in this regard. In contrast, cetuximab and panitumumab are chimeric mouse-human monoclonal IgG1 (cetuximab) and IgG2 (panitumumab) kappa antibodies to the EGFR, which is present on many normal cell types and overexpressed in several forms of cancer.[57] Bevacizumab is a vascular endothelial growth factor (VEGF)-A–specific angiogenesis inhibitor.[58] Lenvatinib is an oral multikinase inhibitor that targets VEGF receptors 1 to 3, fibroblast growth factor receptors 1 to 4, platelet-derived growth factor receptor α, RET, and KIT.[59] For these antibodies to EGFR and VEGF, there has been no association with HBV reactivation to date.

Targeting the Janus Kinase/Signal Transducer and Activator of Transcription Signaling and Complement Pathway

Ruxolitinib is a selective inhibitor of janus kinases (JAKs) 1 and 2 for the treatment of myelofibrosis. JAK1 inhibition disturbs T-cell immune response, which is dependent on cytokines and JAK–signal transducer and activator of transcription (STAT) signaling.[60] Tofacitinib and baricitinib are potent, selective JAK inhibitors that preferentially inhibit JAKs 1/3 and 1/2, respectively. Some reports have shown that ruxolitinib for HBs-positive patients might lead to HBV reactivation.[61,62]

Eculizumab is a recombinant humanized monoclonal antibody targeting complement protein C5 in the treatment of paroxysmal nocturnal hemoglobinuria and atypical hemolytic uremic syndrome–associated thrombotic microangiopathy. Eculizumab prevents the formation of the terminal membrane attack complex C5b-C9,[63] resulting in defective bacterial complement activity. The association between eculizumab and HBV reactivation is not known.

HEPATITIS B VIRUS REACTIVATION FOR HEPATITIS B SURFACE ANTIGEN–NEGATIVE/ ANTI–HEPATITIS B CORE–POSITIVE PATIENTS TREATED WITH BIOLOGICS

Although hepatitis B surface antigen (HBsAg)-negative/anti–hepatitis B core (HBc)-positive patients are at lower risk of HBV reactivation than HBsAg-positive patients, the risk is still considerable with certain classes of biologics and fatal HBV reactivation cases are well documented (**Table 2**).[64] Among the various biologics, anti-CD20 agents, such as rituximab, are considered high risk for reactivation, and patients with resolved HBV infection initiated on anti-CD20 agents should be given antiviral prophylactic therapies. Patients with low risk of HBV reactivation should be monitored carefully every 1 to 3 months, and the decision to monitor or to initiate antiviral prophylactic treatment should probably be individualized for those in the moderate-risk category, balancing the risk of treatment and risk of reactivation. The practicality of frequent monitoring affecting patient adherence also should be taken into consideration.

Tumor Necrosis Factor-α Inhibitors

According to a systematic review and analysis of case reports, HBV reactivation was reported to occur in approximately 5% (9/168) of HBsAg-negative/anti-HBc-positive patients receiving anti-TNF therapy.[65] Subsequent larger reviews have noted lower rates of HBV reactivation (0%–3.1%),[23,66–68] and the latest report suggests that none of the patients in a US cohort (n = 178) had HBV reactivation and none received prophylactic treatment.[69]

Agents Targeting B Cells

As mentioned previously, HBsAg-negative/anti-HBc-positive patients receiving anti-CD20 agents, such as rituximab or ofatumumab, are at high risk and should be offered prophylactic antiviral treatment. Pooled baseline risk estimates without prophylaxis against HBV reactivation during treatment with rituximab revealed a reactivation rate of 16.9% (47/325).[9] Another prospective study showed a 2-year cumulative rate of HBV reactivation of 41.5% among 63 HBsAg-negative/anti-HBc-positive patients with hematologic malignancy who received rituximab without anti-HBV prophylaxis.[26] Of note, HBV reactivation occurred at a median of 23 weeks after the start of rituximab treatment and baseline undetectable anti-HBs was a significant risk factor for HBV reactivation among those with negative HBsAg and positive anti-HBc.[26] Prophylactic antiviral therapy also should be continued for at least 12 months after the end of anti-CD20 therapy.[4]

Other Biologics

The estimate in this population with HBsAg-negative/anti-HBc-positive remains highly uncertain because of the paucity of data regarding HBV reactivation in patients treated with biologics other than TNF-α inhibitors and agents targeting B cells. HBV reactivation has been reported to occur with ustekinumab (anti-IL-12/23 p40),[70] natalizumab (anti-α4 integrin),[40] alemtuzumab (anti-CD52),[71] nivolumab (checkpoint inhibitor),[72] and erlotinib (EGFR-TKI),[37] although the reports of HBV reactivation are restricted to a few case reports. One (4.2%) of 24 HBsAg-negative/anti-HBc-positive patients with psoriasis had HBV reactivation from secukinumab therapy (anti-IL-17).[37] According to a recent review focused on patients receiving TKIs,[73] HBV reactivation can occur even with resolved HBV infection. In another retrospective assessment of HBsAg-negative/anti-HBc-positive patients treated with ibrutinib, the cumulative incidence of HBV reactivation was 9.5%.[74] In the most recent prospective study of HBV reactivation in HBsAg-negative/anti-HBc-positive patients undergoing ruxolitinib (JAK inhibitor), HBV reactivation occurred in 4 (26.7%) of 15 patients.[75] In contrast, a retrospective study on other JAK inhibitors with tofacitinib has shown that none of the HBsAg-negative/anti-HBc-positive patients developed HBV reactivation.[62] Further studies will be needed to confirm the risk of reactivation for patients receiving a JAK inhibitor.

Table 2
Risk of HBV reactivation associated with biologics for hepatitis B surface antigen–negative/ anti-HBc-positive patients

	Reactivation Risk		
	Low (<1%) or Unknown (Probable Low Risk)	Moderate (1 to <10%)	High (≥10%)
TNF-α inhibitors		Infliximab Adalimumab Certolizumab Etanercept Golimumab	
Agents targeting B cells Anti-CD20 Anti-CD38 Anti-CD30 Inhibit B-cell activating factor		Daratumumab Brentuximab Belimumab	Rituximab Ofatumumab Ocrelizumab Obinutuzumab Ibritumomab
Agents targeting T-cell activation Anti-CD80/86 Anti-CD2 IL-23 inhibitors IL-17 inhibitors		Belatacept Abatacept Alefacept Ustekinumab Guselkumab Tildrakizumab Secukinumab Ixekizumab Brodalumab	
Direct T-cell inhibition and agents targeting T-cell migration and chemotaxis Blocking alpha4-integrin Anti-CD52		Natalizumab Vedolizumab Alemtuzumab	
Interleukin inhibitors IL-1 inhibitors IL-6 inhibitors		Anakinra Canakinumab Rilonacept Tocilizumab Sarilumab	
Checkpoint inhibitors	Ipilimumab Atezolizumab Durvalumab Nivolumab Pembrolizumab Cemiplimab Avelumab		
Tyrosine kinase inhibitors for heme malignancies Bruton tyrosine kinase inhibitors Small-molecule Bcr-Abl tyrosine kinase inhibitors		Ibrutinib Acalabrutinib Imatinib Nilotinib Dasatinib Bosutinib Ponatinib Bafetinib	
EGFR inhibitors and other tyrosine kinase inhibitors for solid tumors	Cetuximab Panitumumab Sorafenib	Gefitinib Erlotinib Osimertinib	

(continued on next page)

Table 2 (continued)			
	Reactivation Risk		
	Low (<1%) or Unknown (Probable Low Risk)	Moderate (1 to <10%)	High (≥10%)
EGFR tyrosine kinase inhibitors	Sunitinib	Afatinib	
EGFR inhibiting monoclonal antibody	Bevacizumab Lenvatinib	Dacomitinib	
Other tyrosine kinase inhibitors			
VEGF inhibitors			
VEGF and FGFR inhibitors			
Targeting JAK-STAT signaling and complement pathway	Eculizumab Ravulizumab	Ruxolitinib Tofacitinib Baricitinib	
JAK inhibitors			
C5 inhibitors			

Abbreviations: EGFR, epidermal growth factor receptor; FGFR, fibroblast growth factor receptor; HBV, hepatitis B; IL, interleukin; JAK, janus kinase; STAT, signal transducer and activator of transcription; TNF, tumor necrosis factor; VEGF, vascular endothelial growth factor.

SCREENING, MANAGEMENT, AND PROPHYLAXIS FOR HEPATITIS B VIRUS REACTIVATION

All patients undergoing chemotherapy should be screened for HBsAg, anti-HBc, and HBV DNA before the initiation of biologics (see **Fig. 1**). Testing for the titer of anti-HBs also may be beneficial, because besides those without detectable anti-HBs, those with low titer of anti-HBs are also at higher risk for HBV reactivation, although no recommendations have been made concerning stratified management based on the titer of anti-HBs.[4] A study evaluating the cost-effectiveness of different HBV screening strategies before rituximab-based chemotherapy for lymphoma showed that universal screening reduces the rate of HBV reactivation by 10-fold and that it is less costly than screening only high-risk patients or screening no patients.[76] Moreover, vaccination of HBV seronegative patients is strongly recommended to ensure the achievement of anti-HBs response,[4] especially for immunocompromised patients.

As mentioned previously, the management and prophylaxis of HBV reactivation varies according to the virological profile and biologic used. All CHB and HBsAg-positive patients with high/moderate risk should be urgently referred to either an infectious disease or hepatology specialist, and anti-HBV treatment should be started before the initiation of a biologic. In the case of HBsAg-negative/anti-HBc-positive patients, anti-HBV prophylaxis is recommended only for high-risk patients, although can be considered for selected patients with moderate risk. For patients with low risk and most patients with moderate risk, monitoring for HBsAg, HBV DNA, and ALT level every 1 to 3 months is recommended with on-demand therapy at the first sign of HBV reactivation. As prophylactic treatment of those in the moderate-risk group with prophylaxis is controversial, patients in this group would require an individualized approach depending on comorbidities, duration of biologics, patient willingness, and ability to adhere to monitoring recommendation. In short, the risk of HBV reactivation and its associated morbidity and mortality should be weighed against the risk of antiviral prophylaxis, which is very few if any when new antiviral agents with high genetic barriers for resistance are used.

The antiviral agent lamivudine was initially used for the treatment of HBV reactivation in HBsAg-positive patients with cancer because it was the first oral antiviral to be approved in most locations.[77,78] However, because of its lower potency and high rate of viral resistance, fatal break-through reactivations and disruption in systemic treatment due to HBV reactivation have been reported.[79] Therefore, at present, ETV, TDF, and TAF, as potent antivirals with high genetic resistance barrier are recommended as prophylactic NAs of choice to prevent HBV reactivation. TAF has greater plasma stability, which allows for more efficient uptake by hepatocytes at lower plasma concentration than does TDF.[80,81] TAF also has better bone and renal safety profile, which may become a significant consideration for long-term use, especially for patients with existing renal/bone problems or at risk for them.[81]

Prophylactic anti-HBV treatment should be initiated before biologic therapy, continued throughout the course of biologic use, and continued for at least 6 months following discontinuation of biologic therapy.[4] In the case of anti-CD20, treatment needs to be continued for a minimum of 12 months following discontinuation of anti-CD20 because severely delayed immune reconstitution and severe HBV reactivation have been reported even more than 12 months after CD20 discontinuation.[69]

SPECIAL POPULATION COINFECTED WITH HEPATITIS C VIRUS OR HUMAN IMMUNODEFICIENCY VIRUS

HBV monitoring and treatment should be done in accordance with patient HBV status and the specific biologic used for HBV/hepatitis C virus (HCV) coinfection, as with HBV monoinfection. However, a special situation can arise when HBV/HCV coinfected patients are treated with direct-acting antivirals (DAAs) for HCV infection. Although there are ethnic influences in the pattern of viral dominance,[82] HBV replication often can be inhibited by HCV-induced intrahepatic immune activation.[83] When HCV is eradicated by DAAs, this inhibition is removed, and HBV replication can start leading to HBV reactivation in those with positive HBsAg; therefore, these patients should receive antiviral prophylaxis for HBV during DAA therapy for HCV.[84,85] In HBsAg-positive patients, rises in HBV DNA commonly occur during the first 4 to 8 weeks of DAA therapy.[86] The risk of HBV reactivation is much lower in those with resolved infection (HBsAg-negative/anti-HBc positive). However, fatal reactivation in patients with resolved HBV infection has been reported, so these patients do need to be monitored carefully during DAA therapy with HBsAg and HBV DNA in addition to ALT. It would be prudent to monitor every 4 weeks during DAA therapy and for 3 months after. In summary, testing for HBsAg, anti-HBc, and HBV DNA before starting DAAs is recommended for all patients with chronic hepatitis C being considered for DAA therapy, and HBV-infected and exposed patients should be managed as discussed previously to prevent life-threatening HBV reactivation in this setting.

In the United States, approximately 8% of patients with human immunodeficiency virus (HIV) also have evidence of chronic HBV infection.[87] Current American Association for the Study of Liver Diseases guidelines recommend that all patients with HIV should be started on antiretroviral therapy (ART) regardless of CD4 count.[4] In coinfected patients with HIV/HBV, the ART regimen should include anti-HBV drugs with TDF or TAF, otherwise leading to the potential for HBV reactivation during immune reconstitution with ART.[4]

SUMMARY

All candidates for biologics should be tested with HBsAg, anti-HBc, and HBV DNA before initiations of biologics. All HBsAg-positive patients who initiate biologic therapy but are not otherwise candidates for antiviral for CHB should be offered prophylactic NAs with ETV, TDF, or TAF, except for those treated with very low risk agents. In contrast, HBsAg-negative/anti-HBc positive patients should take NAs if they will initiate on high-risk agents for HBV reactivation such as anti-CD20 biologics. In the case of HBsAg-negative/anti-HBc-positive patients with moderate risk, an individual-ized approach based on comorbidities and duration of biologics will be required, whereas low-risk patients can be safely monitored. The duration of prophylactic anti-HBV treatment is from biologic initiation to at least 6 months (at least 12 months for anti-CD20 agents) after discontinuation of biologics. More precise estimates of the risk of HBV reactivation in response to many classes of biologics, especially newer or lesser used agents, require additional studies. In the meantime, the decision to initiate prophylactic antivirals should be based on the balance between the estimated/pre-sumed risk of HBV reactivation that can be fatal and the risk of prophylactic antivirals, which are few when one of the recommended agents (ETV, TDF or TAF) is used. The practicality of frequent and long-term laboratory monitoring for HBV reactivation also should be considered and discussed with patients.

DISCLOSURE

M.H. Nguyen: Grant/research support: Bristol-Myers Squibb, Gilead Sciences, Jans-sen Pharmaceutical; Advisory board/consultant: Dynavax Laboratories, Gilead Sci-ences, Intercept Pharmaceutical; Anylam Pharmaceutical; Roche Laboratories; and Novartis Pharmaceuticals. The other authors have nothing to disclose.

REFERENCES

1. Schweitzer A, Horn J, Mikolajczyk RT, et al. Estimations of worldwide prevalence of chronic hepatitis B virus infection: a systematic review of data published be-tween 1965 and 2013. Lancet 2015;386:1546–55.
2. Polaris Observatory Collaborators. Global prevalence, treatment, and prevention of hepatitis B virus infection in 2016: a modelling study. Lancet Gastroenterol Hepatol 2018;3:383–403.
3. Yang JD, Roberts LR. Hepatocellular carcinoma: a global view. Nat Rev Gastro-enterol Hepatol 2010;7:448–58.
4. Terrault NA, Lok ASF, McMahon BJ. Update on prevention, diagnosis, and treat-ment of chronic hepatitis B: AASLD 2018 hepatitis B guidance. Hepatology 2018; 67:1560–99.
5. Gordon SC, Lamerato LE, Rupp LB, et al. Antiviral therapy for chronic hepatitis B virus infection and development of hepatocellular carcinoma in a US population. Clin Gastroenterol Hepatol 2014;12:885–93.
6. Lok AS, McMahon BJ, Brown RS Jr, et al. Antiviral therapy for chronic hepatitis B viral infection in adults: a systematic review and meta-analysis. Hepatology 2016; 63:284–306.
7. Hwang JP, Lok AS. Management of patients with hepatitis B who require immu-nosuppressive therapy. Nat Rev Gastroenterol Hepatol 2014;11:209–19.
8. Loomba R, Liang TJ. Hepatitis B reactivation associated with immune suppres-sive and biological modifier therapies: current concepts, management strategies, and future directions. Gastroenterology 2017;152:1297–309.
9. Perrillo RP, Gish R, Falck-Ytter YT. American Gastroenterological Association Institute technical review on prevention and treatment of hepatitis B virus reacti-vation during immunosuppressive drug therapy. Gastroenterology 2015;148: 221–44.

10. Hoofnagle JH. Reactivation of hepatitis B. Hepatology 2009;49:S156–65.
11. Lok AS, Liang RH, Chiu EK, et al. Reactivation of hepatitis B virus replication in patients receiving cytotoxic therapy. Report of a prospective study. Gastroenterology 1991;100:182–8.
12. Yan H, Zhong G, Xu G, et al. Sodium taurocholate cotransporting polypeptide is a functional receptor for human hepatitis B and D virus. Elife 2012;1:e00049.
13. Bock CT, Schwinn S, Locarnini S, et al. Structural organization of the hepatitis B virus minichromosome. J Mol Biol 2001;307:183–96.
14. Seeger C, Mason WS. Hepatitis B virus biology. Microbiol Mol Biol Rev 2000;64: 51–68.
15. Fong TL, Di Bisceglie AM, Gerber MA. Persistence of hepatitis B virus DNA in the liver after loss of HBsAg in chronic hepatitis B. Hepatology 1993;18:1313–8.
16. Rehermann B. Pathogenesis of chronic viral hepatitis: differential roles of T cells and NK cells. Nat Med 2013;19:859–68.
17. Guidotti LG, Chisari FV. Immunobiology and pathogenesis of viral hepatitis. Annu Rev Pathol 2006;1:23–61.
18. Perrillo RP. Acute flares in chronic hepatitis B: the natural and unnatural history of an immunologically mediated liver disease. Gastroenterology 2001;120:1009–22.
19. González-Amaro R, García-Monzón C, García-Buey L, et al. Induction of tumor necrosis factor alpha production by human hepatocytes in chronic viral hepatitis. J Exp Med 1994;179:841–8.
20. Ganem D, Prince AM. Hepatitis B virus infection-natural history and clinical consequences. N Engl J Med 2004;350:1118–29.
21. Lucifora J, Xia Y, Reisinger F, et al. Specific and nonhepatotoxic degradation of nuclear hepatitis B virus cccDNA. Science 2014;343:1221–8.
22. Guidotti LG, Ishikawa T, Hobbs MV, et al. Intracellular inactivation of the hepatitis B virus by cytotoxic T lymphocytes. Immunity 1996;4:25–36.
23. Cantini F, Boccia S, Goletti D, et al. HBV reactivation in patients treated with antitumor necrosis factor-alpha (TNF-α) agents for rheumatic and dermatologic conditions: a systematic review and meta-analysis. Int J Rheumatol 2014;2014: 926836.
24. Xu X, Shang Q, Chen X, et al. Reversal of B-cell hyperactivation and functional impairment is associated with HBsAg seroconversion in chronic hepatitis B patients. Cell Mol Immunol 2015;12:309–16.
25. Evens AM, Jovanovic BD, Su YC, et al. Rituximab-associated hepatitis B virus (HBV) reactivation in lymphoproliferative diseases: meta-analysis and examination of FDA safety reports. Ann Oncol 2011;22:1170–80.
26. Seto WK, Chan TS, Hwang YY, et al. Hepatitis B reactivation in patients with previous hepatitis B virus exposure undergoing rituximab-containing chemotherapy for lymphoma: a prospective study. J Clin Oncol 2014;32:3736–43.
27. Drgona L, Gudiol C, Lanini S, et al. ESCMID study group for infections in compromised hosts (ESGICH) consensus document on the safety of targeted and biological therapies: an infectious diseases perspective (agents targeting lymphoid or myeloid cells surface antigens [II]: CD22, CD30, CD33, CD38, CD40, SLAMF-7 and CCR4). Clin Microbiol Infect 2018;24:S83–94.
28. Vincent FB, Morand EF, Schneider P, et al. The BAFF/APRIL system in SLE pathogenesis. Nat Rev Rheumatol 2014;10:365–73.
29. Vincenti F, Rostaing L, Grinyo J, et al. Belatacept and long-term outcomes in kidney transplantation. N Engl J Med 2016;374:333–43.
30. Blair HA, Deeks ED. Abatacept: a review in rheumatoid arthritis. Drugs 2017;77: 1221–33.

31. Chamian F, Lin SL, Lee E, et al. Alefacept (anti-CD2) causes a selective reduction in circulating effector memory T cells (Tem) and relative preservation of central memory T cells (Tcm) in psoriasis. J Transl Med 2007;5:27.
32. Kim PS, Ho GY, Prete PE, et al. Safety and efficacy of abatacept in eight rheumatoid arthritis patients with chronic hepatitis B. Arthritis Care Res 2012;64:1265–8.
33. Smolen JS, Agarwal SK, Ilivanova E, et al. A randomised phase II study evaluating the efficacy and safety of subcutaneously administered ustekinumab and guselkumab in patients with active rheumatoid arthritis despite treatment with methotrexate. Ann Rheum Dis 2017;76:831–9.
34. Puig L. Paradoxical reactions: anti-tumor necrosis factor alpha agents, ustekinumab, secukinumab, ixekizumab, and others. Curr Probl Dermatol 2018;53:49–63.
35. Huang Z, van Velkinburgh JC, Ni B, et al. Pivotal roles of the interleukin-23/T helper 17 cell axis in hepatitis B. Liver Int 2012;32:894–901.
36. Chiu HY, Chen CH, Wu MS, et al. The safety profile of ustekinumab in the treatment of patients with psoriasis and concurrent hepatitis B or C. Br J Dermatol 2013;169:1295–303.
37. Chiu HY, Hui RC, Huang YH, et al. Safety profile of secukinumab in treatment of patients with psoriasis and concurrent hepatitis B or C: a multicentric prospective cohort study. Acta Derm Venereol 2018;98:829–34.
38. Pagnini C, Arseneau KO, Cominelli F. Natalizumab in the treatment of Crohn's disease patients. Expert Opin Biol Ther 2017;17:1433–8.
39. Wyant T, Fedyk E, Abhyankar B. An overview of the mechanism of action of the monoclonal antibody vedolizumab. J Crohns Colitis 2016;10:1437–44.
40. Hillen ME, Cook SD, Samanta A, et al. Fatal acute liver failure with hepatitis B virus infection during nataluzimab treatment in multiple sclerosis. Neurol Neuroimmunol Neuroinflamm 2015;2:e72.
41. Epstein DJ, Dunn J, Deresinski S. Infectious complications of multiple sclerosis therapies: implications for screening, prophylaxis, and management. Open Forum Infect Dis 2018;5:ofy174.
42. Palomo J, Dietrich D, Martin P, et al. The interleukin (IL)-1 cytokine family–balance between agonists and antagonists in inflammatory diseases. Cytokine 2015;76:25–37.
43. Hunter CA, Jones SA. IL-6 as a keystone cytokine in health and disease. Nat Immunol 2015;16:448–57.
44. Barone M, Notarnicola A, Lopalco G, et al. Safety of long-term biologic therapy in rheumatologic patients with a previously resolved hepatitis B viral infection. Hepatology 2015;62:40–6.
45. Nakamura J, Nagashima T, Nagatani K, et al. Reactivation of hepatitis B virus in rheumatoid arthritis patients treated with biological disease-modifying antirheumatic drugs. Int J Rheum Dis 2016;19:470–5.
46. Maier H, Isogawa M, Freeman GJ, et al. PD-1:PD-L1 interactions contribute to the functional suppression of virus-specific CD8+ T lymphocytes in the liver. J Immunol 2007;178:2714–20.
47. Fisicaro P, Valdatta C, Massari M, et al. Combined blockade of programmed death-1 and activation of CD137 increase responses of human liver T cells against HBV, but not HCV. Gastroenterology 2012;143:1576–85.
48. Gane E, Verdon DJ, Brooks AE, et al. Anti-PD-1 blockade with nivolumab with and without therapeutic vaccination for virally suppressed chronic hepatitis B: a pilot study. J Hepatol 2019. https://doi.org/10.1016/j.jhep.2019.06.028.
49. Wang ML, Rule S, Martin P, et al. Targeting BTK with ibrutinib in relapsed or refractory mantle-cell lymphoma. N Engl J Med 2013;369:507–16.

50. Byrd JC, Furman RR, Coutre SE, et al. Targeting BTK with ibrutinib in relapsed chronic lymphocytic leukemia. N Engl J Med 2013;369:32–42.
51. Treon SP, Tripsas CK, Meid K, et al. Ibrutinib in previously treated Waldenström's macroglobulinemia. N Engl J Med 2015;372:1430–40.
52. Seggewiss R, Loré K, Greiner E, et al. Imatinib inhibits T-cell receptor-mediated T-cell proliferation and activation in a dose-dependent manner. Blood 2005;105: 2473–9.
53. Ikeda K, Shiga Y, Takahashi A, et al. Fatal hepatitis B virus reactivation in a chronic myeloid leukemia patient during imatinib mesylate treatment. Leuk Lymphoma 2006;47:155–7.
54. Kang BW, Lee SJ, Moon JH, et al. Chronic myeloid leukemia patient manifesting fatal hepatitis B virus reactivation during treatment with imatinib rescued by liver transplantation: case report and literature review. Int J Hematol 2009;90:383–7.
55. Temel T, Gunduz E, Sadigova E, et al. Hepatitis B virus reactivation under treatment with nilotinib. Euroasian J Hepatogastroenterol 2015;5:112–4.
56. Yao ZH, Liao WY, Ho CC, et al. Incidence of hepatitis B reactivation during epidermal growth factor receptor tyrosine kinase inhibitor treatment in non-small-cell lung cancer patients. Eur J Cancer 2019;117:107–15.
57. Caratelli S, Arriga R, Sconocchia T, et al. In vitro elimination of EGFR-overexpressing cancer cells by CD32A chimeric receptor T cells in combination with cetuximab or panitumumab. Int J Cancer 2019. https://doi.org/10.1002/ijc.32663.
58. Ferrara N, Hillan KJ, Gerber HP, et al. Discovery and development of bevacizumab, an anti-VEGF antibody for treating cancer. Nat Rev Drug Discov 2004;3: 391–400.
59. Ferrari SM, Bocci G, Di Desidero T, et al. Lenvatinib exhibits antineoplastic activity in anaplastic thyroid cancer in vitro and in vivo. Oncol Rep 2018;39:2225–34.
60. Waldmann TA, Chen J. Disorders of the JAK/STAT pathway in T cell lymphoma pathogenesis: implications for immunotherapy. Annu Rev Immunol 2017;35: 533–50.
61. Shen CH, Hwang CE, Chen YY, et al. Hepatitis B virus reactivation associated with ruxolitinib. Ann Hematol 2014;93:1075–6.
62. Chen YM, Huang WN, Wu YD, et al. Reactivation of hepatitis B virus infection in patients with rheumatoid arthritis receiving tofacitinib: a real-world study. Ann Rheum Dis 2018;77:780–2.
63. Frazer-Abel A, Sepiashvili L, Mbughuni MM, et al. Overview of laboratory testing and clinical presentations of complement deficiencies and dysregulation. Adv Clin Chem 2016;77:1–75.
64. European Association for the Study of the Liver. EASL 2017 clinical practice guidelines on the management of hepatitis B virus infection. J Hepatol 2017; 67:370–98.
65. Pérez-Alvarez R, Díaz-Lagares C, García-Hernández F, et al. Hepatitis B virus (HBV) reactivation in patients receiving tumor necrosis factor (TNF)-targeted therapy: analysis of 257 cases. Medicine (Baltimore) 2011;90:359–71.
66. Mori S, Fujiyama S. Hepatitis B virus reactivation associated with antirheumatic therapy: risk and prophylaxis recommendations. World J Gastroenterol 2015; 21:10274–89.
67. Xuan D, Yu Y, Shao L, et al. Hepatitis reactivation in patients with rheumatic diseases after immunosuppressive therapy-a report of long-term follow-up of serial cases and literature review. Clin Rheumatol 2014;33:577–86.

68. Lee YH, Bae SC, Song GG. Hepatitis B virus (HBV) reactivation in rheumatic patients with hepatitis core antigen (HBV occult carriers) undergoing anti-tumor necrosis factor therapy. Clin Exp Rheumatol 2013;31:118–21.

69. Pauly MP, Tucker LY, Szpakowski JL, et al. Incidence of hepatitis B virus reactivation and hepatotoxicity in patients receiving long-term treatment with tumor necrosis factor antagonists. Clin Gastroenterol Hepatol 2018;16:1964–73.

70. Koskinas J, Tampaki M, Doumba PP, et al. Hepatitis B virus reactivation during therapy with ustekinumab for psoriasis in a hepatitis B surface-antigen-negative anti-HBs-positive patient. Br J Dermatol 2013;168:679–80.

71. Iannitto E, Minardi V, Calvaruso G, et al. Hepatitis B virus reactivation and alemtuzumab therapy. Eur J Haematol 2005;74:254–8.

72. Lake AC. Hepatitis B reactivation in a long-term nonprogressor due to nivolumab therapy. AIDS 2017;31:2115–8.

73. Chang CS, Tsai CY, Yan SL. Hepatitis B reactivation in patients receiving targeted therapies. Hematology 2017;22:592–8.

74. Giammarco S, Peffault de Latour R, Sica S, et al. Transplant outcome for patients with acquired aplastic anemia over the age of 40: has the outcome improved? Blood 2018;131:1989–92.

75. Gill H, Leung GMK, Seto WK, et al. Risk of viral reactivation in patients with occult hepatitis B virus infection during ruxolitinib treatment. Ann Hematol 2019;98:215–8.

76. Zurawska U, Hicks LK, Woo G, et al. Hepatitis B virus screening before chemotherapy for lymphoma: a cost-effectiveness analysis. J Clin Oncol 2012;30:3167–73.

77. Clark FL, Drummond MW, Chambers S, et al. Successful treatment with lamivudine for fulminant reactivated hepatitis B infection following intensive therapy for high-grade non-Hodgkin's lymphoma. Ann Oncol 1998;9:385–7.

78. Ahmed A, Keeffe EB. Lamivudine therapy for chemotherapy-induced reactivation of hepatitis B virus infection. Am J Gastroenterol 1999;94:249–51.

79. Cainelli F, Longhi MS, Concia E, et al. Failure of lamivudine therapy for chemotherapy-induced reactivation of hepatitis B. Am J Gastroenterol 2001;96:1651–2.

80. Ogawa E, Furusyo N, Nguyen MH. Tenofovir alafenamide in the treatment of chronic hepatitis B: design, development, and place in therapy. Drug Des Devel Ther 2017;11:3197–204.

81. Hsu YC, Wei MT, Nguyen MH. Tenofovir alafenamide as compared to tenofovir disoproxil fumarate in the management of chronic hepatitis B with recent trends in patient demographics. Expert Rev Gastroenterol Hepatol 2017;11:999–1008.

82. Nguyen LH, Ko S, Wong SS, et al. Ethnic differences in viral dominance patterns in patients with hepatitis B virus and hepatitis C virus dual infection. Hepatology 2011;53:1839–45.

83. Bini EJ, Perumalswami PV. Hepatitis B virus infection among American patients with chronic hepatitis C virus infection: prevalence, racial/ethnic differences, and viral interactions. Hepatology 2010;51:759–66.

84. Collins JM, Raphael KL, Terry C, et al. Hepatitis B virus reactivation during successful treatment of hepatitis C virus with sofosbuvir and simeprevir. Clin Infect Dis 2015;61:1304–6.

85. Chen G, Wang C, Chen J, et al. Hepatitis B reactivation in hepatitis B and C co-infected patients treated with antiviral agents: a systematic review and meta-analysis. Hepatology 2017;66:13–26.

86. Liu CJ, Chuang WL, Sheen IS, et al. Efficacy of ledipasvir and sofosbuvir treatment of HCV infection in patients coinfected with HBV. Gastroenterology 2018; 154:989–97.

87. Spradling PR, Richardson JT, Buchacz K, et al. Prevalence of chronic hepatitis B virus infection among patients in the HIV Outpatient Study, 1996-2007. J Viral Hepat 2010;17:879–86.

JC Polyomavirus Infection Potentiated by Biologics

Ashrit Multani, MD[a],*, Dora Y. Ho, MD, PhD[b]

KEYWORDS

- John Cunningham virus • JC virus • Polyomavirus
- Progressive multifocal leukoencephalopathy • PML • Biologic agents • Natalizumab
- Rituximab

KEY POINTS

- John Cunningham polyomavirus (JCPyV) is a ubiquitous DNA virus that is the cause of JCPyV encephalopathy, which includes progressive multifocal leukoencephalopathy (PML) and other neurologic diseases.
- The pathogenesis of JCPyV encephalopathy is related to multiple levels of dysfunction in cell-mediated and humoral immune systems.
- The risk for JCPyV encephalopathy varies among biologic classes and among biologics within the same class. Drug-specific causality is difficult to establish because of concomitant or sequential immunomodulator use and/or disease-related immunocompromising conditions.
- The highest risk for JCPyV encephalopathy has been observed with natalizumab (for which estimated risk stratification–based screening algorithms are recommended) followed by rituximab.
- JCPyV encephalopathy carries a poor prognosis with high rates of significant mortality and morbidity because there is no effective prophylaxis or treatment.

INTRODUCTION

JC polyomavirus (JCPyV) is a human polyomavirus that was first identified in 1971 as the cause of progressive multifocal leukoencephalopathy (PML) in the brain of John Cunningham, after whom it is named.[1] Because JCPyV-associated disease in the central nervous system (CNS) may not always be progressive, may present as a unifocal lesion (especially in cases associated with natalizumab), and may involve the gray matter, JCPyV encephalopathy is a more appropriate terminology to cover all associated disease manifestations in the CNS: classic PML,

[a] Division of Infectious Diseases, Department of Medicine, David Geffen School of Medicine at UCLA, 10833 Le Conte Avenue, CHS 37-121, Los Angeles, CA 90095, USA; [b] Division of Infectious Diseases and Geographic Medicine, Department of Medicine, Stanford University School of Medicine, 300 Pasteur Drive, Lane Building L-135, Stanford, CA 94305, USA
* Corresponding author.
E-mail address: amultani@mednet.ucla.edu

Infect Dis Clin N Am 34 (2020) 359–388
https://doi.org/10.1016/j.idc.2020.02.007
0891-5520/20/© 2020 Elsevier Inc. All rights reserved.

id.theclinics.com

inflammatory PML, JCPyV cerebellar granule cell neuronopathy, JCPyV encephalopathy, and JCPyV meningitis.[2-7] JCPyV encephalopathy occurs almost exclusively in immunocompromised hosts, including those with advanced human immunodeficiency virus/AIDS, hematologic malignancies, and solid organ or hematopoietic cell transplantation, and those receiving certain immunomodulatory biologic agents.[8-10] Common clinical manifestations include behavioral and cognitive abnormalities, motor weakness, gait abnormalities, incoordination, visual field deficits, and speech and language disturbances; sensory loss, seizures, headache, diplopia, and signs of pyramidal tract and cerebellar dysfunction are seen less frequently.[11] MRI of the brain is the neuroimaging modality of choice, usually showing multifocal hyperintense lesions of the involved white matter on T2-weighted images and fluid-attenuated inversion recovery images in classic PML.[11] These radiographic findings may not be present in other forms of JCPyV encephalopathy.[4,5,7,12] When combined with clinical and radiographic features, detection of JCPyV DNA by polymerase chain reaction in cerebrospinal fluid (CSF) is sufficient for confirming the diagnosis and averts the need for brain biopsy.[11,13] Because of the lack of reliable therapeutic options, JCPyV encephalopathy is often fatal and most survivors are left with neurologic sequelae resulting in moderate to severe disability.[14,15] Biologic agents are being increasingly adopted for the treatment of autoimmune diseases, hematologic malignancies, solid tumors, and other inflammatory conditions. Their risks for potentiating JCPyV reactivation and encephalopathy are heterogeneous and not well understood.

BIOLOGY OF JC POLYOMAVIRUS
Epidemiology

JCPyV IgG seropositivity is found in 44% to 77% of adults in the United States and higher rates are seen in certain South American, European, and Asian countries.[16-18] Seroprevalence studies have consistently demonstrated increasing seropositivity with age worldwide.[16-18] JCPyV has three superclusters, one major serotype, and 12 subtypes with particular geographic distributions: type 1 in the United States, type 4 in the United States and Europe, type 2 in Asia, and types 3 and 6 in Africa.[19] In contrast with studies from the United States and Europe, JCPyV encephalopathy has a lower reported incidence in India and Africa.[20] Multiple theories have been proposed to explain this phenomenon, including differences in virulence related to JCPyV subtypes, JCPyV and human immunodeficiency virus interviral interactions, and host genetic susceptibility. How these factors might interplay to potentiate the risk of JCPyV encephalopathy has yet to be elucidated.[20]

Virology

JCPyV is one of multiple human polyomavirus species belonging to the Polyomaviridae family. Polyomaviruses are small (40–45 nm diameter), nonenveloped, icosahedral, double-stranded DNA viruses. The circular double-stranded DNA genome is about 5 kbp and has three distinct regions: (1) the early viral gene region, which includes the large T and small t antigens, regulatory proteins responsible for viral transformation, replication, and regulation of gene expression; (2) the late viral gene region, which encodes the capsid proteins VP1, VP2, and VP3 and a small cytoplasmic protein called agnoprotein (which seems to have multiple regulatory functions including regulation of JCPyV transcription and translation and in dysregulation of host cell cycle and DNA repair); and (3) the noncoding control region, which regulates early and late viral gene expression in sync with the differentiation and activation of the host cell.[21-23]

JCPyV uses a linear sialylated pentasaccharide chain as a receptor in addition to the serotonergic 5HT2A receptor, which is present on oligodendrocytes, lymphocytes, renal, and pulmonary cells.[24,25] After JCPyV binds to the cell surface, clathrin-coated pits form and endocytosis ensues.[26,27] The virus travels through the endocytic compartment to the endoplasmic reticulum where the viral capsid is partially uncoated.[27] It then retrotranslocates to the nucleus where viral transcription and replication occur via the three distinct regions previously discussed.[21–23,27]

Transmission

JCPyV has been identified in sewage and in stool, suggesting that fecal-oral transmission may occur.[28–30] JCPyV has also been detected in tonsillar tissue, tendering the possibility of oral and/or respiratory transmission.[31] Transmission has been shown to occur within and outside the family.[32,33] Vertical transmission has also been reported.[34]

Site of Latency

During primary infection of oropharyngeal, respiratory tract, and/or gastrointestinal tract mucosal surfaces, JCPyV spreads to other organs and tissues. After primary infection, JCPyV may remain latent in renal tubular epithelial cells as evidenced by its detection in renal tissue and urine irrespective of host immune status.[18,35–41] The brain and bone marrow may also be important reservoirs.[42–45] JCPyV DNAemia typically only occurs in the setting of immunocompromise but this does not correlate with the presence of JCPyV encephalopathy.[46,47]

Pathogenesis

Multiple levels of deficiency and/or dysfunction in humoral and cellular immune responses may predispose to JCPyV encephalopathy via complex mechanisms.[45,48,49] In the setting of impaired immunity, hematogenous spread of the virions from outside the CNS or reactivation of latent local infection within the CNS may occur.[45,48,49] Neurogenic spread through the axons of infected neurons has also been speculated.[6] JCPyV-infected B cells, CD34 progenitor cells, and/or other peripheral blood leukocyte subsets may be implicated in viral reactivation and transportation to the CNS.[45,48,50,51] Once in the CNS, JCPyV causes a lytic infection of oligodendrocytes and astrocytes (resulting in demyelination) in addition to granule cell neurons (resulting in focal cell loss, neuronopathy, and cerebellar atrophy).[3–6,52] The optic nerves and spinal cord are typically spared.

PATHOGENESIS OF JC POLYOMAVIRUS ENCEPHALOPATHY WITH BIOLOGICS

The risk for JCPyV encephalopathy differs between biologic classes and among different agents within the same class. This risk is difficult to estimate because of multiple confounding variables, including host-related immune defects, concomitant or sequential immunomodulatory use, and other pathogen-specific factors. To help provide guidance to clinicians and patients, a risk classification schema has been proposed and updated over time.[53–55] Three classes of drugs were identified based on the frequency with which JCPyV encephalopathy was observed, the nature of the underlying disease being treated (ie, whether the disease itself predisposed to JCPyV encephalopathy in the absence of the specific drug), and the time between drug initiation and JCPyV encephalopathy development.[54] Class 1 agents have high risk of JCPyV encephalopathy, a long latency period from drug initiation to the development of JCPyV encephalopathy, and are indicated to treat diseases that are not known to predispose to JCPyV encephalopathy.[54] Class 2 agents have low risk of JCPyV encephalopathy, are used for diseases that are known to predispose to JCPyV encephalopathy, and do not have the required latency period seen with class 1 agents.[54] Class 3 agents have low or no risk of JCPyV encephalopathy, with only sporadic cases being reported.[54] The biologics reviewed in this article, their clinical uses, and their risk for JCPyV encephalopathy are summarized in **Table 1**.

Tumor Necrosis Factor-α Inhibitors

Only five cases of tumor necrosis factor (TNF)-α-inhibitor-associated JCPyV encephalopathy have been published but these cases are confounded by concomitant immunomodulator use or underlying disease.[56–61] Two cases were reported in patients who received infliximab in combination with methotrexate.[59,61] Two cases were reported with adalimumab, although both patients also received methotrexate either simultaneously or sequentially.[57,58] Etanercept was associated with JCPyV encephalopathy in a patient who was also taking prednisone.[60] JCPyV encephalopathy has not been described with certolizumab or golimumab use. Multiple patients experienced demyelinating disease after TNF-α inhibitor use and some have speculated that these were undiagnosed cases of JCPyV encephalopathy.[62]

The pathogenesis of TNF-α-inhibitor-associated JCPyV encephalopathy is not well understood. TNF-α inhibitors could influence the frequency of JCPyV infection, viral load, and genotype selection.[63–65] They may interfere with lymphocyte recruitment and decrease interferon-γ levels, thereby alleviating control of the antiviral state and allowing JCPyV reactivation and dissemination.[49,63–66]

Agents Targeting B Cells

Anti-CD20 agents

Rituximab has been associated with JCPyV encephalopathy in several publications, and all of these patients received other immunomodulators or had additional risk factors.[67–71] The risk of JCPyV encephalopathy with rituximab has been estimated to be 1:30,000.[54] It has been classified as a class 2 agent with low risk.[53–55] Ibritumomab tiuxetan has been associated with at least six cases of JCPyV encephalopathy.[72,73] Four cases of JCPyV encephalopathy have been associated with ofatumumab, all in heavily pretreated patients with relapsed or refractory chronic lymphocytic leukemia (CLL).[74,75] Obinutuzumab has been associated with JCPyV encephalopathy in four patients, including three patients who had also received rituximab and one patient with CLL who was treatment-naive.[76,77] No cases have been reported with ocrelizumab.[78–81]

The risk of JCPyV encephalopathy associated with biologics targeting B cells highlights the importance of humoral immune responses in controlling this virus. This may be caused by impaired antibody responses, inefficient clearance of latently JCPyV-infected B cells, or dysfunctional antigen presentation by B cells to T cells.[45,82] Compared with rituximab, obinutuzumab seems to be more potent with B-cell depletion but does not have as high a reported risk of JCPyV encephalopathy.[76,83] It remains to be elucidated if the differences in risk between rituximab and other anti-CD20 biologics are caused by unknown off-target effects of rituximab or the lack of long-term safety data with these newer agents. Many of the cases associated with obinutuzumab and ofatumumab have disproportionately occurred in patients with CLL, suggesting that other host-related immune defects are likely implicated.[84,85]

Other B cell–targeted agents

Brentuximab has been associated with JCPyV encephalopathy in a handful of reports.[67,77,86–91] It has been classified as a class 2 agent.[53,54] The time to onset of

Table 1
Biologic agents, clinical uses, and risk classification for JC polyomavirus encephalopathy

Pharmacologic Agent	Brand Names	Clinical Uses	Risk Classification
TNF-α inhibitors			
Adalimumab	Amjevita Cyltezo Humira	Ankylosing spondylitis Crohn disease Hidradenitis suppurativa Plaque psoriasis Psoriatic arthritis Pyoderma gangrenosum Rheumatoid arthritis Ulcerative colitis Uveitis	Class 3
Certolizumab	Cimzia	Ankylosing spondylitis Axial spondyloarthritis Crohn disease Plaque psoriasis Psoriatic arthritis Rheumatoid arthritis	Class 3
Etanercept	Enbrel	Ankylosing spondylitis Graft vs host disease Plaque psoriasis Psoriatic arthritis Pyoderma gangrenosum Rheumatoid arthritis	Class 3
Golimumab	Simponi	Ankylosing spondylitis Axial spondyloarthritis Psoriatic arthritis Rheumatoid arthritis Ulcerative colitis	Class 3
Infliximab	Inflectra Remicade Renflexis	Ankylosing spondylitis Crohn disease Plaque psoriasis Psoriatic arthritis Pustular psoriasis Rheumatoid arthritis Ulcerative colitis	Class 3
Agents targeting B cells			
Anti-CD20 agents			
Ibritumomab tiuxetan	Zevalin Y-90 Zevalin	Non-Hodgkin lymphoma	Class 3
Obinutuzumab	Gazyva	Chronic lymphocytic leukemia Follicular lymphoma	Class 3
Ocrelizumab	Ocrevus	Multiple sclerosis	Class 3
Ofatumumab	Arzerra	Chronic lymphocytic leukemia	Class 3

(continued on next page)

Table 1 *(continued)*			
Pharmacologic Agent	**Brand Names**	**Clinical Uses**	**Risk Classification**
Rituximab	Rituxan	Antibody-mediated rejection of organ transplant Autoimmune hemolytic anemia Burkitt lymphoma Chronic lymphocytic leukemia CNS lymphoma Graft-vs-host disease Granulomatosis with polyangiitis Hodgkin lymphoma Idiopathic membranous nephropathy Immune thrombocytopenia Lupus nephritis Microscopic polyangiitis Mucosa-associated lymphoid tissue lymphoma Myasthenia gravis Neuromyelitis optica Non-Hodgkin lymphoma Pemphigus vulgaris Post-transplant lymphoproliferative disorder Rheumatoid arthritis Splenic marginal zone lymphoma Thrombotic thrombocytopenic purpura Waldenström macroglobulinemia	Class 2
Other B-cell-targeted agents			
Brentuximab	Adcetris	Anaplastic large cell lymphoma Hodgkin lymphoma Mycoses fungoides Peripheral T-cell lymphoma	Class 2
Daratumumab	Darzalex	Multiple myeloma	Class 3
Epratuzumab	LymphoCide	Acute lymphoblastic leukemia Non-Hodgkin lymphoma Systemic lupus erythematosus	Class 3

(continued on next page)

Table 1
(continued)

Pharmacologic Agent	Brand Names	Clinical Uses	Risk Classification
Gemtuzumab ozogamicin	Mylotarg	Acute myeloid leukemia Acute promyelocytic leukemia	Class 3
Inotuzumab ozogamicin	Besponsa	Acute lymphoblastic leukemia	Class 3
B-cell activating factor inhibitor			
Belimumab	Benlysta	Systemic lupus erythematosus	Class 2
Agents targeting T-cell activation			
CTLA-4 and LFA-3/CD-2 inhibitors			
Abatacept	Orencia	Psoriatic arthritis Rheumatoid arthritis	Class 3
Alefacept[a]	Amevive	Cutaneous T-cell lymphoma Non-Hodgkin lymphoma Plaque psoriasis	Class 3
Belatacept	Nulojix	Prophylaxis of organ rejection	Class 3
IL-23 inhibitors			
Guselkumab	Tremfya	Plaque psoriasis	Class 3
Tildrakizumab	Ilumya	Plaque psoriasis	Class 3
Ustekinumab	Stelara	Crohn disease Plaque psoriasis Psoriatic arthritis	Class 3
IL-17 inhibitors			
Brodalumab	Siliq	Plaque psoriasis	Class 3
Ixekizumab	Taltz	Ankylosing spondylitis Plaque psoriasis Psoriatic arthritis	Class 3
Secukinumab	Cosentyx	Ankylosing spondylitis Plaque psoriasis Psoriatic arthritis	Class 3
Direct T-cell inhibitors and agents targeting T-cell migration and chemotaxis			
α_4-Integrin inhibitors			
Natalizumab	Tysabri	Crohn disease Multiple sclerosis	Class 1
Vedolizumab	Entyvio	Crohn disease Ulcerative colitis	Class 3
LFA-1 inhibitor			
Efalizumab[a]	Raptiva	Plaque psoriasis	Class 1

(continued on next page)

Table 1 (continued)			
Pharmacologic Agent	Brand Names	Clinical Uses	Risk Classification
Anti-CD52 agent			
Alemtuzumab	Campath Lemtrada	Allogeneic stem cell transplant conditioning regimen Aplastic anemia Autoimmune cytopenias Chronic lymphocytic leukemia Graft-vs-host disease Hemophagocytic lymphohistiocytosis Multiple sclerosis Mycosis fungoides Solid organ transplantation induction T-cell large granular lymphocytic leukemia T-cell prolymphocytic leukemia	Class 3
IL-2 receptor inhibitors			
Basiliximab	Simulect	Graft-vs-host disease Prophylaxis of organ rejection	Class 3
Daclizumab[a]	Zinbryta	Multiple sclerosis	Class 3
CD319-targeted agent			
Elotuzumab	Empliciti	Multiple myeloma	Class 3
CCR4-targeted agent			
Mogamulizumab	Poteligeo	Cutaneous T-cell lymphoma Mycoses fungoides	Class 3
Other IL and IgE inhibitors			
IL-1 inhibitors			
Anakinra	Kineret	Familial Mediterranean fever Gout Neonatal-onset multisystem inflammatory disease Pericarditis Rheumatoid arthritis	Class 3
Canakinumab	Ilaris	Cryopyrin-associated periodic syndromes Familial Mediterranean fever Gout Hyperimmunoglobulin D syndrome Mevalonate kinase deficiency Tumor necrosis factor receptor associated periodic syndrome	Class 3

(continued on next page)

Table 1
(continued)

Pharmacologic Agent	Brand Names	Clinical Uses	Risk Classification
Rilonacept	Arcalyst	Cryopyrin-associated periodic syndromes	Class 3
IL-4 inhibitor			
Dupilumab	Dupixent	Asthma Atopic dermatitis Rhinosinusitis with nasal polyposis	Class 3
IL-5 inhibitors			
Benralizumab	Fasenra	Asthma	Class 3
Mepolizumab	Nucala	Asthma Eosinophilic granulomatosis with polyangiitis	Class 3
Reslizumab	Cinqair	Asthma	Class 3
IL-6 inhibitors			
Sarilumab	Kevzara	Rheumatoid arthritis	Class 3
Siltuximab	Sylvant	Multicentric Castleman disease	Class 3
Tocilizumab	Actemra	Cytokine release syndrome Giant cell arteritis Rheumatoid arthritis	Class 3
IL-13 inhibitor			
Lebrikizumab	NA	Asthma Atopic dermatitis	Class 3
IgE inhibitor			
Omalizumab	Xolair	Asthma Chronic idiopathic urticaria	Class 3
Checkpoint inhibitors			
Atezolizumab	Tecentriq	Breast cancer Non–small cell lung cancer Small cell lung cancer Urothelial carcinoma	Class 3
Avelumab	Bavencio	Merkel cell carcinoma Renal cell carcinoma Urothelial carcinoma	Class 3
Cemiplimab	Libtayo	Cutaneous squamous cell carcinoma	Class 3
Durvalumab	Imfinzi	Non–small cell lung cancer Urothelial carcinoma	Class 3
Ipilimumab	Yervoy	Colorectal cancer Melanoma Renal cell carcinoma Small cell lung cancer	Class 3

(continued on next page)

Table 1
(continued)

Pharmacologic Agent	Brand Names	Clinical Uses	Risk Classification
Nivolumab	Opdivo	Colorectal cancer Head and neck squamous cell cancer Hepatocellular carcinoma Hodgkin lymphoma Melanoma Non–small cell lung cancer Renal cell carcinoma Small cell lung cancer Urothelial carcinoma	Class 3
Pembrolizumab	Keytruda	Cervical cancer Endometrial cancer Esophageal cancer Gastric cancer Head and neck squamous cell cancer Hepatocellular carcinoma Hodgkin lymphoma Melanoma Merkel cell carcinoma Microsatellite instability-high cancer Non–small cell lung cancer Primary mediastinal large B-cell lymphoma Renal cell carcinoma Small cell lung cancer Urothelial carcinoma	Class 3
Tremelimumab	NA	NA	Class 3
Tyrosine kinase inhibitors			
Bruton tyrosine kinase inhibitors			
Acalabrutinib	Calquence	Mantle cell lymphoma	Class 3
Ibrutinib	Imbruvica	Chronic lymphocytic leukemia Graft-vs-host disease Mantle cell lymphoma Marginal zone lymphoma Small lymphocytic lymphoma Waldenström macroglobulinemia	Class 3
Small molecule BCR-ABL tyrosine kinase inhibitors			
Bafetinib	NA	Chronic myelogenous leukemia	Class 3
Bosutinib	Bosulif	Chronic myelogenous leukemia	Class 3
Dasatinib	Sprycel	Acute lymphoblastic leukemia Chronic myelogenous leukemia Gastrointestinal stromal tumor	Class 3

(continued on next page)

Table 1
(continued)

Pharmacologic Agent	Brand Names	Clinical Uses	Risk Classification
Imatinib	Gleevec	Acute lymphoblastic leukemia	Class 3
		Aggressive systemic mastocytosis associated with eosinophilia	
		Chordoma	
		Chronic eosinophilic leukemia	
		Chronic myelogenous leukemia	
		Dermatofibrosarcoma protuberans	
		Desmoid tumors	
		Gastrointestinal stromal tumor	
		Hypereosinophilic syndrome	
		Melanoma	
		Myelodysplastic syndrome	
		Myeloproliferative disease	
		Stem cell transplant for chronic myelogenous leukemia	
Nilotinib	Tasigna	Acute lymphoblastic leukemia	Class 3
		Chronic myelogenous leukemia	
		Gastrointestinal stromal tumor	
Ponatinib	Iclusig	Acute lymphoblastic leukemia	Class 3
		Chronic myelogenous leukemia	
Phosphoinositide 3-kinase inhibitors (buparlisib, duvelisib, idelalisib, rigosertib)			
Buparlisib	NA	Breast cancer	Class 3
Duvelisib	Copiktra	Chronic lymphocytic leukemia	Class 3
		Follicular lymphoma	
		Small lymphocytic leukemia	
Idelalisib	Zydelig	Chronic lymphocytic leukemia	Class 3
		Follicular lymphoma	
		Small lymphocytic leukemia	
Rigosertib	Estybon	Chronic myelomonocytic leukemia	Class 3
Other tyrosine kinase inhibitors			
Axitinib	Inlyta	Renal cell carcinoma	Class 3
		Thyroid cancer	

(*continued on next page*)

Table 1
(continued)

Pharmacologic Agent	Brand Names	Clinical Uses	Risk Classification
Cabozantinib	Cabometyx Cometriq	Hepatocellular carcinoma Renal cell carcinoma Thyroid cancer	Class 3
Pazopanib	Votrient	Renal cell carcinoma Soft tissue sarcoma Thyroid cancer	Class 3
Ramucirumab	Cyramza	Colorectal cancer Gastric cancer Hepatocellular carcinoma Non–small cell lung cancer	Class 3
Regorafenib	Stivarga	Colorectal cancer Gastrointestinal stromal tumor Hepatocellular carcinoma	Class 3
Sorafenib	Nexavar	Angiosarcoma Gastrointestinal stromal tumor Hepatocellular carcinoma Renal cell carcinoma Thyroid cancer	Class 3
Sunitinib	Sutent	Gastrointestinal stromal tumor Pancreatic neuroendocrine tumor Renal cell carcinoma Soft tissue sarcoma Thyroid cancer	Class 3
Vandetanib	Caprelsa	Thyroid cancer	Class 3
EGFR inhibitors and VEGF inhibitors			
EGFR tyrosine kinase inhibitors			
Afatinib	Gilotrif	Non–small cell lung cancer	Class 3
Erlotinib	Tarceva	Non–small cell lung cancer Pancreatic cancer	Class 3
Gefitinib	Iressa	Non–small cell lung cancer	Class 3
Lapatinib	Tykerb	Breast cancer	Class 3
Neratinib	Nerlynx	Breast cancer	Class 3
Osimertinib	Tagrisso	Non–small lung cancer	Class 3
EGFR-inhibiting monoclonal antibodies			
Cetuximab	Erbitux	Colorectal cancer Cutaneous squamous cell cancer Head and neck squamous cell cancer Penile squamous cell cancer	Class 3
Panitumumab	Vectibix	Colorectal cancer	Class 3
VEGF inhibitors			

(continued on next page)

Table 1
(continued)

Pharmacologic Agent	Brand Names	Clinical Uses	Risk Classification
Ruxolltlnib	Jakafi	Graft-vs-host disease Myelofibrosis Polycythemia vera	Class 3
Tofacitinib	Xeljanz	Psoriatic arthritis Rheumatoid arthritis Ulcerative colitis	Class 3
C5 inhibitors			
Eculizumab	Soliris	Atypical hemolytic uremic syndrome Myasthenia gravis Neuromyelitis optica Paroxysmal nocturnal hemoglobinuria	Class 3
Ravulizumab	Ultomiris	Paroxysmal nocturnal hemoglobinuria	Class 3
Sphingosine-1-phosphate receptor modulator			
Fingolimod	Gilenya PMS-Fingolimod	Multiple sclerosis	Class 2
Proteasome inhibitors			
Bortezomib	Velcade	Antibody-mediated rejection of organ transplant Cutaneous T-cell lymphoma Follicular lymphoma Mantle cell lymphoma Multiple myeloma Peripheral T-cell lymphoma Systemic light-chain amyloidosis Waldenström macroglobulinemia	Class 3
Carfilzomib	Kyprolis	Multiple myeloma Waldenström macroglobulinemia	Class 3
Ixazomib	Ninlaro	Multiple myeloma	Class 3

Class 1, high risk; class 2, low risk; class 3, very low or no risk.
Abbreviations: EGFR, epidermal growth factor receptor; IL, interleukin; NA, not applicable; VEGF, vascular epidermal growth factor receptor.
[a] No longer available.
Date from Refs.[53–55]

JCPyV encephalopathy and the prior duration of therapy have been described to be much shorter with brentuximab (within 6–9 weeks in some cases) compared with anti-CD20 monoclonal antibodies (median, 63 weeks) or natalizumab (median, 26 months).[67,91] No cases of JCPyV encephalopathy have been reported with the anti-CD22 agents epratuzumab and inotuzumab ozogamicin, the anti-CD33 agent gemtuzumab ozogamicin, and the anti-CD38 agent daratumumab.[91]

Because the cases associated with brentuximab occurred in patients with hematologic malignancies who also received other immunomodulators, its exact risk and mechanism in leading to JCPyV encephalopathy is difficult to determine. The pathogenesis may be caused by depletion of CD30-expressing activated T cells and reduced immune surveillance in the CNS.[67]

B-cell activating factor inhibitor

Belimumab has been associated with JCPyV encephalopathy in two patients with systemic lupus erythematosus who received other immunomodulators previously and concomitantly.[92,93] It has been classified as a class 2 agent.[53,55]

It has been hypothesized that B-cell suppression might lead to proliferation and CNS translocation of infected pre-B cells or indirectly impair T-cell control of JCPyV replication.[92,94] Compared with other rheumatologic diseases, systemic lupus erythematosus seems to particularly predispose to an increased risk for JCPyV encephalopathy irrespective of the nature and degree of iatrogenic immunomodulation, if any.[92,95–97] The reasons for this phenomenon are unclear, but may be caused by low CD4 T-cell counts and CD4/CD8 T-cell ratios.[96,97]

Agents Targeting T-Cell Activation

CTLA-4 and LFA-3/CD2 inhibitors

Belatacept has been associated with JCPyV encephalopathy in two kidney transplant recipients who were also receiving other transplant-related immunosuppressive agents.[98,99] One of the two cases reported with belatacept was suspected to be caused by refractory T-cell anergy.[99] JCPyV encephalopathy has not been reported with abatacept.[100] Alefacept has not been associated with JCPyV encephalopathy despite its reduction of CD4 T cells.[101]

Interleukin-23 inhibitors

JCPyV encephalopathy has not been reported with ustekinumab (which additionally inhibits interleukin [IL]-12), guselkumab, and tildrakizumab.[102]

Interleukin-17 inhibitors

Secukinumab, ixekizumab, and brodalumab have not been associated with JCPyV encephalopathy.[102]

Direct T-Cell Inhibitors and Agents Targeting T-Cell Migration and Chemotaxis

α_4-Integrin inhibitors

Natalizumab (an α_4-integrin inhibitor that acts against α_4/β_1- and α_4/β_7-integrin) was first approved in 2004 and has been the biologic agent most strongly associated with an increased risk of JCPyV encephalopathy. Three cases were first described in 2005, leading to the withdrawal of natalizumab from the market that same year.[103–105] After a careful safety review and no additional deaths, it was reintroduced in 2006 under a special prescription program. Numerous similar reports of JCPyV encephalopathy followed, thereby establishing an indisputable and perilous relationship between the two.[14,68,101,106–111] Nevertheless, it was kept on the market because its clinical benefits outweighed its risks. This is the only currently available class 1 agent with high risk for JCPyV encephalopathy.[53–55,85]

Risk stratification for natalizumab-associated JCPyV encephalopathy is calculated based on anti-JCPyV IgG antibody index, prior immunosuppression, and duration of natalizumab exposure.[84,110,112–114] Cumulative risk estimates are presented in **Table 2**. The estimated risk ranges from less than 1:10,000 in treatment-naive seronegative patients to 1:31 in treatment-experienced seropositive patients with natalizumab exposure of 25 to 48 months.[112] Extended interval dosing may decrease risk of JCPyV encephalopathy and allow a less severe course when it does occur.[111,115,116]

Table 2
Cumulative risk estimates of JC polyomavirus encephalopathy according to number of natalizumab infusions and anti-JC polyomavirus IgG antibody index scores in patients with and without previous immunosuppressant use

Natalizumab Exposure (Number of Infusions)	Patients Without Previous Immunosuppressant Use, per 1000 Patients			Patients with Previous Immunosuppressant Use, per 1000 Patients
	Index ≤0.9	Index >0.9 to ≤1.5	Index >1.5	
0	0.0 (0.0–0.0)	0.0 (0.0–0.0)	0.0 (0.0–0.0)	0.0 (0.0–0.0)
12	0.01 (0.00–0.03)	0.06 (0.00–0.15)	0.2 (0.0–0.5)	0.4 (0.0–1.0)
24	0.06 (0.00–0.17)	0.3 (0.0–0.7)	1.1 (0.4–1.8)	0.8 (0.0–1.8)
36	0.2 (0.0–0.6)	1.1 (0.3–2.0)	3.7 (2.3–5.2)	4.4 (1.5–7.2)
48	0.6 (0.0–1.6)	3.1 (1.2–5.0)	10.4 (7.7–13.2)	12.6 (7.2–18.1)
60	1.1 (0.0–2.8)	5.5 (2.7–8.3)	18.2 (14.1–22.4)	21.3 (14.1–22.3)
72	1.6 (0.0–4.3)	8.5 (4.8–12.2)	28.0 (22.0–34.0)	27.0 (18.4–39.5)

Data are cumulative risk estimates (95% confidence interval) for the pooled cohort. Lengths of natalizumab exposure are given as number of infusions.

Reprinted with permission from Elsevier (Lancet Neurology; Volume 16, Issue 11; Ho PR, Koendgen H, Campbell N, Haddock B, Richman S, Chang I; Risk of natalizumab-associated progressive multifocal leukoencephalopathy in patients with multiple sclerosis: a retrospective analysis of data from four clinical studies; pages 925–933; Copyright 2017.)

In stark contrast, vedolizumab (another α_4-integrin inhibitor that targets only α_4/β_7-integrin) has not been reported to cause even a single case.[101,109,117–123]

The striking difference in risk between these two α_4-integrin inhibitors provides invaluable insights into the pathogenesis of JCPyV encephalopathy. Whereas vedolizumab specifically inhibits interaction of lymphocytes with mucosal addressin cellular adhesion molecule-1 on gut vascular endothelium, natalizumab also inhibits lymphocyte interaction with vascular cell adhesion molecule-1 on tissue vascular endothelium, thereby prohibiting lymphocyte homing to the brain, reducing immune surveillance within the CNS, and promoting JCPyV reactivation.[8,109,120,124] Other supportive evidence for the risk difference between vedolizumab and natalizumab includes the lack of peripheral lymphocytosis with vedolizumab, lack of CD4/CD8 T-cell ratio inversion in CSF with vedolizumab compared with natalizumab, and lack of protection of anti-α_4/β_7 antibody in the primate model of multiple sclerosis.[124] These findings suggest that agents targeting leukocyte trafficking to the gut may avoid systemic infectious diseases, such as JCPyV encephalopathy.[124]

LFA-1 inhibitor
Efalizumab is an LFA-1 inhibitor and anti-CD11a monoclonal antibody that has also been associated with an increased risk of JCPyV encephalopathy.[8,68,101,125–127] Three patients who received efalizumab monotherapy for more than 3 years developed JCPyV encephalopathy.[125,128] A fourth patient died of progressive neurologic decline of unclear cause but was suspected to be related to JCPyV.[125,128] Because of an estimated risk of 1:500 cases of JCPyV encephalopathy, efalizumab was classified as a class 1 agent before being withdrawn from the market in 2009.[8,53–56,126,129]

The pathogenesis of JCPyV encephalopathy with efalizumab is believed to be similar to that of natalizumab in the sense that LFA-1 inhibition also results in downregulation of α_4/β_1-integrin, decreased trafficking of T cells to target organs, reduced intrathecal lymphocyte restimulation with antigen, and impaired target cell lysis.[8,49,68,125,126,130,131]

Anti-CD52 agent

Alemtuzumab has been classified as a class 3 agent with low or unknown risk of JCPyV encephalopathy.[53–55,71,84] Virtually all cases have been reported in patients with CLL or transplant recipients.[73,85,132–137] Because these patients had other concomitant immunocompromising conditions, the actual risk of JCPyV encephalopathy with alemtuzumab is still uncertain.[77,84,85] In fact, alemtuzumab is used as an alternative disease-modifying therapy for patients with relapsing-remitting multiple sclerosis who are at risk for developing JCPyV encephalopathy with natalizumab.[78,138–140]

Alemtuzumab induces a long-lasting loss of CD19 B cells, CD4 T cells, and CD8 T cells that can take months to years to recover.[141] These profound findings were described in the immunologic profiling of a heavily pretreated young woman with relapsing-remitting multiple sclerosis who developed JCPyV encephalopathy after the use of alemtuzumab.[141]

Interleukin-2 receptor inhibitors

Basiliximab has been used to prevent rejection in solid organ transplantation and has only been associated with JCPyV encephalopathy in two individual case safety reports.[98,142] Because these patients received other transplant-related immunosuppression, the risk attributable to basiliximab cannot be assessed. Daclizumab, developed for the treatment of relapsing-remitting multiple sclerosis, has not been associated with JCPyV encephalopathy and was removed from the market in 2018 after reports of immune-mediated encephalitis.[80]

CD319-targeted agent

JCPyV encephalopathy has not been reported with elotuzumab.[91]

CCR4-targeted agent

Mogamulizumab has not been associated with JCPyV encephalopathy.[91]

Other Interleukin and IgE Inhibitors

JCPyV encephalopathy has not been reported with IL-1 inhibitors (anakinra, canakinumab, and rilonacept), IL-4 inhibitors (dupilumab, which also acts on IL-13), IL-5 inhibitors (mepolizumab, reslizumab, and benralizumab), IL-6 inhibitors (tocilizumab, sarilumab, siltuximab), IL-13 inhibitor (lebrikizumab), and IgE inhibitor (omalizumab).[102]

Checkpoint Inhibitors

Ipilimumab, atezolizumab, durvalumab, nivolumab, pembrolizumab, cemiplimab, tremelimumab, and avelumab have not been associated with an increased risk of JCPyV encephalopathy.[101] On the contrary, nivolumab and pembrolizumab have been used for treatment of JCPyV encephalopathy with mixed results.[143–148]

Tyrosine Kinase Inhibitors

Bruton tyrosine kinase inhibitors

Ibrutinib has been associated with the development of JCPyV encephalopathy in patients with CLL, many of whom were previously treated with rituximab.[77,149–152] According to its package insert, acalabrutinib has also been associated with JCPyV encephalopathy, although details and safety data are limited.[149,153]

Ibrutinib's specific risk of JCPyV encephalopathy is difficult to establish because many of these patients had immune defects related to their underlying disease and from prior treatments. The pathogenesis has been proposed to be caused by humoral immune impairment, including the elimination of the B-cell receptor signaling pathway, repression of B-cell proliferation and survival, and IgA deficiency.[150–152]

Small molecule BCR-ABL tyrosine kinase inhibitors
JCPyV encephalopathy has not been reported with imatinib, nilotinib, dasatinib, bosutinib, ponatinib, and bafetinib.[149]

Phosphoinositide 3-kinase inhibitors
Idelalisib has been associated with three cases of JCPyV encephalopathy, all of whom also received rituximab.[77] JCPyV encephalopathy has not been reported with buparlisib, duvelisib, and rigosertib.[149]

Other tyrosine kinase inhibitors
Sorafenib, sunitinib, axitinib, pazopanib, regorafenib, vandetanib, cabozantinib, and ramucirumab have not been associated with JCPyV encephalopathy.[154]

Epidermal Growth Factor Receptor Inhibitors and Vascular Endothelial Growth Factor Inhibitors

Epidermal growth factor receptor tyrosine kinase inhibitors
Gefitinib, erlotinib, osimertinib, afatinib, lapatinib, and neratinib have not been associated with JCPyV encephalopathy.[154]

Epidermal growth factor receptor inhibiting monoclonal antibodies
JCPyV encephalopathy has not been reported with cetuximab and panitumumab.[154]

Vascular endothelial growth factor inhibitors
Bevacizumab and aflibercept have not been associated with JCPyV encephalopathy.[154]

JAK-STAT and Complement Inhibitors

Janus kinase inhibitors
Ruxolitinib, but not baricitinib or tofacitinib, has been associated with JCPyV encephalopathy.[149,155,156] Causality is difficult to prove because this developed in only two patients, both of whom had myelofibrosis and also received hydroxyurea.[155,156] The pathogenesis may be related to T-cell abnormalities.[156]

C5 inhibitors
Eculizumab has only been associated with JCPyV encephalopathy in a single case of an intestine-kidney transplant recipient who was also receiving transplant-related immunosuppression.[102,157] The authors attributed JCPyV encephalopathy development in this patient to eculizumab because of her clinical improvement after the drug was discontinued.[157] They hypothesized that this may be related to the eculizumab's impairment of immune surveillance of viral infections.[157] Ravulizumab has not been associated with JCPyV encephalopathy.

Sphingosine-1-Phosphate Receptor Modulator

Fingolimod has been associated with multiple cases of JCPyV encephalopathy, most of whom also received natalizumab or had lymphopenia.[84,85,101] It has been classified as a class 2 agent.[85]

Proteasome Inhibitors

Ixazomib has been associated with a single case of JCPyV encephalopathy in a patient with multiple myeloma who had also received other immunomodulators.[158] No cases have been reported with bortezomib and carfilzomib.[101]

PREVENTION AND TREATMENT OF JC POLYOMAVIRUS ENCEPHALOPATHY
Screening

The mainstay of prevention of JCPyV encephalopathy is careful vigilance for its development while on an immunomodulatory agent.[159,160] Multiple biologics have been associated with the development of JCPyV encephalopathy but screening has been validated only with natalizumab because the observed incidence is high enough to permit estimated risk stratification in this patient population.[70,114] The screening algorithm should be used in conjunction with risk estimates based on anti-JCPyV IgG antibody index serostatus, prior immunosuppression, and duration of natalizumab exposure.[84,110,112–114] After natalizumab initiation, patients should be monitored closely for development of new neurologic deficits.[84,113] Anti-JCPyV IgG antibody index should be tested before natalizumab treatment initiation, 12 months after treatment initiation, and every 6 months thereafter (except if the antibody index is >1.5, because the risk would be sufficiently high that further testing would not alter management).[84,113,161] Both seroconversion and seroreversion may occur, and risk seems to be unaltered in either scenario.[84,112,162–165] Because radiographic abnormalities are often detected before symptom development, MRI scans of the brain (with consideration for additional imaging of the cervical and thoracic spine in certain circumstances) should be performed before treatment initiation and then at 3- to 12-month intervals depending on the anti-JCPyV IgG antibody index and duration of natalizumab exposure.[84,113,166] MRI abnormalities should prompt clinicians to consider whether additional investigations (eg, lumbar puncture for CSF analysis) or treatment modification are warranted.[113] Monitoring should continue for 6 months after natalizumab discontinuation.[84,113] Serum neurofilament light chains and matrix metalloproteinase-2 and matrix metalloproteinase-9 have been explored as candidate biomarkers for natalizumab-associated JCPyV encephalopathy but further research is required to determine their validity.[167–169]

Because of the increased risk of JCPyV encephalopathy with natalizumab, a comprehensive program for Risk Assessment and Minimization of PML (RAMP) was used during the clinical development of vedolizumab.[123] The RAMP program comprised of patient and study staff education about JCPyV encephalopathy, subjective and objective checklists, case evaluation algorithms for sequential screening and diagnostic evaluation (which incorporated the 2013 American Association of Neurology diagnostic criteria for JCPyV encephalopathy), and post-study telephone follow-up.[11,123]

The utility of screening for JCPyV encephalopathy with other biologics and in other diseases has not been examined but it is unlikely to be cost-effective because of the much lower incidence.[170–173] Many patients have detectable anti-JCPyV IgG antibody and/or detectable JCPyV DNA in the blood and/or urine by polymerase chain reaction, but only a small fraction develop JCPyV encephalopathy.[18,32,36,37,39,46,47,162,169–176] Furthermore, false-negative anti-JCPyV IgG antibody results may underestimate infection rates and limit its usefulness.[177]

Treatment and Prophylaxis

Treatment is challenging, thereby explaining the overall poor prognosis. If JCPyV encephalopathy occurs, immunosuppression should be reduced or discontinued when possible.[159,160] Many drugs including cidofovir, cytarabine, maraviroc, mefloquine, mirtazapine, nivolumab, and pembrolizumab have been explored as treatment options for JCPyV encephalopathy but have demonstrated mixed results.[24,143–147,178–184] They are therefore not considered effective treatment or prophylaxis for JCPyV encephalopathy. Allogeneic BK virus–specific T-cell infusions coincided with improvement in all three patients who received it for JCPyV encephalopathy and seem promising as a potential future therapeutic option.[185]

SUMMARY

The risk of JCPyV encephalopathy varies among biologic classes and among agents within the same class. Of the biologics currently in use, the highest risk is seen with natalizumab followed by rituximab. Multiple other agents have also been implicated. Drug-specific causality is difficult to establish because many patients receive multiple immunomodulatory medications concomitantly or sequentially, and have other immunocompromising factors related to their underlying disease. As the use of biologic therapies continues to expand, further research is needed into the pathogenesis, treatment, and prevention of JCPyV encephalopathy such that the risk for its development is better understood and mitigated, if not eliminated altogether.

DISCLOSURE

This research received no specific grant from any funding agency in the public, commercial, or not-for-profit sectors.

REFERENCES

1. Padgett BL, Walker DL, ZuRhein GM, et al. Cultivation of papova-like virus from human brain with progressive multifocal leucoencephalopathy. Lancet 1971; 1(7712):1257–60.
2. Harrison DM, Newsome SD, Skolasky RL, et al. Immune reconstitution is not a prognostic factor in progressive multifocal leukoencephalopathy. J Neuroimmunol 2011; 238(1–2):81–6.
3. Du Pasquier RA, Corey S, Margolin DH, et al. Productive infection of cerebellar granule cell neurons by JC virus in an HIV+ individual. Neurology 2003;61(6): 775–82.
4. Koralnik IJ, Wüthrich C, Dang X, et al. JC virus granule cell neuronopathy: a novel clinical syndrome distinct from progressive multifocal leukoencephalopathy. Ann Neurol 2005;57(4):576–80.
5. Wüthrich C, Cheng YM, Joseph JT, et al. Frequent infection of cerebellar granule cell neurons by polyomavirus JC in progressive multifocal leukoencephalopathy. J Neuropathol Exp Neurol 2009;68(1):15–25.
6. Wüthrich C, Dang X, Westmoreland S, et al. Fulminant JC virus encephalopathy with productive infection of cortical pyramidal neurons. Ann Neurol 2009;65(6): 742–8.
7. Agnihotri SP, Wuthrich C, Dang X, et al. A fatal case of JC virus meningitis presenting with hydrocephalus in a human immunodeficiency virus-seronegative patient. Ann Neurol 2014;76(1):140–7.
8. Major EO. Progressive multifocal leukoencephalopathy in patients on immunomodulatory therapies. Annu Rev Med 2010;61:35–47.
9. Levy RM, Bredesen DE, Rosenblum ML. Neurological manifestations of the acquired immunodeficiency syndrome (AIDS): experience at UCSF and review of the literature. J Neurosurg 1985;62(4):475–95.
10. Berger JR, Kaszovitz B, Post MJ, et al. Progressive multifocal leukoencephalopathy associated with human immunodeficiency virus infection. A review of the literature with a report of sixteen cases. Ann Intern Med 1987;107(1):78–87.

11. Berger JR, Aksamit AJ, Clifford DB, et al. PML diagnostic criteria: consensus statement from the AAN Neuroinfectious Disease Section. Neurology 2013; 80(15):1430–8.

12. AlTahan AM, Berger T, AlOrainy IA, et al. Progressive multifocal leukoencephalopathy in the absence of typical radiological changes: can we make a diagnosis? Am J Case Rep 2019;20:101–5.

13. Cinque P, Koralnik IJ, Clifford DB. The evolving face of human immunodeficiency virus-related progressive multifocal leukoencephalopathy: defining a consensus terminology. J Neurovirol 2003;9(Suppl 1):88–92.

14. Dahlhaus S, Hoepner R, Chan A, et al. Disease course and outcome of 15 monocentrically treated natalizumab-associated progressive multifocal leukoencephalopathy patients. J Neurol Neurosurg Psychiatry 2013;84(10):1068–74.

15. Engsig FN, Hansen A-BE, Omland LH, et al. Incidence, clinical presentation, and outcome of progressive multifocal leukoencephalopathy in HIV-infected patients during the highly active antiretroviral therapy era: a nationwide cohort study. J Infect Dis 2009;199(1):77–83.

16. Knowles WA. Discovery and epidemiology of the human polyomaviruses BK virus (BKV) and JC virus (JCV). Adv Exp Med Biol 2006;577:19–45.

17. Kean JM, Rao S, Wang M, et al. Seroepidemiology of human polyomaviruses. PLoS Pathog 2009;5(3):e1000363.

18. Egli A, Infanti L, Dumoulin A, et al. Prevalence of polyomavirus BK and JC infection and replication in 400 healthy blood donors. J Infect Dis 2009;199(6): 837–46.

19. Ahsan N. Polyomaviruses and human diseases. New York: Springer; 2006.

20. Shankar SK, Satishchandra P, Mahadevan A, et al. Low prevalence of progressive multifocal leukoencephalopathy in India and Africa: is there a biological explanation? J Neurovirol 2003;9(Suppl 1):59–67.

21. Khalili K, White MK, Sawa H, et al. The agnoprotein of polyomaviruses: a multifunctional auxiliary protein. J Cell Physiol 2005;204(1):1–7.

22. Safak M, Barrucco R, Darbinyan A, et al. Interaction of JC virus agno protein with T antigen modulates transcription and replication of the viral genome in glial cells. J Virol 2001;75(3):1476–86.

23. Unterstab G, Gosert R, Leuenberger D, et al. The polyomavirus BK agnoprotein co-localizes with lipid droplets. Virology 2010;399(2):322–31.

24. Elphick GF, Querbes W, Jordan JA, et al. The human polyomavirus, JCV, uses serotonin receptors to infect cells. Science 2004;306(5700):1380–3.

25. Neu U, Maginnis MS, Palma AS, et al. Structure-function analysis of the human JC polyomavirus establishes the LSTc pentasaccharide as a functional receptor motif. Cell Host Microbe 2010;8(4):309–19.

26. Neu U, Stehle T, Atwood WJ. The Polyomaviridae: contributions of virus structure to our understanding of virus receptors and infectious entry. Virology 2009; 384(2):389–99.

27. Mayberry CL, Nelson CDS, Maginnis MS. JC polyomavirus attachment and entry: potential sites for PML therapeutics. Curr Clin Microbiol Rep 2017;4(3): 132–41.

28. Vanchiere JA, Abudayyeh S, Copeland CM, et al. Polyomavirus shedding in the stool of healthy adults. J Clin Microbiol 2009;47(8):2388–91.

29. Bofill-Mas S, Formiga-Cruz M, Clemente-Casares P, et al. Potential transmission of human polyomaviruses through the gastrointestinal tract after exposure to virions or viral DNA. J Virol 2001;75(21):10290–9.

30. Bofill-Mas S, Pina S, Girones R. Documenting the epidemiologic patterns of polyomaviruses in human populations by studying their presence in urban sewage. Appl Environ Microbiol 2000;66(1):238–45.

31. Monaco MC, Jensen PN, Hou J, et al. Detection of JC virus DNA in human tonsil tissue: evidence for site of initial viral infection. J Virol 1998;72(12):9918–23.

32. Kitamura T, Kunitake T, Guo J, et al. Transmission of the human polyomavirus JC virus occurs both within the family and outside the family. J Clin Microbiol 1994; 32(10):2359–63.

33. Kunitake T, Kitamura T, Guo J, et al. Parent-to-child transmission is relatively common in the spread of the human polyomavirus JC virus. J Clin Microbiol 1995;33(6):1448–51.

34. Boldorini R, Allegrini S, Miglio U, et al. Serological evidence of vertical transmission of JC and BK polyomaviruses in humans. J Gen Virol 2011;92(Pt 5): 1044–50.

35. Chesters PM, Heritage J, McCance DJ. Persistence of DNA sequences of BK virus and JC virus in normal human tissues and in diseased tissues. J Infect Dis 1983;147(4):676–84.

36. Polo C, Pérez JL, Mielnichuck A, et al. Prevalence and patterns of polyomavirus urinary excretion in immunocompetent adults and children. Clin Microbiol Infect 2004;10(7):640–4.

37. Markowitz RB, Thompson HC, Mueller JF, et al. Incidence of BK virus and JC virus viruria in human immunodeficiency virus-infected and -uninfected subjects. J Infect Dis 1993;167(1):13–20.

38. Markowitz RB, Eaton BA, Kubik MF, et al. BK virus and JC virus shed during pregnancy have predominantly archetypal regulatory regions. J Virol 1991; 65(8):4515–9.

39. Kitamura T, Sugimoto C, Kato A, et al. Persistent JC virus (JCV) infection is demonstrated by continuous shedding of the same JCV strains. J Clin Microbiol 1997;35(5):1255–7.

40. Doerries K. Human polyomavirus JC and BK persistent infection. Adv Exp Med Biol 2006;577:102–16.

41. Caldarelli-Stefano R, Vago L, Omodeo-Zorini E, et al. Detection and typing of JC virus in autopsy brains and extraneural organs of AIDS patients and non-immunocompromised individuals. J Neurovirol 1999;5(2):125–33.

42. Tan CS, Dezube BJ, Bhargava P, et al. Detection of JC virus DNA and proteins in the bone marrow of HIV-positive and HIV-negative patients: implications for viral latency and neurotropic transformation. J Infect Dis 2009;199(6):881–8.

43. Marzocchetti A, Wuthrich C, Tan CS, et al. Rearrangement of the JC virus regulatory region sequence in the bone marrow of a patient with rheumatoid arthritis and progressive multifocal leukoencephalopathy. J Neurovirol 2008;14(5): 455–8.

44. Tan CS, Ellis LC, Wüthrich C, et al. JC virus latency in the brain and extraneural organs of patients with and without progressive multifocal leukoencephalopathy. J Virol 2010;84(18):9200–9.

45. Jelcic I, Jelcic I, Faigle W, et al. Immunology of progressive multifocal leukoencephalopathy. J Neurovirol 2015;21(6):614–22.

46. Koralnik IJ, Schmitz JE, Lifton MA, et al. Detection of JC virus DNA in peripheral blood cell subpopulations of HIV-1-infected individuals. J Neurovirol 1999;5(4): 430–5.

47. Tornatore C, Berger JR, Houff SA, et al. Detection of JC virus DNA in peripheral lymphocytes from patients with and without progressive multifocal leukoencephalopathy. Ann Neurol 1992;31(4):454–62.
48. Durali D, de Goër de Herve M-G, Gasnault J, et al. B cells and progressive multifocal leukoencephalopathy: search for the missing link. Front Immunol 2015; 6:241.
49. Bellizzi A, Anzivino E, Rodio DM, et al. New insights on human polyomavirus JC and pathogenesis of progressive multifocal leukoencephalopathy. Clin Dev Immunol 2013;2013:839719.
50. Marshall LJ, Dunham L, Major EO. Transcription factor Spi-B binds unique sequences present in the tandem repeat promoter/enhancer of JC virus and supports viral activity. J Gen Virol 2010;91(Pt 12):3042–52.
51. Chapagain ML, Nerurkar VR. Human polyomavirus JC (JCV) infection of human B lymphocytes: a possible mechanism for JCV transmigration across the blood-brain barrier. J Infect Dis 2010;202(2):184–91.
52. Dang L, Dang X, Koralnik IJ, et al. JC polyomavirus granule cell neuronopathy in a patient treated with rituximab. JAMA Neurol 2014;71(4):487–9.
53. Chahin S, Berger JR. A risk classification for immunosuppressive treatment-associated progressive multifocal leukoencephalopathy. J Neurovirol 2015; 21(6):623–31.
54. Zaheer F, Berger JR. Treatment-related progressive multifocal leukoencephalopathy: current understanding and future steps. Ther Adv Drug Saf 2012;3(5): 227–39.
55. Calabrese LH, Molloy E, Berger J. Sorting out the risks in progressive multifocal leukoencephalopathy. Nat Rev Rheumatol 2015;11(2):119–23.
56. Lin EJ, Reddy S, Shah VV, et al. A review of neurologic complications of biologic therapy in plaque psoriasis. Cutis 2018;101(1):57–60.
57. Babi M-A, Pendlebury W, Braff S, et al. JC virus PCR detection is not infallible: a fulminant case of progressive multifocal leukoencephalopathy with false-negative cerebrospinal fluid studies despite progressive clinical course and radiological findings. Case Rep Neurol Med 2015;2015:643216. Available at: https://www.hindawi.com/journals/crinm/2015/643216/abs/.
58. Ray M, Curtis JR, Baddley JW. A case report of progressive multifocal leucoencephalopathy (PML) associated with adalimumab. Ann Rheum Dis 2014;73(7): 1429–30.
59. Kumar D, Bouldin TW, Berger RG. A case of progressive multifocal leukoencephalopathy in a patient treated with infliximab. Arthritis Rheum 2010;62(11): 3191–5.
60. Graff-Radford J, Robinson MT, Warsame RM, et al. Progressive multifocal leukoencephalopathy in a patient treated with etanercept. Neurologist 2012; 18(2):85–7.
61. Sammut L, Wallis D, Holroyd C. Progressive multifocal leukoencephalopathy associated with infliximab. J R Coll Physicians Edinb 2016;46(3):163–5.
62. Magnano MD, Robinson WH, Genovese MC. Demyelination and inhibition of tumor necrosis factor (TNF). Clin Exp Rheumatol 2004;22(5 Suppl 35):S134–40.
63. Comar M, Delbue S, Lepore L, et al. Latent viral infections in young patients with inflammatory diseases treated with biological agents: prevalence of JC virus genotype 2. J Med Virol 2013;85(4):716–22.
64. Bellizzi A, Anzivino E, Ferrari F, et al. Polyomavirus JC reactivation and noncoding control region sequence analysis in pediatric Crohn's disease patients treated with infliximab. J Neurovirol 2011;17(4):303–13.

65. Nardis C, Anzivino E, Bellizzi A, et al. Reactivation of human polyomavirus JC in patients affected by psoriasis vulgaris and psoriatic arthritis and treated with biological drugs: preliminary results. J Cell Physiol 2012;227(12):3796–802.

66. Bellizzi A, Anzivino E, Rodio DM, et al. Human Polyomavirus JC monitoring and noncoding control region analysis in dynamic cohorts of individuals affected by immune-mediated diseases under treatment with biologics: an observational study. Virol J 2013;10:298.

67. Carson KR, Newsome SD, Kim EJ, et al. Progressive multifocal leukoencephalopathy associated with brentuximab vedotin therapy: a report of 5 cases from the Southern Network on Adverse Reactions (SONAR) project. Cancer 2014; 120(16):2464–71.

68. Carson KR, Focosi D, Major EO, et al. Monoclonal antibody-associated progressive multifocal leucoencephalopathy in patients treated with rituximab, natalizumab, and efalizumab: a Review from the Research on Adverse Drug Events and Reports (RADAR) Project. Lancet Oncol 2009;10(8):816–24.

69. Carson KR, Evens AM, Richey EA, et al. Progressive multifocal leukoencephalopathy after rituximab therapy in HIV-negative patients: a report of 57 cases from the Research on Adverse Drug Events and Reports project. Blood 2009; 113(20):4834–40.

70. Berger JR, Malik V, Lacey S, et al. Progressive multifocal leukoencephalopathy in rituximab-treated rheumatic diseases: a rare event. J Neurovirol 2018;24(3): 323–31.

71. Mikulska M, Lanini S, Gudiol C, et al. ESCMID Study Group for Infections in Compromised Hosts (ESGICH) Consensus Document on the safety of targeted and biological therapies: an infectious diseases perspective (agents targeting lymphoid cells surface antigens [I]: CD19, CD20 and CD52). Clin Microbiol Infect 2018;24(Suppl 2):S71–82.

72. Lane MA, Renga V, Pachner AR, et al. Late occurrence of PML in a patient treated for lymphoma with immunomodulatory chemotherapies, bendamustine, rituximab, and ibritumomab tiuxetan. Case Rep Neurol Med 2015;2015:892047.

73. Keene DL, Legare C, Taylor E, et al. Monoclonal antibodies and progressive multifocal leukoencephalopathy. Can J Neurol Sci 2011;38(4):565–71.

74. Moreno C, Montillo M, Panayiotidis P, et al. Ofatumumab in poor-prognosis chronic lymphocytic leukemia: a phase IV, non-interventional, observational study from the European Research Initiative on Chronic Lymphocytic Leukemia. Haematologica 2015;100(4):511–6.

75. Jones JA, Robak T, Brown JR, et al. Efficacy and safety of idelalisib in combination with ofatumumab for previously treated chronic lymphocytic leukaemia: an open-label, randomised phase 3 trial. Lancet Haematol 2017;4(3):e114–26.

76. Pejsa V, Lucijanic M, Jonjic Z, et al. Progressive multifocal leukoencephalopathy developing after obinutuzumab treatment for chronic lymphocytic leukemia. Ann Hematol 2019;98(6):1509–10.

77. Raisch DW, Rafi JA, Chen C, et al. Detection of cases of progressive multifocal leukoencephalopathy associated with new biologicals and targeted cancer therapies from the FDA's adverse event reporting system. Expert Opin Drug Saf 2016;15(8):1003–11.

78. Vargas DL, Tyor WR. Update on disease-modifying therapies for multiple sclerosis. J Investig Med 2017;65(5):883–91.

79. Grebenciucova E, Pruitt A. Infections in patients receiving multiple sclerosis disease-modifying therapies. Curr Neurol Neurosci Rep 2017;17(11):88.

80. Faissner S, Gold R. Efficacy and safety of the newer multiple sclerosis drugs approved since 2010. CNS Drugs 2018;32(3):269–87.
81. Baber U, Bouley A, Egnor E, et al. Anti-JC virus antibody index changes in rituximab-treated multiple sclerosis patients. J Neurol 2018;265(10):2342–5.
82. Cooper N, Arnold DM. The effect of rituximab on humoral and cell mediated immunity and infection in the treatment of autoimmune diseases. Br J Haematol 2010;149(1):3–13.
83. Edelmann J, Gribben JG. Obinutuzumab for the treatment of indolent lymphoma. Future Oncol 2016;12(15):1769–81.
84. Epstein DJ, Dunn J, Deresinski S. Infectious complications of multiple sclerosis therapies: implications for screening, prophylaxis, and management. Open Forum Infect Dis 2018;5(8):ofy174.
85. Berger JR. Classifying PML risk with disease modifying therapies. Mult Scler Relat Disord 2017;12:59–63.
86. Lai C-M, Horowitz S. Brentuximab vedotin: treatment role for relapsed refractory systemic anaplastic large-cell lymphoma. Expert Rev Hematol 2013;6(4): 361–73.
87. Wagner-Johnston ND, Bartlett NL, Cashen A, et al. Progressive multifocal leukoencephalopathy in a patient with Hodgkin lymphoma treated with brentuximab vedotin. Leuk Lymphoma 2012;53(11):2283–6.
88. von Geldern G, Pardo CA, Calabresi PA, et al. PML-IRIS in a patient treated with brentuximab. Neurology 2012;79(20):2075–7.
89. Jalan P, Mahajan A, Pandav V, et al. Brentuximab associated progressive multifocal leukoencephalopathy. Clin Neurol Neurosurg 2012;114(10):1335–7.
90. Newland AM, Li JX, Wasco LE, et al. Brentuximab vedotin: a CD30-directed antibody-cytotoxic drug conjugate. Pharmacotherapy 2013;33(1):93–104.
91. Drgona L, Gudiol C, Lanini S, et al. ESCMID Study Group for Infections in Compromised Hosts (ESGICH) Consensus Document on the safety of targeted and biological therapies: an infectious diseases perspective (agents targeting lymphoid or myeloid cells surface antigens [II]: CD22, CD30, CD33, CD38, CD40, SLAMF-7 and CCR4). Clin Microbiol Infect 2018;24(Suppl 2):S83–94.
92. Fredericks CA, Kvam KA, Bear J, et al. A case of progressive multifocal leukoencephalopathy in a lupus patient treated with belimumab. Lupus 2014;23(7): 711–3.
93. Leblanc-Trudeau C, Masetto A, Bocti C. Progressive multifocal leukoencephalopathy associated with belimumab in a patient with systemic lupus erythematosus. J Rheumatol 2015;42(3):551–2.
94. Tavazzi E, Ferrante P, Khalili K. Progressive multifocal leukoencephalopathy: an unexpected complication of modern therapeutic monoclonal antibody therapies. Clin Microbiol Infect 2011;17(12):1776–80.
95. Molloy ES, Calabrese LH. Progressive multifocal leukoencephalopathy in patients with rheumatic diseases: are patients with systemic lupus erythematosus at particular risk? Autoimmun Rev 2008;8(2):144–6.
96. Berntsson SG, Katsarogiannis E, Lourenço F, et al. Progressive multifocal leukoencephalopathy and systemic lupus erythematosus: focus on etiology. Case Rep Neurol 2016;8(1):59–65.
97. Brandão M, Damásio J, Marinho A, et al. Systemic lupus erythematosus, progressive multifocal leukoencephalopathy, and T-CD4+ lymphopenia. Clin Rev Allergy Immunol 2012;43(3):302–7.

98. Grinyó J, Charpentier B, Pestana JM, et al. An integrated safety profile analysis of belatacept in kidney transplant recipients. Transplantation 2010;90(12): 1521–7.
99. Dekeyser M, de Goër de Herve M-G, Hendel-Chavez H, et al. Refractory T-cell anergy and rapidly fatal progressive multifocal leukoencephalopathy after prolonged CTLA4 therapy. Open Forum Infect Dis 2017;4(2):ofx100.
100. Aringer M, Smolen JS. Safety of off-label biologicals in systemic lupus erythematosus. Expert Opin Drug Saf 2015;14(2):243–51.
101. Redelman-Sidi G, Michielin O, Cervera C, et al. ESCMID Study Group for Infections in Compromised Hosts (ESGICH) Consensus Document on the safety of targeted and biological therapies: an infectious diseases perspective (immune checkpoint inhibitors, cell adhesion inhibitors, sphingosine-1-phosphate receptor modulators and proteasome inhibitors). Clin Microbiol Infect 2018; 24(Suppl 2):S95–107.
102. Winthrop KL, Mariette X, Silva JT, et al. ESCMID Study Group for Infections in Compromised Hosts (ESGICH) Consensus Document on the safety of targeted and biological therapies: an infectious diseases perspective (soluble immune effector molecules [II]: agents targeting interleukins, immunoglobulins and complement factors). Clin Microbiol Infect 2018;24(Suppl 2):S21–40.
103. Langer-Gould A, Atlas SW, Green AJ, et al. Progressive multifocal leukoencephalopathy in a patient treated with natalizumab. N Engl J Med 2005;353(4): 375–81.
104. Van Assche G, Van Ranst M, Sciot R, et al. Progressive multifocal leukoencephalopathy after natalizumab therapy for Crohn's disease. N Engl J Med 2005;353(4):362–8.
105. Kleinschmidt-DeMasters BK, Tyler KL. Progressive multifocal leukoencephalopathy complicating treatment with natalizumab and interferon beta-1a for multiple sclerosis. N Engl J Med 2005;353(4):369–74.
106. Wenning W, Haghikia A, Laubenberger J, et al. Treatment of progressive multifocal leukoencephalopathy associated with natalizumab. N Engl J Med 2009; 361(11):1075–80.
107. Lindå H, von Heijne A, Major EO, et al. Progressive multifocal leukoencephalopathy after natalizumab monotherapy. N Engl J Med 2009;361(11):1081–7.
108. Bloomgren G, Richman S, Hotermans C, et al. Risk of natalizumab-associated progressive multifocal leukoencephalopathy. N Engl J Med 2012;366(20): 1870–80.
109. Chandar AK, Singh S, Murad MH, et al. Efficacy and safety of natalizumab and vedolizumab for the management of Crohn's disease: a systematic review and meta-analysis. Inflamm Bowel Dis 2015;21(7):1695–708.
110. Ho P-R, Koendgen H, Campbell N, et al. Risk of natalizumab-associated progressive multifocal leukoencephalopathy in patients with multiple sclerosis: a retrospective analysis of data from four clinical studies. Lancet Neurol 2017; 16(11):925–33.
111. Scarpazza C, De Rossi N, Tabiadon G, et al. Four cases of natalizumab-related PML: a less severe course in extended interval dosing? Neurol Sci 2019. https://doi.org/10.1007/s10072-019-03959-4.
112. Schwab N, Schneider-Hohendorf T, Melzer N, et al. Natalizumab-associated PML: challenges with incidence, resulting risk, and risk stratification. Neurology 2017;88(12):1197–205.
113. McGuigan C, Craner M, Guadagno J, et al. Stratification and monitoring of natalizumab-associated progressive multifocal leukoencephalopathy risk:

recommendations from an expert group. J Neurol Neurosurg Psychiatry 2016; 87(2):117–25.

114. Lee P, Plavina T, Castro A, et al. A second-generation ELISA (STRATIFY JCV DxSelect) for detection of JC virus antibodies in human serum and plasma to support progressive multifocal leukoencephalopathy risk stratification. J Clin Virol 2013;57(2):141–6.

115. Baldassari LE, Jones SE, Clifford DB, et al. Progressive multifocal leukoencephalopathy with extended natalizumab dosing. Neurol Clin Pract 2018;8(3): e12–4.

116. Zhovtis Ryerson L, Frohman TC, Foley J, et al. Extended interval dosing of natalizumab in multiple sclerosis. J Neurol Neurosurg Psychiatry 2016;87(8): 885–9.

117. Colombel J-F, Sands BE, Rutgeerts P, et al. The safety of vedolizumab for ulcerative colitis and Crohn's disease. Gut 2017;66(5):839–51.

118. Bye WA, Jairath V, Travis SPL. Systematic review: the safety of vedolizumab for the treatment of inflammatory bowel disease. Aliment Pharmacol Ther 2017; 46(1):3–15.

119. Card T, Xu J, Liang H, et al. What is the risk of progressive multifocal leukoencephalopathy in patients with ulcerative colitis or Crohn's disease treated with vedolizumab? Inflamm Bowel Dis 2018;24(5):953–9.

120. Ng SC, Hilmi IN, Blake A, et al. Low frequency of opportunistic infections in patients receiving vedolizumab in clinical trials and post-marketing setting. Inflamm Bowel Dis 2018;24(11):2431–41.

121. Battat R, Ma C, Jairath V, et al. Benefit-risk assessment of vedolizumab in the treatment of Crohn's disease and ulcerative colitis. Drug Saf 2019;42(5):617–32.

122. Sands BE, Peyrin-Biroulet L, Loftus EV Jr, et al. Vedolizumab versus adalimumab for moderate-to-severe ulcerative colitis. N Engl J Med 2019;381(13): 1215–26.

123. Parikh A, Stephens K, Major E, et al. A programme for risk assessment and minimisation of progressive multifocal leukoencephalopathy developed for vedolizumab clinical trials. Drug Saf 2018;41(8):807–16.

124. Sands BE. Leukocyte anti-trafficking strategies: current status and future directions. Dig Dis 2017;35(1–2):13–20.

125. Berger JR. Progressive multifocal leukoencephalopathy and newer biological agents. Drug Saf 2010;33(11):969–83.

126. Talamonti M, Spallone G, Di Stefani A, et al. Efalizumab. Expert Opin Drug Saf 2011;10(2):239–51.

127. Schmedt N, Andersohn F, Garbe E. Signals of progressive multifocal leukoencephalopathy for immunosuppressants: a disproportionality analysis of spontaneous reports within the US Adverse Event Reporting System (AERS). Pharmacoepidemiol Drug Saf 2012;21(11):1216–20.

128. Korman BD, Tyler KL, Korman NJ. Progressive multifocal leukoencephalopathy, efalizumab, and immunosuppression: a cautionary tale for dermatologists. Arch Dermatol 2009;145(8):937–42.

129. Di Lernia V. Progressive multifocal leukoencephalopathy and antipsoriatic drugs: assessing the risk of immunosuppressive treatments. Int J Dermatol 2010;49(6):631–5.

130. Berger JR, Houff SA, Major EO. Monoclonal antibodies and progressive multifocal leukoencephalopathy. MAbs 2009;1(6):583–9.

131. Schwab N, Ulzheimer JC, Fox RJ, et al. Fatal PML associated with efalizumab therapy: insights into integrin αLβ2 in JC virus control. Neurology 2012;78(7): 458–67 [discussion: 465].

132. Uppenkamp M, Engert A, Diehl V, et al. Monoclonal antibody therapy with CAMPATH-1H in patients with relapsed high- and low-grade non-Hodgkin's lymphomas: a multicenter phase I/II study. Ann Hematol 2002;81(1):26–32.

133. Martin SI, Marty FM, Fiumara K, et al. Infectious complications associated with alemtuzumab use for lymphoproliferative disorders. Clin Infect Dis 2006;43(1): 16–24.

134. Waggoner J, Martinu T, Palmer SM. Progressive multifocal leukoencephalopathy following heightened immunosuppression after lung transplant. J Heart Lung Transplant 2009;28(4):395–8.

135. Isidoro L, Pires P, Rito L, et al. Progressive multifocal leukoencephalopathy in a patient with chronic lymphocytic leukaemia treated with alemtuzumab. BMJ Case Rep 2014;2014. https://doi.org/10.1136/bcr-2013-201781.

136. Zent CS, Victoria Wang X, Ketterling RP, et al. A phase II randomized trial comparing standard and low dose rituximab combined with alemtuzumab as initial treatment of progressive chronic lymphocytic leukemia in older patients: a trial of the ECOG-ACRIN cancer research group (E1908). Am J Hematol 2016;91(3):308–12.

137. Faulkner M. Risk of progressive multifocal leukoencephalopathy in patients with multiple sclerosis. Expert Opin Drug Saf 2015;14(11):1737–48.

138. Giovannoni G, Marta M, Davis A, et al. Switching patients at high risk of PML from natalizumab to another disease-modifying therapy. Pract Neurol 2016; 16(5):389–93.

139. Pfeuffer S, Schmidt R, Straeten FA, et al. Efficacy and safety of alemtuzumab versus fingolimod in RRMS after natalizumab cessation. J Neurol 2019;266(1): 165–73.

140. Sellner J, Rommer PS. A review of the evidence for a natalizumab exit strategy for patients with multiple sclerosis. Autoimmun Rev 2019;18(3):255–61.

141. Gerevini S, Capra R, Bertoli D, et al. Immune profiling of a patient with alemtuzumab-associated progressive multifocal leukoencephalopathy. Mult Scler 2019;25(8):1196–201.

142. Melis M, Biagi C, Småbrekke L, et al. Drug-induced progressive multifocal leukoencephalopathy: a comprehensive analysis of the WHO adverse drug reaction database. CNS Drugs 2015;29(10):879–91.

143. Cortese I, Muranski P, Enose-Akahata Y, et al. Pembrolizumab treatment for progressive multifocal leukoencephalopathy. N Engl J Med 2019;380(17): 1597–605.

144. Rauer S, Marks R, Urbach H, et al. Treatment of progressive multifocal leukoencephalopathy with pembrolizumab. N Engl J Med 2019;380(17):1676–7.

145. Hoang E, Bartlett NL, Goyal MS, et al. Progressive multifocal leukoencephalopathy treated with nivolumab. J Neurovirol 2019;25(2):284–7.

146. Walter O, Treiner E, Bonneville F, et al. Treatment of progressive multifocal leukoencephalopathy with nivolumab. N Engl J Med 2019;380(17):1674–6.

147. Martinot M, Ahle G, Petrosyan I, et al. Progressive multifocal leukoencephalopathy after treatment with nivolumab. Emerg Infect Dis 2018;24(8):1594–6.

148. Koralnik IJ. Can immune checkpoint inhibitors keep JC virus in check? N Engl J Med 2019;380(17):1667–8.

149. Reinwald M, Silva JT, Mueller NJ, et al. ESCMID Study Group for Infections in Compromised Hosts (ESGICH) Consensus Document on the safety of targeted

and biological therapies: an infectious diseases perspective (intracellular signaling pathways: tyrosine kinase and mTOR inhibitors). Clin Microbiol Infect 2018;24(Suppl 2):S53–70.

150. Bennett CL, Berger JR, Sartor O, et al. Progressive multi-focal leucoencephalopathy among ibrutinib-treated persons with chronic lymphocytic leukaemia. Br J Haematol 2018;180(2):301–4.

151. Hsiehchen D, Arasaratnam R, Raj K, et al. Ibrutinib use complicated by progressive multifocal leukoencephalopathy. Oncology 2018;95(5):319–22.

152. Lutz M, Schulze AB, Rebber E, et al. Progressive multifocal leukoencephalopathy after ibrutinib therapy for chronic lymphocytic leukemia. Cancer Res Treat 2017;49(2):548–52.

153. Calquence (acalabrutinib) [package insert]. Wilmington (DE): AstraZeneca Pharmaceuticals LP; 2017. Available at: https://www.azpicentral.com/calquence/calquence.pdf#page=1.

154. Aguilar-Company J, Fernández-Ruiz M, García-Campelo R, et al. ESCMID Study Group for Infections in Compromised Hosts (ESGICH) Consensus Document on the safety of targeted and biological therapies: an infectious diseases perspective (cell surface receptors and associated signaling pathways). Clin Microbiol Infect 2018;24:S41–52.

155. Wathes R, Moule S, Milojkovic D. Progressive multifocal leukoencephalopathy associated with ruxolitinib. N Engl J Med 2013;369(2):197–8.

156. Ballesta B, González H, Martín V, et al. Fatal ruxolitinib-related JC virus meningitis. J Neurovirol 2017;23(5):783–5.

157. Gómez-Cibeira E, Ivanovic-Barbeito Y, Gutiérrez-Martínez E, et al. Eculizumab-related progressive multifocal leukoencephalopathy. Neurology 2016;86(4):399–400.

158. Sawicki CP, Climans SA, Hsia CC, et al. Progressive multifocal leukoencephalopathy during ixazomib-based chemotherapy. Curr Oncol 2018;25(1):e99–102.

159. Tan CS, Koralnik IJ. Progressive multifocal leukoencephalopathy and other disorders caused by JC virus: clinical features and pathogenesis. Lancet Neurol 2010;9(4):425–37.

160. Calabrese L. A rational approach to PML for the clinician. Cleve Clin J Med 2011;78(Suppl 2):S38–41.

161. Kolcava J, Hulova M, Benesova Y, et al. The value of anti-JCV antibody index assessment in multiple sclerosis patients treated with natalizumab with respect to demographic, clinical and radiological findings. Mult Scler Relat Disord 2019; 30:187–91.

162. Auer M, Hegen H, Sellner J, et al. Conversion and reversion of anti-John Cunningham virus antibody serostatus: a prospective study. Brain Behav 2019; 9(7):e01332.

163. Fragoso YD, Brooks JBB, Eboni ACB, et al. Seroconversion of JCV antibodies is strongly associated to natalizumab therapy. J Clin Neurosci 2019;61:112–3.

164. Peters J, Williamson E. Natalizumab therapy is associated with changes in serum JC virus antibody indices over time. J Neurol 2017;264(12):2409–12.

165. Plavina T, Subramanyam M, Bloomgren G, et al. Anti-JC virus antibody levels in serum or plasma further define risk of natalizumab-associated progressive multifocal leukoencephalopathy. Ann Neurol 2014;76(6):802–12.

166. Scarpazza C, Signori A, Cosottini M, et al. Should frequent MRI monitoring be performed in natalizumab-treated MS patients? A contribution to a recent debate. Mult Scler 2019. https://doi.org/10.1177/1352458519854162.

167. Loonstra FC, Verberk IMW, Wijburg MT, et al. Serum neurofilaments as candidate biomarkers of natalizumab associated progressive multifocal leukoencephalopathy. Ann Neurol 2019;86(2):322–4.
168. Dalla Costa G, Martinelli V, Moiola L, et al. Serum neurofilaments increase at progressive multifocal leukoencephalopathy onset in natalizumab-treated multiple sclerosis patients. Ann Neurol 2019;85(4):606–10.
169. Iannetta M, Zingaropoli MA, Latronico T, et al. Dynamic changes of MMP-9 plasma levels correlate with JCV reactivation and immune activation in natalizumab-treated multiple sclerosis patients. Sci Rep 2019;9(1):311.
170. Molloy ES, Calabrese CM, Calabrese LH. The risk of progressive multifocal leukoencephalopathy in the biologic era: prevention and management. Rheum Dis Clin North Am 2017;43(1):95–109.
171. Reuwer AQ, Heron M, van der Dussen D, et al. The clinical utility of JC virus antibody index measurements in the context of progressive multifocal leukoencephalopathy. Acta Neurol Scand 2017;136(Suppl 201):37–44.
172. Bellaguarda E, Keyashian K, Pekow J, et al. Prevalence of antibodies against JC virus in patients with refractory crohn's disease and effects of natalizumab therapy. Clin Gastroenterol Hepatol 2015;13(11):1919–25.
173. Borie D, Kremer JM. Considerations on the appropriateness of the John Cunningham virus antibody assay use in patients with rheumatoid arthritis. Semin Arthritis Rheum 2015;45(2):163–6.
174. Delbue S, Ferraresso M, Elia F, et al. Investigation of polyomaviruses replication in pediatric patients with nephropathy receiving rituximab. J Med Virol 2012; 84(9):1464–70.
175. Domínguez-Mozo MI, Toledano-Martínez E, Rodríguez Rodríguez L, et al. JC virus reactivation in patients with autoimmune rheumatic diseases treated with rituximab. Scand J Rheumatol 2016;45(6):507–11.
176. Verheyen J, Maizus K, Feist E, et al. Increased frequency of JC-polyomavirus detection in rheumatoid arthritis patients treated with multiple biologics. Med Microbiol Immunol 2015;204(5):613–8.
177. Berger JR, Houff SA, Gurwell J, et al. JC virus antibody status underestimates infection rates. Ann Neurol 2013;74(1):84–90.
178. Brickelmaier M, Lugovskoy A, Kartikeyan R, et al. Identification and characterization of mefloquine efficacy against JC virus in vitro. Antimicrob Agents Chemother 2009;53(5):1840–9.
179. Bsteh G, Auer M, Iglseder S, et al. Severe early natalizumab-associated PML in MS: effective control of PML-IRIS with maraviroc. Neurol Neuroimmunol Neuroinflamm 2017;4(2):e323.
180. Cettomai D, McArthur JC. Mirtazapine use in human immunodeficiency virus-infected patients with progressive multifocal leukoencephalopathy. Arch Neurol 2009;66(2):255–8.
181. Hodecker SC, Stürner KH, Becker V, et al. Maraviroc as possible treatment for PML-IRIS in natalizumab-treated patients with MS. Neurol Neuroimmunol Neuroinflamm 2017;4(2):e325.
182. Loignon M, Toma E. Treatment options for progressive multifocal leukoencephalopathy in HIV-infected persons: current status and future directions. Expert Rev Anti Infect Ther 2016;14(2):177–91.
183. Pavlovic D, Patera AC, Nyberg F, et al, Progressive Multifocal Leukeoncephalopathy Consortium. Progressive multifocal leukoencephalopathy: current treatment options and future perspectives. Ther Adv Neurol Disord 2015;8(6):255–73.

184. Yokoyama H, Watanabe T, Maruyama D, et al. Progressive multifocal leukoence-phalopathy in a patient with B-cell lymphoma during rituximab-containing chemotherapy: case report and review of the literature. Int J Hematol 2008; 88(4):443–7.

185. Muftuoglu M, Olson A, Marin D, et al. Allogeneic BK virus–specific T cells for progressive multifocal leukoencephalopathy. N Engl J Med 2018;379(15): 1443–51.

Fungal Infections Potentiated by Biologics

Matthew R. Davis, PharmD[a],*, George R. Thompson III, MD[b,c],
Thomas F. Patterson, MD[d]

KEYWORDS

- Monoclonal antibodies • Tyrosine kinase inhibitors • Fungal infections • Biologic
- TNF-α inhibitors

KEY POINTS

- Biologic therapies affect the immune system in intentional and unintentional ways, which can predispose patients to the development of fungal infections.
- TNF-α are used in the treatment of several autoimmune conditions and have been historically implicated in the development of opportunistic fungal infections prompting a black box warning for this commonly used biologic class.
- Ibrutinib, a Bruton kinase inhibitor, certain monoclonal interleukin inhibitors (IL), and cluster of differentiation (CD) inhibitors have also been associated with an elevated risk of fungal infections.

INTRODUCTION

The advent of targeted biologic therapy has had a dramatic impact in the treatment of a wide variety of diseases including immune-mediated inflammatory diseases, cancer, allergy, and infectious diseases with the pipeline continuing to expand as new targets are identified.[1] Because of the ability of many of these agents to directly or indirectly impact immune function, there is a pressing need to understand the scope of fungal infections associated with their use. This review summarizes the published literature regarding fungal infections associated with the use of biologic agents in adult patients with a targeted focus on fungal infections associated with the tumor necrosis factor (TNF)-α inhibitor class given their Food and Drug Administration (FDA) black box warning.[2]

---

[a] Department of Pharmacy, University of California, Los Angeles Ronald Reagan Medical Center, 757 Westwood Plaza, Los Angeles, CA 90095, USA; [b] Division of Infectious Diseases, Department of Internal Medicine, University of California Davis Health, 4150 V Street, Sacramento, CA 95817, USA; [c] Department of Medical Microbiology and Immunology, University of California Davis Health, 4150 V Street, Sacramento, CA 95817, USA; [d] Division of Infectious Diseases, Department of Medicine, University of Texas Health Science Center at San Antonio, South Texas Veterans Health Care System, 7703 Floyd Curl Drive, San Antonio, TX 78229, USA
* Corresponding author.
E-mail address: mrdavis@mednet.ucla.edu

Infect Dis Clin N Am 34 (2020) 389–411
https://doi.org/10.1016/j.idc.2020.02.010
0891-5520/20/© 2020 Elsevier Inc. All rights reserved.

TUMOR NECROSIS FACTOR-α INHIBITORS

TNF-α is a pleiotropic cytokine synthesized by immune cells including activated macrophages and T cells and acts as a central mediator in inflammation and immune regulation. Mechanistically, TNF-α functions through the stimulation of the transmembrane receptors tumor necrosis factor receptor (TNFR)-1 and TNFR-2.[3] In humans, TNFR-1 is constitutively expressed on membranes for most mammalian tissues and binds TNF-α irreversibly with subsequent activation of intracellular signaling cascades. In contrast to this, TNFR-2 expression is regulated and expressed predominantly on immune cells with rapid on and off binding to TNF-α. This rapid on and off binding allows immune cells to "ligand pass" TNF-α to TNFR-1 expressed on tissues.[4] Additionally, TNFR-2 stimulation has resulted in the proliferation of certain immune cells including thymocytes and peripheral cytotoxic T cells.[5] The primary net immune effects of TNF-α are monocyte differentiation, migration of inflammatory cells to infection site, regulation of the macrophage life cycle, and the formation of granulomas.[6,7] Additionally, TNF-α action leads to the production of cytokines including interleukin (IL)-1, IL-6, IL-8, monocyte chemoattractant protein type-1, and adhesion molecules.[8] Importantly, TNF-α stimulates production of interferon (IFN)-γ by T helper 1 cells, which primes mononuclear cells to express toll-like receptor-2 and -4 on cell membranes.[8–12] Toll-like receptor-2 and -4 function as pattern recognition receptors on host immune cells, which trigger immune responses in the presence of ligands on fungal cells including *Candida albicans*, *Aspergillus fumigatus*, *Coccidioides* spp, *Cryptococcus neoformans*, and agents of mucormycosis.[13–18]

TNF-α blockade has proven to be a useful therapeutic approach in numerous autoimmune conditions because of its far-reaching effects on inflammatory processes. Monoclonal antibodies targeting TNF-α are used in the treatment of rheumatoid arthritis, juvenile idiopathic arthritis, psoriatic arthritis, ankylosing spondylitis, plaque psoriasis, and inflammatory bowel diseases.[8,19–26]

The TNF-α inhibitors currently in use include the following:

- Infliximab: Chimeric (mouse/human) antibody, approved 1998
- Adalimumab: Fully human antibody, approved 2002
- Etanercept: Human TNFR-2 receptor fused to Fc portion of human IgG1, approved 2002
- Certolizumab pegol: Pegylated Fab of a human antibody, approved 2008
- Golimumab: Fully human antibody, approved 2009

Blockade of TNF-α produces a potent anti-inflammatory effect leading to decreased cytokine production,[8,27] impairment of monocyte recruitment,[8] prevention of granuloma formation,[8,28] and apoptotic and nonapoptotic cell death of TNFR expressing cells.[8,29,30] This can impair immune response against invading fungal pathogens and increase the risk of fungal infections. There have been numerous reviews characterizing fungal infections associated with TNF-α inhibitors,[8,31–34] and in 2008 the FDA assigned the class a black box warning for their increased risk of invasive fungal infections following 240 reported cases of histoplasmosis.[2] Next is a summary of the published literature surrounding fungal infections associated with the use of TNF-α inhibitor therapy.

Tumor Necrosis Factor-α Inhibitors and Fungal Infections

Several difficulties arise when attempting to accurately compare the incidence of fungal infections secondary to TNF-α inhibitors and other biologic agents. Notable difficulties include heterogeneous study design and fungal infections monitored, geographic considerations with endemic mycoses, baseline predisposition to fungal infections in patients with immune dysregulation from autoimmune disorders, and concomitant immunosuppressant therapy.[31] In a report characterizing fungal infections occurring in patients taking infliximab, adalimumab, and etanercept, the authors identified risk factors for the development of fungal infections including graft-versus-host disease, history of invasive mold infections, colonization with pathogenic fungi, environmental exposure, high-risk travel in endemic area (eg, histoplasmosis, coccidioidomycosis, and blastomycosis), high-risk outdoor activities (eg, spelunking), and construction work.[8]

Most of the experience characterizing fungal infections in TNF-α inhibitor therapy pertains to the older agents, infliximab, etanercept, and adalimumab. However, newer agents including certolizumab pegol and golimumab have also been associated with fungal infections.[35,36] Serious infection rates analyzed within the first year of initiating certolizumab pegol were not found to be significantly higher than other TNF-α inhibitors.[37] For golimumab, a follow-up of randomized controlled trials reported opportunistic infections (OIs) to occur more frequently in the patients receiving higher dose (100 mg) compared with the lower dose (50 mg).[38]

Candida and Cryptococcus

Invasive candidiasis has been reported with the use of TNF-α inhibitor therapy. Tsiodras and colleagues8,[39–45] report on 64 cases of Candida infections associated with infliximab, adalimumab, and etanercept. Three of these cases presented with coinfection with Aspergillus spp and Pneumocystis jirovecii,[44] Salmonella spp,[13] and a mixed intra-abdominal abscess.[46] The reported incidence of candidiasis associated with TNF-α in the FDA Adverse Events Reporting System (AERS) from 1998 to 2002 was 5.31 cases/100,000 persons with etanercept to 10.15 cases/100,000 persons with infliximab.[42,47] Data from 10 pooled randomized controlled trials of certolizumab pegol for rheumatoid arthritis reported seven cases of oral and esophageal candidiasis with an event rate of 0.08/100 person-years (PY).[48] Five-year safety follow-up of five clinical trials assessing golimumab including 2228 patients documented six cases of esophageal and gastrointestinal candidiasis and one case of mixed Candida and Aspergillus esophagitis. The overall OI occurrence across all trials was 0.22/100 PY.[49]

Cryptococcosis, predominantly pulmonary cryptococcosis, has been identified in patients receiving monoclonal TNF-α inhibitor therapy.[50–54] However, extrapulmonary disease has occurred including disseminated cryptococcosis[55] and tenosynovitis.[56] In their AERS review, Wallis and colleagues[42] identified a cryptococcosis case incidence of 5.08/100,000 persons on infliximab.

Aspergillus

Tsiodras and colleagues[8] identified 64 cases of aspergillosis in their review. Of these, 50 occurred in patients receiving monoclonal TNF-α inhibitors (infliximab, n = 48; adalimumab, n = 2) and 14 occurred in patients receiving etanercept. Eighteen out of 24 cases with information available were in patients with graft-versus-host disease after hematopoietic stem cell transplant, a patient demographic with a high baseline risk for aspergillosis, and all patients were on concomitant immunosuppressant therapy. However, 6/24 (25%) of patients were receiving TNF-α inhibitor therapy for other inflammatory conditions including inflammatory bowel disease in two patients and rheumatoid arthritis in four patients. Aspergillosis has also been reported with newer monoclonal TNF-α inhibitors golimumab[36] and certolizumab pegol.[35,48] The reported incidence of aspergillosis in patients on TNF-α inhibitor therapy ranges from 6.19 to 8.63 cases/100,000 persons.[42,47]

Agents of Mucormycosis

Although not as common as other reported fungal infections, there have been reports of mucormycosis in patients on TNF-α inhibitor therapy. Two cases have been reported in hematopoietic stem cell recipients receiving infliximab for severe graft-versus-host disease.[57] A case of mucormycosis presenting as recurrent gastric perforation was observed in a patient on infliximab, 6-mercaptopurine, and glucocorticoid therapy for the treatment of Crohn's disease.[58] A separate case reported a patient on adalimumab in combination with methotrexate and prednisone for rheumatoid arthritis who succumbed to disseminated mucormycosis.[59]

Endemic Mycoses

In an early report from the German Biologics Register, infliximab demonstrated an overall increased risk of serious infections compared with placebo in randomized controlled trials (relative risk [RR], 3.0; 95% confidence interval [CI], 1.8–5.1). In the identifiable infections, 2 of the 10 identifiable granulomatous infections were caused by histoplasmosis and coccidioidomycosis.[60,61] The 2008 FDA warning for increased risk of invasive fungal infections was prompted by 240 cases of histoplasmosis in patients treated with TNF-αinhibitor therapy and it warns providers to remain vigilant in monitoring patients on TNF-α inhibitors.[2] A separate multicenter retrospective review of 98 patients diagnosed with histoplasmosis from 2000 to 2011 while on TNF-α inhibitor therapy sought to determine the need for long-term antifungals and the safety of resuming TNF-α inhibitors. Most patients were on infliximab (n = 66; 67%), followed by adalimumab (n = 23; 23.5%), and etanercept (n = 9; 9.5%). The authors concluded that discontinuation of antifungal treatment after a favorable clinical response and an appropriate duration of therapy, probably at least 12 months, seems to be safe if pharmacologic immunosuppression has been held. Resumption of TNF-α inhibitor therapy also seems to be safe assuming that the initial antifungal therapy was administered for an appropriate duration. A comparison of infliximab and adalimumab versus etanercept did not demonstrate a significantly higher propensity for severe disease in patients on infliximab or adalimumab.[62] When reviewing 13 coccidioidomycosis cases in patients with rheumatoid arthritis in endemic areas, Nevada, Arizona, and California, the use of TNF-α inhibitors significantly increased risk of developing coccidioidomycosis compared with other therapies (RR, 5.23; 95% CI, 1.54–17.71). Although it is prudent to consider holding TNF-α inhibitor therapy during treatment of active coccidioidomycosis, it seems TNF-α inhibitors can be resumed after coccidioidomycosis disease control has been achieved in carefully selected patients based on disease activity.[63] Blastomycosis has not been reported with the same frequency as the other endemic mycoses, but there have been case reports associated with the use of TNF-α inhibitors.[8,31,64,65]

Pneumocystis

In a database review of 33,324 new TNF-α inhibitor patients, 80 nonviral OIs were identified with *P jirovecii* pneumonia (PJP) being the most common (n = 16). There was a significantly higher crude rate of nonviral OI among new users of TNF-α inhibitors compared with those initiating nonbiologic disease-modifying antirheumatic drug (2.7 vs 1.7 per 1000 PY; adjusted hazard ratio, 1.6; 95% CI, 1.0–2.6). Baseline corticosteroid use was also significantly associated with nonviral OI (adjusted hazard ratio, 2.5; 95% CI, 1.5–4.0).[65] Eighty-four cases of PJP were identified in the FDA AERS from 1998 to 2003 associated with infliximab therapy. Patients receiving infliximab also had concomitant immunosuppressive medications including methotrexate, prednisone, azathioprine, 6-mercaptopurine, and cyclosporine. The mean time between infliximab infusion and onset of symptoms, when reported, was 21 days.[66] High-dose glucocorticoid use was identified as risk factor for development of PJP in a case-control study and prophylaxis is indicated in patients receiving high doses for prolonged courses.[67]

IBRUTINIB AND TYROSINE KINASE INHIBITORS

The small molecule tyrosine kinase inhibitor (TKI) class represents a monumental step forward in the search for targeted therapy in the treatment of various oncologic and autoimmune disorders. The agents in the TKI class exert their effects on target cells through competing with ATP at its binding site on protein tyrosine kinase preventing phosphorylation and subsequent cellular proliferation. Ibrutinib, a Bruton TKI for B-cell cancers, is perhaps the most notable agent in this class with respect to opportunistic fungal infections. In a review of fungal infections associated with TKIs, Chamilos and colleagues[68] describe 41 reported cases of fungal infections in patients on ibrutinib therapy (**Table 1**). A considerable number of these cases presented with atypical manifestations of diseases including central nervous system aspergillosis, extrapulmonary P jirovecii infection, and disseminated cryptococcosis with a high overall mortality rate. This atypical presentation of disease in an exceptionally vulnerable population requires providers to maintain a high clinical suspicion for opportunistic fungal infections with a low threshold to initiate empiric treatment in patients on ibrutinib. It is theorized that increased susceptibility to fungal infections, particularly to A fumigatus, could be facilitated by decreased macrophage fungal immune surveillance.[69] Other TKIs that have been implicated in the development of opportunistic fungal infections include dasatinib,[70,71] imatinib,[72,73] idelasilib,[18] ruxolitinib,[74] sunitinib,[75,76] sorafenib,[77] and tofacitinib[78] (see **Table 1**).

MONOCLONAL CHECKPOINT INHIBITORS

Programmed cell death-1 (PD-1, CD270) is an immune inhibitory receptor belonging to the CD28:B7 family of costimulatory molecules. Expressed on active B cells, T cells, and myeloid cells, PD-1 binds to two ligands (PD-L1 and PD-L2) and because PD-1 upregulation occurs after many costimulatory pathways have been engaged, one possible role for this inhibitory receptor is to help attenuate or shut off developing effector T-cell responses.[79] Similar effects have also been observed for anti–cytotoxic T-lymphocyte-association protein 4 (CTLA-4) antibodies.[80]

Most of the work on the role of PD-1 in infectious diseases has focused on chronic viral infections where it has been shown to regulate $CD8^+$ T-cell function and with overexpression has been associated with disease progression during persistent viral infections.[81] Of note, in virus-infected patients, $CD8^+$ T cells overexpressing PD-1 (in comparison with healthy volunteers) exhibit a so-called "exhaustion profile" because they produced less IFN-γ following antigen stimulation, had reduced cytotoxic activity, and had decreased proliferation in response to specific antigens.

Blockade of the PD-1 pathway during lymphocytic choriomeningitis virus and simian immunodeficiency virus enhances viral control in mice and primates, respectively.[82,83] In humans, in vitro PD-1 blockade enhances virus-specific T-cell responses against human immunodeficiency virus,[84–86] hepatitis C,[87] and hepatitis B.[88] On the contrary, PD-1 knockout mice seem to display markedly increased susceptibility to Mycobacterium tuberculosis.[89] Presumably, this higher death rate was caused by unregulated clonal expansion of the T-cell response with an accompanying

Table 1
Reported fungal infections with monoclonal antibody therapy

Drug	Infection	Reference
TNF-α Inhibitors		
Adalimumab	17 Histoplasmosis 8 Coccidioidomycosis 2 Cryptococcosis 2 Aspergillosis 1 Disseminated mucormycosis 1 Candidiasis	2,8,43,56,59,63,131
Certolizumab pegol	7 Oral/esophageal candidiasis 0.08/100 PY 3 Bronchopulmonary aspergillosis 0.03/100 PY 2 Fungal esophageal/gastrointestinal infections 0.02/100 PY 2 Histoplasmosis 0.02/100 PY 1 PJP 0.01/100 PY 1 Aspergillosis 1 Oral candidiasis	35,48
Etanercept	14 Aspergillosis 7 Coccidioidomycosis 10 Cryptococcosis	8,63,141
Golimumab	6 Oral/esophageal candidiasis 2 *Histoplasma* infections 1 Aspergilloma 1 Mixed *Candida/Aspergillus* esophagitis 1 PJP 1 Aspergillosis	36,49
Infliximab	8.63 Aspergillosis/100,000 persons 10.15 Candidiasis/100,000 persons 5.58 Coccidioidomycosis/100,000 persons 5.08 Cryptococcosis/100,000 persons 18.78 Histoplasmosis/100,000 persons 307 Histoplasmosis 84 PJP 55 Aspergillosis 34 Coccidioidomycosis 17 Candidiasis 6 Cryptococcosis 3 Mucormycosis 2 Unspecified fungal infections 1 PJP	2,8,39–42,44–46,50–55,57,58,61–63,66,141
Infliximab Adalimumab Etanercept	16 PJP 9 Histoplasmosis 3 Cryptococcosis 1 Unspecified endemic fungal infection 1 Coccidioidomycosis 1 Blastomycosis 1 Aspergillosis	65
TNF-α Inhibitor	2 Blastomycosis	64
Tyrosine Kinase Inhibitors		

(continued on next page)

Table 1
(*continued*)

Drug	Infection	Reference
Dasatinib	2 PJP 1 Candidemia	70,71
Ibrutinib	13 Invasive aspergillosis (3 CNS, 4 lung, 5 CNS/lung, 1 CNS/sinusitis) 5 PJP 4 Disseminated cryptococcosis 2 Mucormycosis 1 Cryptococcosis 1 Extrapulmonary *Pneumocystis* infection 1 Histoplasmosis 1 Pulmonary mucormycosis/ aspergillosis 1 Disseminated fusariosis	68,72
Ruxolitinib	2 PJP	74
Sorafenib	1 Invasive pulmonary aspergillosis	77
Sunitinib	2 Invasive pulmonary aspergillosis	75,76
Tofacitinib	9 Esophageal candidiasis 4 PJP 3 Cryptococcosis (2 pulmonary, 1 meningitis)	78
Ustekinumab	3 Candidiasis 1 Pulmonary blastomycosis	101,142
Checkpoint Inhibitors		
Durvalumab	1 Pulmonary aspergillosis	143
Ipilimumab Nivolumab Pembrolizumab	3 Invasive pulmonary aspergillosis 2 PJP 1 Candidemia	92
Interleukin Inhibitors		
Brodalumab	29 Candidiasis	101
Canakinumab	1 Fungal infection	97
Ixekizumab	16 Mucocutaneous candidiasis	105
Mogamulizumab	1 Oral candidiasis	144
Reslizumab	1 Disseminated aspergillosis	99
Sarilumab	1 Candida bronchitis	108
Secukinumab	6 Candidiasis	104
Tocilizumab	0.13 Opportunistic infections/100 PY (tocilizumab) 1 PJP	106,107
CD Inhibitors		
Alemtuzumab	47 Candidiasis 30 Aspergillosis 15 Superficial fungal infections 12 Cryptococcosis 3 Mucormycosis 3 Histoplasmosis 1 Fusariosis 10 Unidentified fungal infections	123,124,145

(*continued on next page*)

Table 1 (continued)		
Drug	**Infection**	**Reference**
Basiliximab	4 Aspergillosis 20 Unidentified fungal infections	126,128
Daclizumab	66 Aspergillosis 14 *Candida albicans* 10 Nonalbicans *Candida* spp 10 Other yeasts 7 Aspergillosis 5 *Torulopsis glabrata (Candida glabrata)* 1 Cunninghamella 1 *Scedosporium apiospermum*	129,130
Ocrelizumab	2 Candidiasis 1 Histoplasmosis 1 PJP	146
Rituximab	1.51%–2.97% PJP incidence 17 PJP 7 Candidiasis and candidemia 4 Aspergillosis 1 Scedosporiosis	31,111–114
Agents Targeting T-Cell Activation		
Abatacept	3 Oral candidiasis 2 Histoplasmosis	131,132
Belatacept	Tinea versicolor 2.19/100 PY Onychomycosis 2.13/100 PY Fungal infection 1.28/100 PY Fungal skin infection 0.85/100 PY Body tinea 0.85/100 PY Vulvovaginal candidiasis 0.84/100 PY 1 Histoplasmosis 1 PJP	134,135,147
Complement C5 Inhibitors		
Eculizumab	1 *Aspergillus niger* peritonitis (+*Escherichia coli* and *Enterococcus faecium*)	137
Alpha-4 Integrin Inhibitors		
Natalizumab	1 Cutaneous candidiasis	138
VEGFR Inhibitors		
Bevacizumab	1 *Fusarium*-associated nasal septum perforation	139

Abbreviations: CNS, central nervous system; VEGFR, vascular endothelial growth factor receptor.

increase in tissue necrosis suggesting a need for careful dosing for PD-1 antagonists rather than complete inhibition and unchecked T-cell proliferation.

Checkpoint Inhibitors and Fungal Infections

Limited data regarding the role of PD-1 and PD-1 inhibition exist for invasive fungal infections and upregulation in human infection has been evaluated only in paracoccidioidomycosis, an infection endemic to Central and South America.[90] However, a precedent for improvements in mortality with PD-1 blockade in invasive fungal infections has been observed in *Histoplasma capsulatum*–infected mice.[91] In this study, PD-1 knockout mice and mice treated with PD-1-blocking antibody showed less signs of disease and more rapidly cleared infection than wild-type and untreated mice, which all eventually died of disseminated histoplasmosis. It is apparent from these studies that the infectious agent and the target tissue may vary greatly in their responsiveness to PD-1 blockade. In one retrospective review of 740 patients prescribed checkpoint inhibitors for treatment of melanoma, 54 patients (7.3%) developed serious infections after an average of 135 days (range, 6–491 days) postinitiation. Six proven or probable fungal infections were reported with three patients diagnosed with invasive pulmonary aspergillosis, two with PJP, and one candidemia.[92] In a case report of a patient prescribed ipilimumab for melanoma, the patient developed invasive pulmonary aspergillosis 3 months after starting therapy. The clinical picture was complicated by the administration of infliximab and corticosteroids for active colitis after the initiation of ipilimumab and before diagnosis of aspergillosis.[93] PD-1 checkpoint inhibitor therapy has been used as salvage therapy in conjunction with IFN-γ for the treatment of intractable mucormycosis in an immunocompromised patient with lymphocytopenia and high T-cell PD-1 expression.[94]

INTERLEUKIN INHIBITORS
IL-1β Inhibitors

Several monoclonal antibodies have been developed that target ILs, proteins involved in the regulation of cell growth, differentiation, motility, and stimulation of immune responses.[95] Canakinumab, a human monoclonal targeting IL-1B involved in proinflammatory responses, demonstrated a nonsignificant increase in the incidence rate of infections relative to placebo in a dose-finding study, but fungal infections were not described in these data.[96] A single, unspecified fungal infection was reported in an open-label study of canakinumab for neonatal-onset multisystem inflammatory disease.[97]

IL-5 Inhibitors

Long-term safety data for the humanized monoclonal IL-5 inhibitor mepolizumab used for severe eosinophilic asthma identified seven OIs (two herpesvirus infections, five unidentified), but no fungal infections were reported.[98] A case of disseminated aspergillosis has been reported in a patient with a history of allergic bronchopulmonary aspergillosis and severe asthma treated with reslizumab, another humanized monoclonal IL-5 inhibitor. The patient developed several skin nodules that grew *Aspergillus* spp after initiation of therapy. The authors highlight that although IL-5 inhibitors are used for their inhibition of eosinophilic function, IL-5 neutralization also affects macrophage, T-lymphocyte, and B-lymphocyte function.[99]

IL-17 and IL-23 Inhibitors

Ustekinumab is a human monoclonal antibody inhibitor of proinflammatory cytokines IL-12 and IL-23 used in the treatment of plaque psoriasis. Its use resulted in a lower overall incidence of serious infections (0.83/100 PY) compared with adalimumab (1.97/100 PY) and infliximab (2.47/100 PY) in a follow-up study of biologic agents used for psoriasis therapy.[100] Infections caused by *Candida* spp occurred in similar rates in the ustekinumab and placebo arms in two phase III trials comparing ustekinumab with an IL-17 inhibitor, brodalumab, for the treatment of psoriasis.[101] In these trials, infections consistent with mild to moderate candidiasis occurred approximately twice as frequently with brodalumab (1.3% in 140-mg arm; 1.6% in 210-mg arm) than placebo (0.6%).[101] Secukinumab and ixekizumab, monoclonal inhibitors of IL-17A indicated in the treatment of psoriasis, were also associated with increased rates of candidiasis. Patients treated with secukinumab developed oral, esophageal, skin, or vaginal candidiasis at a rate of 1% to 5%.[31,102–104] Patients given ixekizumab developed mucocutaneous candidiasis twice as frequently when compared with placebo in two phase III trials, but there were no invasive fungal infections reported.[105] This predisposition for candidiasis in patients receiving IL-17 and IL-17A inhibitor therapy supports the belief that IL-17A plays a role in host defenses against fungal pathogens, particularly at mucosal membranes.[103]

IL-6 Inhibitors

Tocilizumab is a humanized monoclonal inhibitor of the IL-6 receptor, which leads to a reduction in cytokine and acute phase reactant production. Tocilizumab is used in the treatment of cytokine release syndrome caused by CAR-T cell therapy and in autoimmune conditions, such as rheumatoid arthritis and giant cell arteritis. Risk factors for serious infections in patients prescribed tocilizumab for rheumatoid arthritis compared with other biologics were reported in a review of the French Registry REGATE.[106] Among the 1491 patients, 125 serious infections requiring hospitalization and/or intravenous therapy occurred in 122 patients (incidence rate, 4.7/100 PY). Of the two OIs identified, there was one case of PJP. The mean corticosteroid dose prescribed for evaluated subjects was 10.9 mg/d with 8.4% of patients on a dose of greater than 15 mg/d. The probability of remaining free of serious infections during at 36-month follow-up was 87.3% (95% CI, 84.9–89.7). In a multidatabase review of serious infections in tocilizumab versus other biologic therapies for patients with rheumatoid arthritis from 2010 to 2015, the incidence rate of OIs with tocilizumab was 0.13/100 PY (95% CI, 0.07–0.20) compared with 0.13/100 PY (95% CI, 0.09–0.17) with TNF-α inhibitor therapy.[107] OIs have been described in patients taking sarilumab,[108] a newer IL-6 inhibitor, but long-term safety data are needed to fully characterize its impact on fungal infections.

CLUSTER OF DIFFERENTIATION INHIBITORS

Cluster of differentiation (CD) receptors are cell surface molecules present on lymphoid and myeloid lineage cells in the immune system with diverse immunologic and biologic functions including cellular signaling, cellular adhesion, cellular activation, and immune regulation.[109] Several monoclonal antibody therapies have been developed to selectively target CD proteins expressed on various immune cell lines primarily in the treatment of autoimmune conditions and malignancies, such as leukemia, lymphoma, and multiple myeloma. Directly attributing fungal infections to monoclonal antibody therapy is challenging in this patient population given common exposure to concomitant immunosuppression, neutropenia, and effect of underlying disease on infection risk.

Agents Targeting B Cells: Anti-CD20, Anti-CD22, and Anti-CD30 Monoclonals

CD20 antigen is expressed on normal and malignant B cells, with expression gradually increasing as these cells mature. Despite targeting B cells, anti-CD20 monoclonal inhibitors do not immediately impair production of immunoglobulin because CD20 antigens are not expressed on B-cell precursors or plasma cells.[110] Rituximab is a first-generation CD20 inhibitor and is the most extensively studied monoclonal in its class. Rituximab has been used in the treatment of various CD20-positive malignancies affecting B cells and autoimmune conditions. Kelesidis and colleagues[111] have characterized fungal infections that have been reported with the use of rituximab. When used with the regimen of cyclophosphamide, doxorubicin, vincristine, and prednisone (CHOP) for human immunodeficiency virus–associated non-Hodgkin lymphoma, there was an increased risk of opportunistic fungal infections compared with CHOP alone with three patients suffering from PJP, one candidemia, and one esophageal candidiasis. All patients received mandatory PJP prophylaxis.[112] They summarize additional case reports of fungal infections temporally associated with the onset of rituximab therapy, which are found in **Table 1**. A meta-analysis of 11 cohort studies of patients with lymphoma suggested an increased risk for PJP (RR, 3.65; $P = .001$), but with a low overall incidence (rituximab 2.97% vs nonrituximab 0.51%). Patients treated with biweekly rituximab-containing regimens were at a nonsignificant higher risk than those treated with triweekly regimens and prophylaxis with trimethoprim-sulfamethoxazole reduced occurrence of infection by 91%.[113] A consensus statement from the European Society of Clinical Microbiology and Infectious Diseases Study Group for Infections in Compromised Hosts does not recommend universal PJP prophylaxis with rituximab therapy because of the low overall incidence of infection, which is below the conventional threshold for necessitating prophylaxis (3.5%). However, if a patient has additional indications for prophylaxis ($\geq$20 mg prednisone for 4 or more weeks), it is warranted.[110,114] Long-term follow-up safety data are needed to characterize the opportunistic fungal infection risk with second-generation (ofatumumab, ocrelizumab, veltuzumab) and third-generation (obinutuzumab, ocaratuzumab, ublituximab) CD20 inhibitors.[115]

CD22 is a surface protein expressed on mature B cells that facilitates cellular adhesion, cellular activation, and cell survival. Currently approved monoclonal inhibitors of CD22 include epratuzumab, inotuzumab ozogamicin, and moxetumomab. It is believed that increased susceptibility to infection with these agents would closely resemble that seen with CD20 inhibitor rituximab. Despite this theoretic risk, rates of serious infections caused by epratuzumab with background standard therapy were nearly identical to placebo (51.7%–60.6% vs 59.7%–60.6%) in two phase III trials for the treatment of systemic lupus erythematous. No fungal infections were described in either of the two trials.[116] In a study comparing inotuzumab ozogamicin with standard therapy for acute lymphoblastic leukemia, no fungal infections occurred in the inotuzumab arm, but two cases of fungal pneumonia were observed in the standard therapy arm.[117] A consensus statement by the European Society of Clinical Microbiology and Infectious Diseases states that no benefit is to be expected from universal PJP prophylaxis in patients on CD22 inhibitors, but concomitant immunosuppression and comorbidities should be considered.[109]

CD30 is expressed on various cell types including T cells, B cells, monocytes, and activated natural killer cells. Its functions are not fully understood, but it is implicated in the regulation of memory and effector cell production and is a part of the TNF/nerve growth factor receptor superfamily.[109] No increased risk for fungal infections was appreciated in clinical trials for the CD30 inhibitor brentuximab vedotin, a chimeric antibody-drug conjugate used in the treatment of relapsed or refractory Hodgkin lymphoma and cutaneous anaplastic large cell lymphoma.[118,119] However, PJP prophylaxis was used in these trials and is recommended in recipients of hematopoietic stem cell transplants on brentuximab vedotin therapy.

Agents for Rejection Prevention: Anti-CD52 and Anti-CD25 Monoclonals

The CD52 antigen is highly expressed on mature lymphocytes including T cells, B cells, monocytes, and natural killer cells, and it is densely expressed on malignant

T cells. Alemtuzumab is a humanized monoclonal antibody that binds to CD52 antigen leading to antibody-dependent lysis, which can manifest in significant lymphopenia.[120,121] Alemtuzumab has been used in the induction for solid organ transplant and stem cell transplant and in the treatment of lymphoproliferative disorders and relapsing forms of multiple sclerosis. Alemtuzumab therapy has been associated with various opportunistic and fungal infections.[122] In a single-center study characterizing the infectious complications of patients receiving alemtuzmab therapy for lymphoproliferative disorders over a period of 2.5 years, 15 of 27 (56%) patients were diagnosed with an OI. Of those, there were three patients with invasive pulmonary aspergillosis and one patient each with disseminated histoplasmosis and disseminated cryptococcosis.[123] A systematic review was conducted on fungal infections following alemtuzumab use, which included 38 trials and 1225 patients. Antifungal prophylaxis was provided in 13 trials (n = 472; 38.5%) and PJP prophylaxis with sulfamethoxazole/trimethoprim in 27 trials (n = 1107; 90.3%). Overall, 730 infections were diagnosed in 1225 patients (59.6%). The cause of these infections was viral in (n = 385; 52.7%), bacterial (n = 155; 21.2%), fungal (n = 90; 12.3%), PJP (n = 18; 2.5%), protozoal (n = 2; 0.3%), and unknown (n = 80; 11%). The causes of fungal infections are listed in **Table 1**.[124]

Basiliximab is a monoclonal antibody directed against the α-chain of the IL-2 receptor (IL-2Rα or CD25) to prevent CD25-mediated T-cell activation.[125] In a trial comparing basiliximab with rabbit anti-thymocyte globulin (rATG) for induction therapy in renal transplant recipients, there were 20 fungal infections observed in the basiliximab and rATG arms (14.6% vs 14.2%; P = 1.0). Antifungal prophylaxis was administered based on the standard protocols at each center.[126] There were no fungal infections observed with basiliximab induction in an observational study of 46 consecutive liver transplant recipients compared with one case of fungemia in the historical control group.[127] Invasive aspergillosis occurred at comparable rates in another comparative trial between basiliximab and rATG in lung transplant recipients (4/21 [19%] vs 3/16 [18.8%]), a patient population that is disproportionately afflicted by invasive pulmonary aspergillosis compared with other solid organ transplant groups.[128,129]

Daclizumab is also an anti-CD25 antibody with the same mechanism of action as basiliximab used in induction therapy for rejection prevention in solid organ transplant recipients. In a retrospective review of a single-lung, double-lung, and heart-lung transplants at a single center from 1992 to 2003, the use of daclizumab was an independent risk factor for *Aspergillus* colonization and invasive disease when compared with polyclonal induction (odds ratio [OR], 2.05; 95% CI, 1.14–3.75). Additional independent risk factors identified were donor age (OR, 1.40 per decade; 95% CI, 1.10–1.80), and ischemia time (OR, 1.17 per hour increase; 95% CI, 1.01–1.39). Patients with cystic fibrosis as their underlying lung pathology were noted to have an elevated risk of *Aspergillus* colonization and invasive disease compared with patients without cystic fibrosis (53% vs 29%; P = .01).[129] Daclizumab use in combination with other immunosuppressive therapy was associated with a higher overall OI rate with fungal pathogens including *Aspergillus*, *Scedosporium*, *Cunninghamella*, *Candida* spp, and other yeasts.[130]

AGENTS TARGETING T-CELL ACTIVATION

Abatacept is a fusion protein consisting of the Fc domain of human IgG1 protein and the extracellular domain of CTLA-4. Abatacept produces its immunomodulatory effects through inhibition of T-cell activation and is used clinically in the treatment of rheumatoid arthritis and psoriatic arthritis. Fungal infections have been reported following abatacept treatment including candidiasis[131] and histoplasmosis.[131,132]

Despite this, abatacept therapy seems to be linked to lower serious infections compared with TNF-α inhibitor therapy, particularly infliximab.[133]

Belatacept, similar to abatacept, is a soluble fusion protein consisting of the modified extracellular domain of CTLA-4 fused to a portion of a human IgG antibody. It functions similarly to abatacept through blocking costimulation of T-lymphocytes and is used in the prevention of solid organ transplant rejection. In a 3-year follow-up study of the safety of belatacept compared with calcineurin inhibitor therapy in the prevention of rejection for kidney transplant recipients, more patients had fungal infections in the belatacept group than those receiving calcineurin inhibitors (9.73/100 PY vs 2.58/100 PY). The most common types of fungal infections were onychomycosis and tinea versicolor. Additional fungal infections have been reported with belatacept therapy including invasive fungal infections, such as mediastinal histoplasmosis[134] and PJP.[135]

OTHER MONOCLONAL ANTIBODIES

Eculizumab is a humanized monoclonal antibody that blocks the cleavage and activity of complement factor 5 impairing complement-mediated cell lysis. It is approved for use in paroxysmal nocturnal hemoglobinuria, atypical hemolytic uremic syndrome, generalized myasthenia gravis, and neuromyelitis optica spectrum disorder. Eculizumab therapy is associated with an increased risk of infections because of its direct antagonism on the complement system. Because of their thick cell wall, fungi are resistant to membrane attack complex–mediated cell lysis. However, secondary effects including complement factor 3 mediated-opsonization leading to phagocyte recruitment and inflammatory response may provide protection against fungal infections.[136] A case of polymicrobial (*Escherichia coli*, *Enterococcus faecium*, and *Aspergillus niger*) peritonitis has been reported in a patient on peritoneal dialysis on long-term eculizumab therapy for atypical hemolytic uremic syndrome.[137]

Natalizumab is a humanized recombinant monoclonal antibody targeting the α-4 subunit of integrin proteins, which facilitate adhesion and migration of cells from the vasculature into inflamed tissue. Natalizumab blocks integrin association with vascular receptors preventing transmigration of leukocytes and it carries indications for the treatment of Crohn's disease and multiple sclerosis. The FDA issued a black box warning of progressive multifocal leukoencephalopathy after several patients developed the disease in clinical trials leading to its approval, which is covered in greater depth in elsewhere in this issue. Fungal infections attributed to natalizumab include PJP, aspergillosis, and candidiasis.[125,138]

Bevacizumab is a humanized monoclonal targeting vascular epithelial growth factor receptor, which prevents angiogenesis in the treatment of various advanced cancers. Infections while on therapy have been predominantly seen in the setting of concomitant immunosuppressive chemotherapy with severe neutropenia. Because of its disruptive effects on angiogenesis and endothelial cell proliferation, there is an increased risk of intestinal perforation with or without abscess formation with bevacizumab therapy. Most infections reported with bevacizumab are caused by bacterial pathogens, but there has been a case report of *Fusarium solani* nasal septal perforation following initiation of bevacizumab for advanced colorectal cancer.[139] Bevacizumab, in combination with triamcinolone, is injected intravitreally for the treatment of exudative age-related macular degeneration. There have been reported infectious complications of this practice including an outbreak of *Candida* endophthalmitis caused by contaminated mixtures.[140]

Table 2
Agents without apparent increased risk of fungal infection or insufficient data

Agent	Class	Reference
Abciximab	Glycoprotein IIb/IIIa inhibitor	125
Alefacept	T-cell costimulation modulator	148,149
Avelumab	PD-L1 inhibitor	150
Belimumab	BLyS inhibitor	151
Blinatumomab	CD19 inhibitor	110
Bosutinib	BCR-ABL inhibitor	152,153
Brentuximab vedotin	CD30 inhibitor	118
Cabozantinib	c-MET, VEGFR2, and AXL inhibitor	68
Cemiplimab	PD-1 inhibitor	154
Cetuximab	EGFR inhibitor	125
Dabrafenib	B-raf inhibitor	68
Daratumumab	CD38 inhibitor	125
Dupilumab	IL-4 inhibitor	155
Elotuzumab	SLAMF7 inhibitor	109
Epratuzumab	CD22 inhibitor	116
Gemtuzumab ozogamicin	CD33 inhibitor	125
Inotuzumab ozogamicin	CD22 inhibitor	117
Omalizumab	IgE receptor antibody	125
Palivizumab	RSV fusion protein inhibitor	125
Panitumumab	EGFR inhibitor	125
Ponatinib	BCR-ABL, PDGFR, EGFR, KIT, and FLT3 inhibitor	68
Ravulizumab	Complement C5 inhibitor	156
Trastuzumab	HER-2 inhibitor	125
Vedolizumab	Anti-integrin antibody	31

Abbreviations: AXL, axl tyrosine kinase receptor; BLyS, B-lymphocyte stimulator; EGFR, epidermal growth factor receptor; FLT3, fms-like tyrosine receptor 3; HER-2, human epidermal growth factor receptor 2; KIT, c-kit tyrosine kinase receptor; PDGFR, platelet-derived growth factor receptor; RSV, human respiratory syncytial virus; SLAMF7, signaling lymphocytic activation molecule F7; VEGFR2, vascular growth factor receptor 2.

SUMMARY

With an ever-growing armamentarium of novel biologic agents exerting known and unforeseen effects on the immune system, it is imperative that clinicians maintain awareness of the associated risks these therapies pose for development of fungal infections (**Table 2**). Careful screening of baseline risk factors before initiation, targeted preventive measures, and vigilant monitoring while on active biologic therapy can help mitigate these risks as the use of these agents becomes increasingly more commonplace.

REFERENCES

1. Geng X, Kong X, Hu H, et al. Research and development of therapeutic mabs: an analysis based on pipeline projects. Hum Vaccin Immunother 2015;11(12): 2769–76.
2. Information for healthcare professionals: Cimzia (certolizumab pegol), Enbrel (etanercept), Humira (adalimumab), and Remicade (infliximab). U.S. Food

and Drug Administration. 2008. Available at: https://wayback.archive-it.org/ 7993/20170112032015/http://www.fda.gov/Drugs/DrugSafety/PostmarketDrugSafety-InformationforPatientsandProviders/ucm124185.htm. Accessed September 10, 2019.

3. Parameswaran N, Patial S. Tumor necrosis factor-alpha signaling in macrophages. Crit Rev Eukaryot Gene Expr 2010;20(2):87–103.

4. Tartaglia LA, Pennica D, Goeddel DV. Ligand passing: the 75-kda tumor necrosis factor (TNF) receptor recruits TNF for signaling by the 55-kda TNF receptor. J Biol Chem 1993;268(25):18542–8.

5. Tartaglia LA, Weber RF, Figari IS, et al. The two different receptors for tumor necrosis factor mediate distinct cellular responses. Proc Natl Acad Sci U S A 1991; 88(20):9292–6.

6. Deepe GS Jr, Smelt S, Louie JS. Tumor necrosis factor inhibition and opportunistic infections. Clin Infect Dis 2005;41(Suppl 3):S187–8.

7. Wajant H, Siegmund D. Tnfr1 and tnfr2 in the control of the life and death balance of macrophages. Front Cell Dev Biol 2019;7:91.

8. Tsiodras S, Samonis G, Boumpas DT, et al. Fungal infections complicating tumor necrosis factor alpha blockade therapy. Mayo Clin Proc 2008;83(2):181–94.

9. Mosmann TR, Sad S. The expanding universe of T-cell subsets: Th1, th2 and more. Immunol Today 1996;17(3):138–46.

10. Bosisio D, Polentarutti N, Sironi M, et al. Stimulation of toll-like receptor 4 expression in human mononuclear phagocytes by interferon-gamma: a molecular basis for priming and synergism with bacterial lipopolysaccharide. Blood 2002; 99(9):3427–31.

11. Syed MM, Phulwani NK, Kielian T. Tumor necrosis factor-alpha (TNF-alpha) regulates toll-like receptor 2 (TLR2) expression in microglia. J Neurochem 2007; 103(4):1461–71.

12. Hermoso MA, Matsuguchi T, Smoak K, et al. Glucocorticoids and tumor necrosis factor alpha cooperatively regulate toll-like receptor 2 gene expression. Mol Cell Biol 2004;24(11):4743–56.

13. Netea MG, Ferwerda G, van der Graaf CA, et al. Recognition of fungal pathogens by toll-like receptors. Curr Pharm Des 2006;12(32):4195–201.

14. Netea MG, Van Der Graaf CA, Vonk AG, et al. The role of toll-like receptor (TLR) 2 and TLR4 in the host defense against disseminated candidiasis. J Infect Dis 2002;185(10):1483–9.

15. Meier A, Kirschning CJ, Nikolaus T, et al. Toll-like receptor (TLR) 2 and TLR4 are essential for aspergillus-induced activation of murine macrophages. Cell Microbiol 2003;5(8):561–70.

16. Dubourdeau M, Athman R, Balloy V, et al. *Aspergillus fumigatus* induces innate immune responses in alveolar macrophages through the MAPK pathway independently of TLR2 and TLR4. J Immunol 2006;177(6):3994–4001.

17. Viriyakosol S, Fierer J, Brown GD, et al. Innate immunity to the pathogenic fungus *Coccidioides posadasii* is dependent on toll-like receptor 2 and dectin-1. Infect Immun 2005;73(3):1553–60.

18. Chamilos G, Lewis RE, Lamaris G, et al. Zygomycetes hyphae trigger an early, robust proinflammatory response in human polymorphonuclear neutrophils through toll-like receptor 2 induction but display relative resistance to oxidative damage. Antimicrob Agents Chemother 2008;52(2):722–4.

19. Lis K, Kuzawinska O, Balkowiec-Iskra E. Tumor necrosis factor inhibitors: state of knowledge. Arch Med Sci 2014;10(6):1175–85.

20. Maini RN, Feldmann M. How does infliximab work in rheumatoid arthritis? Arthritis Res 2002;4(Suppl 2):S22–8.
21. Tracey D, Klareskog L, Sasso EH, et al. Tumor necrosis factor antagonist mechanisms of action: a comprehensive review. Pharmacol Ther 2008;117(2):244–79.
22. Ford AC, Sandborn WJ, Khan KJ, et al. Efficacy of biological therapies in inflammatory bowel disease: systematic review and meta-analysis. Am J Gastroenterol 2011;106(4):644–59 [quiz: 60].
23. Cimzia (certolizumab pegol) [package insert]. Brussels: UCB I and. Available at: http://www.cimzia.com. Accessed September 10, 2019.
24. Humira (adalimumab) [package insert]. Chicago IA, Inc. 2019. Available at: http://www.humira.com. Accessed September 10.
25. Remicade (infliximab) [package insert]. Horsham PJ, Inc. 2019. Available at: http://www.remicade.com. Accessed September 10.
26. Simponi (golimumab) [package insert]. Beerse BJB, Inc. 2019. Available at: http://www.simponi.com. Accessed September 10.
27. van der Meer JW, Popa C, Netea MG. Side effects of anticytokine strategies. Neth J Med 2005;63(3):78–80.
28. Tubach F, Salmon D, Ravaud P, et al. Risk of tuberculosis is higher with anti-tumor necrosis factor monoclonal antibody therapy than with soluble tumor necrosis factor receptor therapy: the three-year prospective French research axed on tolerance of biotherapies registry. Arthritis Rheum 2009;60(7):1884–94.
29. Ueda N, Tsukamoto H, Mitoma H, et al. The cytotoxic effects of certolizumab pegol and golimumab mediated by transmembrane tumor necrosis factor alpha. Inflamm Bowel Dis 2013;19(6):1224–31.
30. Mitoma H, Horiuchi T, Tsukamoto H, et al. Molecular mechanisms of action of anti-TNF-alpha agents: comparison among therapeutic TNF-alpha antagonists. Cytokine 2018;101:56–63.
31. Vallabhaneni S, Chiller TM. Fungal infections and new biologic therapies. Curr Rheumatol Rep 2016;18(5):29.
32. Gundacker ND, Baddley JW. Fungal infections in the era of biologic therapies. Curr Clin Microbiol Rep 2015;2(76).
33. Smith JA, Kauffman CA. Endemic fungal infections in patients receiving tumour necrosis factor-a inhibitor therapy. Drugs 2009;69(11):1403–15.
34. Ali T, Kaitha S, Mahmood S, et al. Clinical use of anti-TNF therapy and increased risk of infections. Drug Healthc Patient Saf 2013;5:79–99.
35. Curtis JR, Mariette X, Gaujoux-Viala C, et al. Long-term safety of certolizumab pegol in rheumatoid arthritis, axial spondyloarthritis, psoriatic arthritis, psoriasis and Crohn's disease: a pooled analysis of 11 317 patients across clinical trials. RMD Open 2019;5(1):e000942.
36. Alonso-Sierra M, Calvo M, Gonzalez-Lama Y. Nocardia and aspergillus coinfection in a patient with ulcerative colitis during golimumab therapy. J Crohns Colitis 2016;10(9):1127–8.
37. Harrold LR, Litman HJ, Saunders KC, et al. One-year risk of serious infection in patients treated with certolizumab pegol as compared with other TNF inhibitors in a real-world setting: Data from a national U.S. Rheumatoid arthritis registry. Arthritis Res Ther 2018;20(1):2.
38. Kay J, Fleischmann R, Keystone E, et al. Golimumab 3-year safety update: an analysis of pooled data from the long-term extensions of randomised, double-blind, placebo-controlled trials conducted in patients with rheumatoid arthritis, psoriatic arthritis or ankylosing spondylitis. Ann Rheum Dis 2015; 74(3):538–46.

39. Ricart E, Panaccione R, Loftus EV, et al. Infliximab for Crohn's disease in clinical practice at the Mayo Clinic: the first 100 patients. Am J Gastroenterol 2001; 96(3):722–9.
40. Patriarca F, Sperotto A, Damiani D, et al. Infliximab treatment for steroid-refractory acute graft-versus-host disease. Haematologica 2004;89(11):1352–9.
41. Couriel D, Saliba R, Hicks K, et al. Tumor necrosis factor-alpha blockade for the treatment of acute GVHD. Blood 2004;104(3):649–54.
42. Wallis RS, Broder MS, Wong JY, et al. Granulomatous infectious diseases associated with tumor necrosis factor antagonists. Clin Infect Dis 2004;38(9):1261–5.
43. Burmester GR, Mariette X, Montecucco C, et al. Adalimumab alone and in combination with disease-modifying antirheumatic drugs for the treatment of rheumatoid arthritis in clinical practice: the research in active rheumatoid arthritis (REACT) trial. Ann Rheum Dis 2007;66(6):732–9.
44. Kaur N, Mahl TC. Pneumocystis carinii pneumonia with oral candidiasis after infliximab therapy for Crohn's disease. Dig Dis Sci 2004;49(9):1458–60.
45. Belda A, Hinojosa J, Serra B, et al. [systemic candidiasis and infliximab therapy]. Gastroenterol Hepatol 2004;27(6):365–7.
46. Colombel JF, Loftus EV Jr, Tremaine WJ, et al. The safety profile of infliximab in patients with Crohn's disease: the Mayo Clinic experience in 500 patients. Gastroenterology 2004;126(1):19–31.
47. Filler SG, Yeaman MR, Sheppard DC. Tumor necrosis factor inhibition and invasive fungal infections. Clin Infect Dis 2005;41(Suppl 3):S208–12.
48. Bykerk VP, Cush J, Winthrop K, et al. Update on the safety profile of certolizumab pegol in rheumatoid arthritis: an integrated analysis from clinical trials. Ann Rheum Dis 2015;74(1):96–103.
49. Kay J, Fleischmann R, Keystone E, et al. Five-year safety data from 5 clinical trials of subcutaneous golimumab in patients with rheumatoid arthritis, psoriatic arthritis, and ankylosing spondylitis. J Rheumatol 2016;43(12):2120–30.
50. Takazono T, Sawai T, Tashiro M, et al. Relapsed pulmonary cryptococcosis during tumor necrosis factor alpha inhibitor treatment. Intern Med 2016;55(19): 2877–80.
51. Shrestha RK, Stoller JK, Honari G, et al. Pneumonia due to Cryptococcus neoformans in a patient receiving infliximab: possible zoonotic transmission from a pet cockatiel. Respir Care 2004;49(6):606–8.
52. Starett W, Czachor J, Dallal M, et al. Cryptococcal pneumonia following treatment with infliximab for rheumatoid arthritis. 40th annual meeting of the Infectious Diseases Society of America. Chicago, IL October 24th-27th, 2002. . Poster #374:110; 2002.
53. Hage CA, Wood KL, Winer-Muram HT, et al. Pulmonary cryptococcosis after initiation of anti-tumor necrosis factor-alpha therapy. Chest 2003;124(6):2395–7.
54. Arend SM, Kuijper EJ, Allaart CF, et al. Cavitating pneumonia after treatment with infliximab and prednisone. Eur J Clin Microbiol Infect Dis 2004;23(8): 638–41.
55. True DG, Penmetcha M, Peckham SJ. Disseminated cryptococcal infection in rheumatoid arthritis treated with methotrexate and infliximab. J Rheumatol 2002;29(7):1561–3.
56. Horcajada JP, Pena JL, Martinez-Taboada VM, et al. Invasive cryptococcosis and adalimumab treatment. Emerg Infect Dis 2007;13(6):953–5.
57. Marty FM, Lee SJ, Fahey MM, et al. Infliximab use in patients with severe graft-versus-host disease and other emerging risk factors of non-candida invasive

fungal infections in allogeneic hematopoietic stem cell transplant recipients: a cohort study. Blood 2003;102(8):2768–76.

58. Devlin SM, Hu B, Ippoliti A. Mucormycosis presenting as recurrent gastric perforation in a patient with Crohn's disease on glucocorticoid, 6-mercaptopurine, and infliximab therapy. Dig Dis Sci 2007;52(9):2078–81.

59. Singh P, Taylor SF, Murali R, et al. Disseminated mucormycosis and orbital ischaemia in combination immunosuppression with a tumour necrosis factor alpha inhibitor. Clin Exp Ophthalmol 2007;35(3):275–80.

60. Bongartz T, Sutton AJ, Sweeting MJ, et al. Anti-TNF antibody therapy in rheumatoid arthritis and the risk of serious infections and malignancies: systematic review and meta-analysis of rare harmful effects in randomized controlled trials. JAMA 2006;295(19):2275–85.

61. Listing J, Strangfeld A, Kary S, et al. Infections in patients with rheumatoid arthritis treated with biologic agents. Arthritis Rheum 2005;52(11):3403–12.

62. Vergidis P, Avery RK, Wheat LJ, et al. Histoplasmosis complicating tumor necrosis factor-alpha blocker therapy: a retrospective analysis of 98 cases. Clin Infect Dis 2015;61(3):409–17.

63. Taroumian S, Knowles SL, Lisse JR, et al. Management of coccidioidomycosis in patients receiving biologic response modifiers or disease-modifying antirheumatic drugs. Arthritis Care Res (Hoboken) 2012;64(12):1903–9.

64. Ruderman E and Markenson J. Granulomatous infections and tumor necrosis factor antagonist therapies. European Congress of Rheumatology (EULAR). Lisbon, Portugal. Abstract #THU0209; 2003.

65. Baddley JW, Winthrop KL, Chen L, et al. Non-viral opportunistic infections in new users of tumour necrosis factor inhibitor therapy: results of the safety assessment of biologic therapy (SABER) study. Ann Rheum Dis 2014;73(11):1942–8.

66. Kaur N, Mahl TC. *Pneumocystis jirovecii* (*carinii*) pneumonia after infliximab therapy: a review of 84 cases. Dig Dis Sci 2007;52(6):1481–4.

67. Harigai M, Koike R, Pneumocystis Pneumonia under Anti-Tumor Necrosis Factor Therapy (PAT) Study Group. *Pneumocystis pneumonia* associated with infliximab in Japan. N Engl J Med 2007;357(18):1874–6.

68. Chamilos G, Lionakis MS, Kontoyiannis DP. Call for action: invasive fungal infections associated with ibrutinib and other small molecule kinase inhibitors targeting immune signaling pathways. Clin Infect Dis 2018;66(1):140–8.

69. Lionakis MS, Dunleavy K, Roschewski M, et al. Inhibition of B cell receptor signaling by ibrutinib in primary CNS lymphoma. Cancer Cell 2017;31(6):833–843 e5.

70. Chang H, Hung YS, Chou WC. *Pneumocystis jirovecii* pneumonia in patients receiving dasatinib treatment. Int J Infect Dis 2014;25:165–7.

71. El-Dabh A, Acharya D. Express: pulmonary hypertension with dasatinib and other tyrosine kinase inhibitors. Pulm Circ 2019. 2045894019865704.[Epub ahead of print].

72. Crisan AM, Ghiaur A, Stancioaca MC, et al. Mucormycosis during imatinib treatment: case report. J Med Life 2015;8(3):365–70.

73. Mughal TI, Schrieber A. Principal long-term adverse effects of imatinib in patients with chronic myeloid leukemia in chronic phase. Biologics 2010;4:315–23.

74. Lussana F, Cattaneo M, Rambaldi A, et al. Ruxolitinib-associated infections: a systematic review and meta-analysis. Am J Hematol 2018;93(3):339–47.

75. Kim YW, Lee HW, Cho J, et al. Conversion of aspergilloma to chronic necrotizing pulmonary aspergillosis following treatment with sunitinib: a case report. Oncol Lett 2016;12(5):3472–4.

76. Visvardis EE, Gao F, Paes MN, et al. Lung aspergillosis in renal cell carcinoma patient treated with sunitinib. QJM 2012;105(7):689–92.

77. Bazaz R, Denning DW. Subacute invasive aspergillosis associated with sorafenib therapy for hepatocellular carcinoma. Clin Infect Dis 2018;67(1):156–7.

78. Winthrop KL, Park SH, Gul A, et al. Tuberculosis and other opportunistic infections in tofacitinib-treated patients with rheumatoid arthritis. Ann Rheum Dis 2016;75(6):1133–8.

79. Brown KE, Freeman GJ, Wherry EJ, et al. Role of PD-1 in regulating acute infections. Curr Opin Immunol 2010;22(3):397–401.

80. Inoue S, Bo L, Bian J, et al. Dose-dependent effect of anti-CTLA-4 on survival in sepsis. Shock 2011;36(1):38–44.

81. La Rosa C, Krishnan A, Longmate J, et al. Programmed death-1 expression in liver transplant recipients as a prognostic indicator of cytomegalovirus disease. J Infect Dis 2008;197(1):25–33.

82. Barber DL, Wherry EJ, Masopust D, et al. Restoring function in exhausted CD8 T cells during chronic viral infection. Nature 2006;439(7077):682–7.

83. Velu V, Titanji K, Zhu B, et al. Enhancing SIV-specific immunity in vivo by PD-1 blockade. Nature 2009;458(7235):206–10.

84. Day CL, Kaufmann DE, Kiepiela P, et al. PD-1 expression on HIV-specific T cells is associated with T-cell exhaustion and disease progression. Nature 2006; 443(7109):350–4.

85. Trautmann L, Janbazian L, Chomont N, et al. Upregulation of PD-1 expression on HIV-specific CD8+ T cells leads to reversible immune dysfunction. Nat Med 2006;12(10):1198–202.

86. Petrovas C, Casazza JP, Brenchley JM, et al. PD-1 is a regulator of virus-specific CD8+ T cell survival in HIV infection. J Exp Med 2006;203(10):2281–92.

87. Urbani S, Amadei B, Tola D, et al. PD-1 expression in acute hepatitis C virus (HCV) infection is associated with HCV-specific CD8 exhaustion. J Virol 2006; 80(22):11398–403.

88. Boni C, Fisicaro P, Valdatta C, et al. Characterization of hepatitis B virus (HBV)-specific T-cell dysfunction in chronic HBV infection. J Virol 2007;81(8):4215–25.

89. Barber DL, Mayer-Barber KD, Feng CG, et al. CD4 T cells promote rather than control tuberculosis in the absence of PD-1-mediated inhibition. J Immunol 2011;186(3):1598–607.

90. Cacere CR, Mendes-Giannini MJ, Fontes CJ, et al. Altered expression of the costimulatory molecules CD80, CD86, CD152, PD-1 and icos on T-cells from paracoccidioidomycosis patients: lack of correlation with T-cell hyporesponsiveness. Clin Immunol 2008;129(2):341–9.

91. Lazar-Molnar E, Gacser A, Freeman GJ, et al. The PD-1/PD-l costimulatory pathway critically affects host resistance to the pathogenic fungus histoplasma capsulatum. Proc Natl Acad Sci U S A 2008;105(7):2658–63.

92. Del Castillo M, Romero FA, Arguello E, et al. The spectrum of serious infections among patients receiving immune checkpoint blockade for the treatment of melanoma. Clin Infect Dis 2016;63(11):1490–3.

93. Kyi C, Hellmann MD, Wolchok JD, et al. Opportunistic infections in patients treated with immunotherapy for cancer. J Immunother Cancer 2014;2:19.

94. Grimaldi D, Pradier O, Hotchkiss RS, et al. Nivolumab plus interferon-gamma in the treatment of intractable mucormycosis. Lancet Infect Dis 2017;17(1):18.

95. Akdis M, Aab A, Altunbulakli C, et al. Interleukins (from IL-1 to IL-38), interferons, transforming growth factor beta, and TNF-alpha: receptors, functions, and roles in diseases. J Allergy Clin Immunol 2016;138(4):984–1010.

96. Howard C, Noe A, Skerjanec A, et al. Safety and tolerability of canakinumab, an IL-1beta inhibitor, in type 2 diabetes mellitus patients: a pooled analysis of three randomised double-blind studies. Cardiovasc Diabetol 2014;13:94.

97. Sibley CH, Chioato A, Felix S, et al. A 24-month open-label study of canakinumab in neonatal-onset multisystem inflammatory disease. Ann Rheum Dis 2015;74(9):1714–9.

98. Khatri S, Moore W, Gibson PG, et al. Assessment of the long-term safety of mepolizumab and durability of clinical response in patients with severe eosinophilic asthma. J Allergy Clin Immunol 2019;143(5):1742–17451 e7.

99. Wood C, Im Y, Millard M. Disseminated aspergillosis after IL-5 therapy for severe asthma. American Thoracic Society. San Diego, CA, May 18th-23rd, 2018. Poster #A31.

100. Kalb RE, Fiorentino DF, Lebwohl MG, et al. Risk of serious infection with biologic and systemic treatment of psoriasis: results from the psoriasis longitudinal assessment and registry (PSOLAR). JAMA Dermatol 2015;151(9):961–9.

101. Lebwohl M, Strober B, Menter A, et al. Phase 3 studies comparing brodalumab with ustekinumab in psoriasis. N Engl J Med 2015;373(14):1318–28.

102. Langley RG, Elewski BE, Lebwohl M, et al. Secukinumab in plaque psoriasis: results of two phase 3 trials. N Engl J Med 2014;371(4):326–38.

103. Mease PJ, McInnes IB, Kirkham B, et al. Secukinumab inhibition of interleukin-17a in patients with psoriatic arthritis. N Engl J Med 2015;373(14):1329–39.

104. Baeten D, Sieper J, Braun J, et al. Secukinumab, an interleukin-17a inhibitor, in ankylosing spondylitis. N Engl J Med 2015;373(26):2534–48.

105. Griffiths CE, Reich K, Lebwohl M, et al. Comparison of ixekizumab with etanercept or placebo in moderate-to-severe psoriasis (UNCOVER-2 and UNCOVER-3): results from two phase 3 randomised trials. Lancet 2015;386(9993):541–51.

106. Morel J, Constantin A, Baron G, et al. Risk factors of serious infections in patients with rheumatoid arthritis treated with tocilizumab in the French registry REGATE. Rheumatology (Oxford) 2017;56(10):1746–54.

107. Pawar A, Desai RJ, Solomon DH, et al. Risk of serious infections in tocilizumab versus other biologic drugs in patients with rheumatoid arthritis: a multidatabase cohort study. Ann Rheum Dis 2019;78(4):456–64.

108. Genovese MC, Fleischmann R, Kivitz AJ, et al. Sarilumab plus methotrexate in patients with active rheumatoid arthritis and inadequate response to methotrexate: results of a phase III study. Arthritis Rheumatol 2015;67(6):1424–37.

109. Drgona L, Gudiol C, Lanini S, et al. ESCMID study group for infections in compromised hosts (ESGICH) consensus document on the safety of targeted and biological therapies: an infectious diseases perspective (agents targeting lymphoid or myeloid cells surface antigens [II]: CD22, CD30, CD33, CD38, CD40, slamf-7 and ccr4). Clin Microbiol Infect 2018;24(Suppl 2):S83–94.

110. Mikulska M, Lanini S, Gudiol C, et al. ESCMID study group for infections in compromised hosts (ESGICH) consensus document on the safety of targeted and biological therapies: an infectious diseases perspective (agents targeting lymphoid cells surface antigens [I]: CD19, CD20 and CD52). Clin Microbiol Infect 2018;24(Suppl 2):S71–82.

111. Kelesidis T, Daikos G, Boumpas D, et al. Does rituximab increase the incidence of infectious complications? A narrative review. Int J Infect Dis 2011;15(1): e2–16.

112. Kaplan LD, Lee JY, Ambinder RF, et al. Rituximab does not improve clinical outcome in a randomized phase 3 trial of chop with or without rituximab in patients with HIV-associated non-Hodgkin lymphoma: AIDS-Malignancies Consortium Trial 010. Blood 2005;106(5):1538–43.

113. Jiang X, Mei X, Feng D, et al. Prophylaxis and treatment of Pneumocystis jirovecii pneumonia in lymphoma patients subjected to rituximab-contained therapy: a systemic review and meta-analysis. PLoS One 2015;10(4):e0122171.

114. Barreto JN, Ice LL, Thompson CA, et al. Low incidence of pneumocystis pneumonia utilizing PCR-based diagnosis in patients with B-cell lymphoma receiving rituximab-containing combination chemotherapy. Am J Hematol 2016;91(11): 1113–7.

115. Du FH, Mills EA, Mao-Draayer Y. Next-generation anti-CD20 monoclonal antibodies in autoimmune disease treatment. Auto Immun Highlights 2017;8(1):12.

116. Clowse ME, Wallace DJ, Furie RA, et al. Efficacy and safety of epratuzumab in moderately to severely active systemic lupus erythematosus: results from two phase III randomized, double-blind, placebo-controlled trials. Arthritis Rheumatol 2017;69(2):362–75.

117. Kantarjian HM, DeAngelo DJ, Stelljes M, et al. Inotuzumab ozogamicin versus standard therapy for acute lymphoblastic leukemia. N Engl J Med 2016; 375(8):740–53.

118. Younes A, Gopal AK, Smith SE, et al. Results of a pivotal phase II study of brentuximab vedotin for patients with relapsed or refractory Hodgkin's lymphoma. J Clin Oncol 2012;30(18):2183–9.

119. Pro B, Advani R, Brice P, et al. Brentuximab vedotin (SGN-35) in patients with relapsed or refractory systemic anaplastic large-cell lymphoma: results of a phase II study. J Clin Oncol 2012;30(18):2190–6.

120. Dearden CE, Matutes E, Cazin B, et al. High remission rate in T-cell prolymphocytic leukemia with campath-1h. Blood 2001;98(6):1721–6.

121. Rawstron AC, Kennedy B, Moreton P, et al. Early prediction of outcome and response to alemtuzumab therapy in chronic lymphocytic leukemia. Blood 2004;103(6):2027–31.

122. Thursky KA, Worth LJ, Seymour JF, et al. Spectrum of infection, risk and recommendations for prophylaxis and screening among patients with lymphoproliferative disorders treated with alemtuzumab. Br J Haematol 2006;132(1):3–12.

123. Martin SI, Marty FM, Fiumara K, et al. Infectious complications associated with alemtuzumab use for lymphoproliferative disorders. Clin Infect Dis 2006;43(1): 16–24.

124. Cornely O, Heidecke C. Fungal infections following alemtuzumab treatment. 15th Annual Focus on Fungal Infections. Abstract #14; March 16-18,2005.

125. Salvana EM, Salata RA. Infectious complications associated with monoclonal antibodies and related small molecules. Clin Microbiol Rev 2009;22(2): 274–90. Table of Contents.

126. Brennan DC, Daller JA, Lake KD, et al. Rabbit antithymocyte globulin versus basiliximab in renal transplantation. N Engl J Med 2006;355(19):1967–77.

127. Ramirez CB, Doria C, di Francesco F, et al. Basiliximab induction in adult liver transplant recipients with 93% rejection-free patient and graft survival at 24 months. Transplant Proc 2006;38(10):3633–5.

128. Clinckart F, Bulpa P, Jamart J, et al. Basiliximab as an alternative to antithymocyte globulin for early immunosuppression in lung transplantation. Transplant Proc 2009;41(2):607–9.

129. Iversen M, Burton CM, Vand S, et al. Aspergillus infection in lung transplant patients: incidence and prognosis. Eur J Clin Microbiol Infect Dis 2007;26(12): 879–86.
130. Perales MA, Ishill N, Lomazow WA, et al. Long-term follow-up of patients treated with daclizumab for steroid-refractory acute graft-vs-host disease. Bone Marrow Transplant 2007;40(5):481–6.
131. Schiff M, Weinblatt ME, Valente R, et al. Head-to-head comparison of subcutaneous abatacept versus adalimumab for rheumatoid arthritis: two-year efficacy and safety findings from ample trial. Ann Rheum Dis 2014;73(1):86–94.
132. Jain N, Doyon JB, Lazarus JE, et al. A case of disseminated histoplasmosis in a patient with rheumatoid arthritis on abatacept. J Gen Intern Med 2018;33(5): 769–72.
133. Chen SK, Liao KP, Liu J, et al. Risk of hospitalized infection and initiation of abatacept versus TNF inhibitors among patients with rheumatoid arthritis: a propensity score-matched cohort study. Arthritis Care Res (Hoboken) 2020;72(1):9–17.
134. Trimarchi H, Rengel T, Andrews J, et al. Belatacept and mediastinal histoplasmosis in a kidney transplant patient. J Nephropathol 2016;5(2):84–7.
135. Haidinger M, Hecking M, Memarsadeghi M, et al. Late onset pneumocystis pneumonia in renal transplantation after long-term immunosuppression with belatacept. Transpl Infect Dis 2009;11(2):171–4.
136. Benamu E, Montoya JG. Infections associated with the use of eculizumab: recommendations for prevention and prophylaxis. Curr Opin Infect Dis 2016;29(4): 319–29.
137. Bonfante L, Nalesso F, Cara M, et al. Aspergillus fumigatus peritonitis in ambulatory peritoneal dialysis: a case report and notes on the therapeutic approach. Nephrology (Carlton) 2005;10(3):270–3.
138. Gutwinski S, Erbe S, Munch C, et al. Severe cutaneous candida infection during natalizumab therapy in multiple sclerosis. Neurology 2010;74(6):521–3.
139. Ruiz N, Fernandez-Martos C, Romero I, et al. Invasive fungal infection and nasal septum perforation with bevacizumab-based therapy in advanced colon cancer. J Clin Oncol 2007;25(22):3376–7.
140. Sheyman AT, Cohen BZ, Friedman AH, et al. An outbreak of fungal endophthalmitis after intravitreal injection of compounded combined bevacizumab and triamcinolone. JAMA Ophthalmol 2013;131(7):864–9.
141. Bergstrom L, Yocum DE, Ampel NM, et al. Increased risk of coccidioidomycosis in patients treated with tumor necrosis factor alpha antagonists. Arthritis Rheum 2004;50(6):1959–66.
142. Ammar A, Zahia E, Ruiz-Rodriquez O, et al. A case of pulmonary blastomycosis in an nonendemic area after initiation of an interleukin monoclonal antibody. Chest. San Antonio, TX. Poster #212-A; October 6th-10th,2018.
143. Gupta A, Tun A, Ticona K, et al. Invasive aspergillosis in a patient with stage III (or 3a or 3b) non-small-cell lung cancer treated with durvalumab. Case Rep Oncol Med 2019;2019:2178925.
144. Ogura M, Ishida T, Hatake K, et al. Multicenter phase II study of mogamulizumab (kw-0761), a defucosylated anti-cc chemokine receptor 4 antibody, in patients with relapsed peripheral T-cell lymphoma and cutaneous T-cell lymphoma. J Clin Oncol 2014;32(11):1157–63.
145. Nath DS, Kandaswamy R, Gruessner R, et al. Fungal infections in transplant recipients receiving alemtuzumab. Transplant Proc 2005;37(2):934–6.
146. Emery P, Rigby W, Tak PP, et al. Safety with ocrelizumab in rheumatoid arthritis: results from the ocrelizumab phase III program. PLoS One 2014;9(2):e87379.

147. Grinyo JM, Del Carmen Rial M, Alberu J, et al. Safety and efficacy outcomes 3 years after switching to belatacept from a calcineurin inhibitor in kidney transplant recipients: results from a phase 2 randomized trial. Am J Kidney Dis 2017;69(5):587–94.
148. Jenneck C, Novak N. The safety and efficacy of alefacept in the treatment of chronic plaque psoriasis. Ther Clin Risk Manag 2007;3(3):411–20.
149. Gade JN. Clinical update on alefacept: consideration for use in patients with psoriasis. J Manag Care Pharm 2004;10(3 Suppl B):S33–7.
150. Bavencio (avelumab) [package insert]. Rockland, MA: EMD Serono, Inc; 2019.
151. Danza A, Ruiz-Irastorza G. Infection risk in systemic lupus erythematosus patients: S\susceptibility factors and preventive strategies. Lupus 2013;22(12): 1286–94.
152. Cortes JE, Apperley JF, DeAngelo DJ, et al. Management of adverse events associated with bosutinib treatment of chronic-phase chronic myeloid leukemia: Expert panel review. J Hematol Oncol 2018;11(1):143.
153. Isfort S, Brummendorf TH. Bosutinib in chronic myeloid leukemia: patient selection and perspectives. J Blood Med 2018;9:43–50.
154. Migden MR, Rischin D, Schmults CD, et al. PD-1 blockade with cemiplimab in advanced cutaneous squamous-cell carcinoma. N Engl J Med 2018;379(4): 341–51.
155. Eichenfield LF, Bieber T, Beck LA, et al. Infections in dupilumab clinical trials in atopic dermatitis: a comprehensive pooled analysis. Am J Clin Dermatol 2019; 20(3):443–56.
156. Lee JW, Sicre de Fontbrune F, Wong Lee L, et al. Ravulizumab (alxn1210) vs eculizumab in adult patients with PNH naive to complement inhibitors: the 301 study. Blood 2019;133(6):530–9.

Mycobacterial Infections Potentiated by Biologics

Cassandra Calabrese, DO[a],*, Kevin L. Winthrop, MD, MPH[b]

KEYWORDS

- Mycobacteria • Tuberculosis • Biologics • Opportunistic infection

KEY POINTS

- The risk of tuberculosis (TB) is increased with most biologic therapies, in particular with the tumor necrosis factor-α inhibitors (TNFi), and least likely with rituximab, a monoclonal antibody targeting CD20 on the surface of B cells.
- Screening for latent tuberculosis before starting biologic therapy is critical.
- The risk of nontuberculous mycobacterial (NTM) infections is increased with biologic therapy, and is more common than TB in areas of low TB prevalence, such as the United States.
- There are no recommendations to screen for NTM before starting biologic therapy, so a heightened awareness of this infection is key.

INTRODUCTION

The introduction of biologic therapies has revolutionized the treatment of immune-mediated inflammatory diseases (IMIDs). With this advantage comes an increased risk of infection that varies across biologic classes. The list of approved biologic agents is ever-growing and encompasses numerous drug classes with unique mechanisms of action that are used to treat a wide array of autoimmune disease, and span many different subspecialties (rheumatology, dermatology, gastroenterology, neurology, and others). Numerous studies have shown that some biologics carry an increased risk of serious infections and opportunistic infections, compared with use of traditional disease-modifying antirheumatic drugs (DMARDs).[1] Infectious risk is also dependent on host factors, such as underlying disease type and disease activity, and it is well known that a diagnosis of rheumatoid arthritis (RA) is associated with an increased risk of routine bacterial and opportunistic infections at baseline.[2] Since the

[a] Department of Rheumatologic & Immunologic Disease, Cleveland Clinic Foundation, 9500 Euclid Avenue, Desk A50, Cleveland, OH 44195, USA; [b] Division of Infectious Diseases, Schools of Medicine and Public Health, Oregon Health and Science University, OHSU, 3181 Sam Jackson Road, Mail Code: Gaines Hall, Portland, OR 97239, USA
* Corresponding author.
E-mail address: calabrc@ccf.org
Twitter: @CCalabrese (C.C.)

Infect Dis Clin N Am 34 (2020) 413–423
https://doi.org/10.1016/j.idc.2020.02.011
0891-5520/20/© 2020 Elsevier Inc. All rights reserved.

id.theclinics.com

approval of the first biologic therapy to treat IMIDs, tuberculous and nontuberculous mycobacterial (NTM) infections have become well-known infectious complications of these therapies. Herein, the authors review the risk of tuberculous and NTM infections in the setting of biologic therapy.

TUBERCULOSIS
Incidence and Drug-specific Risk

Infection with *Mycobacterium tuberculosis* remains one of the leading causes of death worldwide, infecting an estimated 10 million people in 2017, with approximately one-third of exposed patients developing latent tuberculosis infection (LTBI).[3] Prevalence of tuberculosis (TB) infection varies by geographic region, with 30 countries accounting for 87% of the world's TB burden. The lifetime risk of reactivation of LTBI is estimated to be 5% to 10%, but the risk is significantly higher in the presence of certain risk factors, including in patients with IMIDs receiving biologic therapies and other forms of immunosuppression. For this reason, screening patients for latent TB before starting biologic therapy has become the standard of care.[4]

The first biologic approved for treatment of IMIDs was etanercept, a tumor necrosis factor-α inhibitor (TNFi), in 1998, followed quickly by approval of infliximab. Currently there are five approved drugs in this class, with the addition of adalimumab, golimumab, and certolizumab pegol. Soon after the approval of etanercept and infliximab, a signal for increased risk of TB became apparent and was first reported in the setting of infliximab. A single case of TB was reported in the first randomized control trial (RCT) of TNFi.[5] Since this first case, a significant amount has been learned about this risk through registry data, long-term extension and pharmacovigilance studies, and real-life experiences. Within 3 years of infliximab approval, 70 cases of TB occurred in about 147,000 patients, as reported through the Food and Drug Administration spontaneous reporting system, prompting the addition of a black box warning, recommending patients be screened for latent TB before starting infliximab.[6]

The most frequently used class of biologics are the TNFi, because they carry treatment indications for a wide variety of autoimmune disease including RA, psoriasis, psoriatic arthritis, ankylosing spondylitis, inflammatory bowel disease, and off-label use in a variety of other autoimmune/autoinflammatory diseases. TNF-α plays a key role in host control of TB infection, providing mechanistic explanation as to why TNFi promote TB reactivation, which was demonstrated in many studies early on (**Table 1**). Among the different TNFi, numerous studies have shown a higher TB risk with the monoclonal TNFi (adalimumab, infliximab, golimumab, certolizumab pegol) compared with etanercept, a soluble receptor fusion protein.[13] This difference is most likely related to the unique pharmacologic properties of etanercept, and its differential effects on granulomatous inflammatory conditions, because etanercept causes less complement-dependent cytotoxicity and apoptosis of affected cells compared with the monoclonal TNFi.[14] Also, infliximab has been shown to suppress antigen-induced interferon-γ responses in vitro to a greater degree compared with etanercept.[15] In a murine model of TB, Plessner and colleagues[16] demonstrated that granuloma penetration by infliximab was more robust compared with etanercept.

Tuberculosis Incidence in Tumor Necrosis Factor-α Inhibitors Users

TB incidence among TNFi users strongly varies according to the background prevalence of TB in the region. Most studies evaluating risk have been done in low-prevalence regions, although as such therapies have become more commonly used throughout the world, recent data exist from higher prevalence areas. In North

Table 1
Studies reporting risk of tuberculosis from TNF inhibitors

Reference/Study	Study Type	Location	Study Period	TB Rate/ 100,000 PYs
Seong et al,[10] 2007	Retrospective cohort	South Korea	2001–2005	2258 INF
Kim et al,[11] 2011	Retrospective cohort	South Korea	2002–2009	540 INF 490 ADA
Tubach et al,[8] 2009 RATIO	Prospective cohort	France	2004–2006	116.7
Dixon et al,[9] 2010 BSRBR	Prospective cohort	United Kingdom	2001–2008	136 INF 144 ADA 39 ETN
Winthrop et al,[7] 2013	Retrospective cohort	United States	2000–2008	74
Baddley et al,[12] 2014 SABER	Retrospective cohort	United States	1998–2007	36

Abbreviations: ADA, adalimumab; ETN, etanercept; INF, infliximab; PY, person-year.
Adapted from Bryant PA, Baddley JW. Opportunistic infections in biologic therapy, risk and prevention. Rheumatic Disease Clinics of North America 2017; 43:27-41; with permission.

America, a retrospective cohort study by Winthrop and colleagues[7] using US health care claims data examined more than 8000 patients receiving TNFi, most of which had RA, and reported a TB rate of 74/100,000 person-years, compared with a background rate of 8.7/100,000 person-years in patients with RA not receiving TNFi. In Europe, Tubach, and colleagues[8] created the French registry RATIO to prospectively collect cases of TB occurring in patients receiving TNFi between 2004 and 2007. The incidence rate of TB was 116.7/100,000 patient-years, and rates were higher in patients receiving infliximab or adalimumab versus etanercept. Data from the British Society for Rheumatology Biologics Register (BSRBR), a national prospective observational study, were used to address the risk of TB in patients with RA receiving infliximab, adalimumab, or etanercept versus DMARDs.[9] Out of 13,739 patients (10,712 receiving TNFi, 3232 receiving DMARDs), there were 40 episodes of TB, all occurring in patients receiving TNFi, for a rate of 144 and 136 cases/100,000 person-years for infliximab and adalimumab, respectively, compared with 39/100,000 person-years for etanercept users.

Tuberculosis and Other Biologics

Beyond the TNFi, there exist many other biologics with different molecular targets that are used in the treatment of IMIDs. These biologics are associated with variable risks of LTBI reactivation, which in general has reported to be lower compared with the TNF-inhibitors. In 2014, Souto and colleagues[17] published a systematic review and meta-analysis of RCTs and long-term extension studies, looking at risk of TB in patients on biologics and tofacitinib, a Janus kinase (JAK) inhibitor used for the treatment of RA, ulcerative colitis, and psoriasis. Out of 75,000 patients in 100 RCTs, there were 31 TB cases with TNFi, one with abatacept and none with rituximab, tocilizumab, ustekinumab, or tofacitinib. However, in the long-term extension studies (80,774.45 patient-years), the incidence of TB was greater than 40/100,000 for patients receiving tofacitinib and other biologics except for rituximab. It is important to recognize the limitations of RCT data when considering TB risk (and other uncommon infections), and these findings should be interpreted with caution. Patients in RCTs are routinely screened for TB, unlike in early TNFi trials. Also, many of these trials were conducted in areas of low TB risk. There exist little real-world data for many of the non-TNFi biologics. In a Japanese postmarketing surveillance of 3881 patients with RA receiving tocilizumab, an interleukin (IL)-6 inhibitor, four patients developed TB (0.22/100 patient-years), all of whom had been appropriately screened before starting therapy.[18]

The JAK/signal transducers and activators of transcription pathway has become increasingly recognized as playing a critical role in the pathogenesis of several IMIDs including RA, spondylarthritis, and inflammatory bowel disease. Tofacitinib was the first JAK inhibitor to be approved and is used in the treatment of RA, psoriatic arthritis, and ulcerative colitis. There are three currently approved JAK inhibitors (tofacitinib, baricitinib, and upadacitinib) and although they preferentially inhibit different combinations of JAKs, their infectious safety profiles are similar. These kinases mediate interferon responses against nonviral pathogens, such as *M tuberculosis*, and TB cases have been reported with use of tofacitinib.[19,20] In an analysis of data from phase II, phase III, and long-term extension studies, Winthrop and colleagues[21] examined risk of opportunistic infections in patients with RA treated with tofacitinib, finding 26 cases of active TB out of 5671 subjects, with most occurring in patients receiving tofacitinib, 10 mg twice daily. The median time between start of tofacitinib and diagnosis of TB was 64 weeks, and 58% of cases were extrapulmonary.

Abatacept, a fusion protein consisting of the Fc region of IgG1 fused to the extracellular domain of CTLA-4, is used in treatment of RA and its TB risk is considered to be low. Like many of the non-TNFi biologics, real-world data on TB risk are limited. Data pooled from eight clinical trials of intravenous abatacept examined 4149 patients with 12,132 patient-years and found a TB incidence rate of 0.07/100 patient-years.[22] The ATTEST trial was a multicenter randomized double-blind control trial examining efficacy and safety of abatacept or infliximab versus placebo in patients with RA and found the incidence of serious infections to be significantly lower in the abatacept group (1.3%) versus infliximab (4.2%).[23] No cases of TB were reported in the abatacept group.

Of all the biologics used to treat IMIDs, rituximab seems to be associated with the lowest risk of TB, and is often considered first line for the management of IMIDs in patients who are high risk for TB reactivation. Rituximab is a monoclonal antibody targeting the B-cell surface molecule CD20 and is approved for treatment of the ANCA-associated vasculitides, RA, and several malignancies including non-Hodgkin lymphoma and chronic lymphocytic leukemia. In a prospective observational cohort study by Winthrop and colleagues[24] (SUNSTONE), the safety of rituximab in patients with RA who had previous exposure to TNFi was examined. Out of 989 patients who received at least one dose of rituximab, with 3844 patient-years of follow-up, no incident cases of TB were reported. Although the 2015 American College of Rheumatology guidelines for treatment of RA do recommend screening for LTBI before starting rituximab, an international consensus statement on use of rituximab in patients with RA states there is no evidence indicating the necessity to systematically screen patients for LTBI before rituximab initiation.[1,25] Data from mouse models have suggested that B cells may play a greater role in host defenses against *M tuberculosis* than previously thought, with one study demonstrating that B cell–deficient mice had enhanced susceptibility to infection.[26]

We have scant data from real-life clinical practice on newer biologics, such as inhibitors of IL-17 and IL-12/23 in terms of TB reactivation; however, no cases of TB have been reported in clinical studies, and these biologics may represent a good option for patients who are at increased risk of TB.

Screening and Prevention

Identifying individuals with LTBI is problematic because there is no gold standard for diagnosing LTBI, and current tests capture only immunologic responses to prior exposure. There are two available testing modalities for LTBI screening: the tuberculin skin test (TST) and interferon-γ release assays (IGRAs) (**Box 1**). For more than a century, clinicians have relied on the TST to detect immunologic memory to *M tuberculosis* through a delayed type hypersensitivity reaction, but the test has limited sensitivity in immunosuppressed patients, and limited specificity in patients who were previously vaccinated with bacille Calmette-Guérin (BCG).[27]

IGRA tests detect interferon-γ production by peripheral blood T cells in response to activation by specific TB antigens, and have become increasingly used because of their superior specificity given they do not cross-react with *Mycobacterium bovis* strains used in the BCG vaccine. IGRAs, however, also have disadvantages, including uncertainty generated by "indeterminate" results, which occur more frequently in patients with IMIDs.[28] Indeterminate results pose a challenge to clinicians, generally leading them to repeat LTBI testing and/or to rely on other clinical and radiologic factors to help interpret the test result. Also, neither test can differentiate between LTBI and active TB. Current Centers for Disease Control and Prevention (CDC) guidelines recommend that IGRAs be used in all situations in which TST is currently used to screen for LTBI in adults.[29]

There remains a degree of uncertainty surrounding the value of TST and IGRAs in the setting of immunosuppression, and their relative sensitivity has been difficult to determine. In general, studies have shown that IGRAs are likely more sensitive than TST for detecting LTBI in immunosuppressed patients.[30,31] Sensitivity of both test types is limited in the setting of immunosuppression, but IGRAs are likely affected to a lesser degree.[32,33] Thus, screening with only one testing method may lead to false-negative results, and for this reason various testing algorithms have been recommended to increase sensitivity in the setting of biologic therapy.[34]

The American College of Rheumatology Guidelines for the management of RA include recommendations for LTBI screening before starting biologics (**Fig. 1**).[1] Before initiation of biologic therapy (which includes tofacitinib), it is recommended to check a TST or IGRA. Screening for latent TB need not be repeated yearly, but only if a new TB

Box 1
Advantages and disadvantages of TB testing modalities

Tuberculin skin test
  Advantages
  • Lower cost
  Disadvantages
  • Requires two clinic visits
  • Possibility of variability among observers
  • False-positive results in the setting of prior BCG
  • Subject to false-negative results in the setting of immunosuppression

Interferon-γ release assay (preferred over TST)
  Advantages
  • Does not give false-positive results in the setting of prior BCG
  • Requires a single clinic visit
  • Improved sensitivity over TST in the setting of immunosuppression
  Disadvantages
  • Possibility of indeterminate results
  • Subject to false-negative results in the setting of immunosuppression, although to a lesser degree than TST
  • Higher cost

Abbreviation: BCG, bacille Calmette-Guérin.

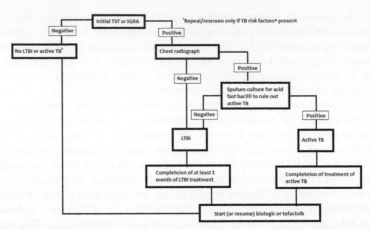

Fig. 1. American College of Rheumatology TB screening algorithm for biologics and tofacitinib. [a] TB risk factors: history of contact with active TB; birth or greater than 3-month stay in regions where TB is prevalent; history of incarceration or working in jail/prison, health care facilities, or homeless shelters; intravenous drug use. [b] False-negative results more likely with immunosuppressed patients; consider repeating TST or IGRA. (*Adapted from* Singh, J. A. *et al.* 2015 American College of Rheumatology Guideline for the Treatment of Rheumatoid Arthritis. *Arthritis Rheumatol.* **68**, 1–26 (2016); with permission.)

risk factor has been identified. If testing is positive, a chest radiograph should be obtained. If chest radiograph is negative, the patient is considered to have LTBI. If chest radiograph is abnormal, sputum should be sent for acid-fast bacilli to evaluate for active TB. In either scenario, the patient should be referred to an infectious disease specialist. If a positive IGRA results in a patient without TB risk factors, we recommend repeat testing, which has been adopted based on health care worker LTBI screening data and experiences.[34,35]

The need to rescreen patients for LTBI while on biologic therapy has been a subject of debate. Patients with new or ongoing risk factors (eg, living in an endemic area, health care worker) should be screened yearly; however, for patients without these risk factors, the need for yearly screening is unnecessary.

Treatment Issues

Patients with IMIDs receiving biologic therapy who require LTBI treatment can receive a CDC-recommended regimen; however, drug-drug interactions should be considered.[36] For example, there is a significant drug interaction between rifampin and tofacitinib, such that concurrent use can decrease the bioavailability of tofacitinib by 80%.[37] Isoniazid should be the drug of choice for tofacitinib-treated patients requiring treatment of LTBI. Daily isoniazid monotherapy is most widely used, with recommended courses of either 6 or 9 month's duration; however, rifampin-based regimens are preferred over isoniazid-based regiments, with a 4-month regimen of daily rifampin being most preferable. At present, the shortest LTBI treatment course recommended by the CDC is a combination regiment of once-weekly isoniazid and rifapentine for 12 weeks.[36] Recently, a randomized, phase III trial demonstrated noninferiority of a 1-month regimen of daily rifapentine plus isoniazid with 9 months of daily isoniazid monotherapy in patients with human immunodeficiency virus with LTBI.[38] A Similar study in patients without human immunodeficiency virus is ongoing, but it is likely that such a regimen would be equally effective in the IMID setting. Moving forward, it is likely that shorter LTBI treatment regimens will become standard.

If a patient receives treatment of LTBI, the question of when it is safe to start or resume biologic therapy has been an area of controversy. According to the American College of Rheumatology treatment guidelines, at least 1 month of LTBI treatment should be completed before starting or resuming biologic (or tofacitinib) therapy.[1] However, several studies have suggested that it is unnecessary to delay starting or resuming biologic therapy In the setting of LTBI treatment.[39] Experts still recommend a delay of at least 1 to 2 weeks to ensure the patient is tolerating their LTBI treatment. In an analysis of clinical trial data of tofacitinib-treated patients, in phase III studies, of 263 patients diagnosed with LTBI treated concurrently with isoniazid and tofacitinib, none developed active TB, none developed clinically significant hepatitis, and all completed isoniazid therapy.[21] For a patient requiring treatment of active TB, biologic therapy should not be started or resumed until after completion of antimicrobial treatment.

For treatment of active TB, patients with IMIDs can receive any standard treatment regimen, barring any prohibitive comorbidities. Most guidelines recommend cessation of biologic therapy during active TB treatment, and resumption after completion; however, the British Thoracic Society recommends that patients could resume anti-TNF-α treatment after completing 2 months of TB treatment.[40,41] These data are all expert opinion and there is a lack of prospective studies on whether it is safe to resume biologics during TB treatment. Regardless, close monitoring of retreated patients is crucial.

Immune Reconstitution Syndrome

Immune reconstitution syndrome (IRIS), or a paradoxic worsening of symptoms, can occur after starting TB treatment in patients who discontinue biologic therapy. In a case control study including patients from the French RATIO biologics registry, 14 cases of TNFi-associated TB-IRIS out of 56 total TB cases were described.[42] IRIS developed within a median of 45 days after starting TB treatment and 110 days after the last TNFi dose. Nine out of 14 patients received glucocorticoids, and IRIS symptoms disappeared within a median of 5 months after IRIS diagnosis. There were no fatalities. They found that exposure to glucocorticoids after stopping TNFi at the time of diagnosis was associated with IRIS risk. The optimal treatment of TB-IRIS in this setting is unclear, but glucocorticoids are used most often. Rarely, TNFi have been used to treat glucocorticoid-refractory mycobacterial IRIS.[43]

NONTUBERCULOUS MYCOBACTERIA

NTM infections encompass a large group of ubiquitous, environmental organisms that can also complicate biologic therapy. Although risk of NTM infections is recognized with use of TNFi, scant population-based data regarding incidence and risk factors in this setting have been published. One reason for this may be that NTM disease is not reportable in the United States. Diseases caused by NTM are being diagnosed with increasing frequency worldwide including in the United States and in regions of low TB prevalence, such as the United States, it is likely that NTM are a more important complication of TNFi.[44,45] Through a public health surveillance project using Oregon statewide laboratory data from 2007 to 2012, Henkle and colleagues[45] identified 1146 incident pulmonary NTM cases. The subjects were more likely to be female, with a median age of 67 years. Most cases were *Mycobacterium avium/intracellulare*. Furthermore, in a nationwide survey of infectious disease physicians that queried responders to identify mycobacterial infections in patients receiving biologics, NTM infections were reported twice as often as TB.[46]

RA is considered to be a risk factor for NTM infection and several studies have highlighted this important association. In a population-based study using health care data from a large Northern California health system, Winthrop and colleagues[7] reported an incidence rate of NTM of 106/100,000 among patients with RA exposed to TNFi, which was double that of patients with RA unexposed to TNFi.

Rates were higher with the monoclonal antibodies, infliximab and adalimumab, and underlying lung disease and RA were independent risk factors. Chronic lung disease as a result of RA is common, so it is not surprising that RA is a risk factor for NTM disease. Similarly, a case control study conducted at a single center in Taiwan investigated the associated between RA and NTM disease.[47] They reported the following to be predisposing factors for NTM disease in RA: prior TB history; preexisting hypertension, diabetes, interstitial lung disease, or obstructive pulmonary disease; and use of oral glucocorticoids greater than or equal to 5 mg/d.

Although NTM disease in the setting of biologics is most often attributed to use of TNFi, there have been case reports with use of other biologics, including ustekinumab, an inhibitor of the p40 subunit of IL-12/23 that is used in the treatment of psoriasis, psoriatic arthritis, and inflammatory bowel disease.[48] No cases have been reported to date with the IL-17 inhibitors.

There are no formal recommendations to screen for NTM before starting a biologic; however, given that NTM disease may be a more commonly encountered infectious complication than TB in low-prevalence areas, such as the United States, it is important to maintain a heightened awareness. Clinical suspicion for NTM infection should be raised in patients with a chronic unexplained cough, and further evaluation with sputum culture and/or chest computerized tomography should be considered.[49] In terms of management, similar to management of active TB in this setting, biologics should be stopped. If and when biologics are reintroduced during NTM treatment remains a gray area with only case reports and expert opinion as guidance.

SUMMARY

The era of biologic therapies has transformed the lives of patients with IMIDs. Since their introduction in the 1990s there has been a tidal wave of biologics with different immunologic targets and this number is going to continue to grow at a rapid pace. Although biologics are associated with an increased risk of serious and opportunistic infections, such as TB and NTM infections, the overall risk-benefit ratio remains favorable with appropriate screening and risk assessment. Screening for TB before starting biologic therapy remains a cornerstone of infection prevention, although we acknowledge that the available screening tools (TST and IGRAs) are suboptimal. Screening for NTM disease remains an area of uncertainty, but given its increasing incidence it is important to remain vigilant for its presence or development in the setting of biologic therapy, especially with TNFi. Further population-based studies are needed to establish the risk of TB and NTM with the new biologics.

DISCLOSURE

C. Calabrese, nothing to disclose. K.L. Winthrop, scientific consulting and/or research grants from Pfizer, BMS, AbbVie, UCB, Lilly, Gilead, Roche, and Insmed.

REFERENCES

1. Singh JA, Saag KG, Bridges SL Jr, et al. 2015 American College of Rheumatology guideline for the treatment of rheumatoid arthritis. Arthritis Rheumatol 2016; 68:1–26.

2. Listing J, Gerhold K, Zink A. The risk of infections associated with rheumatoid arthritis, with its comorbidity and treatment. Rheumatol 2013;52:53–61.

3. World Health Organization (WHO). Global tuberculosis report 2019. Available at: https://www.who.int/tb/publications/global_report/en/. Accessed September 12, 2019.

4. Furst DE, Cush J, Kaufmann S, et al. Preliminary guidelines for diagnosing and treating tuberculosis in patients with rheumatoid arthritis in immunosuppressive trials or being treated with biological agents. Ann Rheum Dis 2002;61:ii61–3.

5. Maini R, Clair EW St, Breedveld F, et al. Infliximab (chimeric anti-tumour necrosis factor alpha monoclonal antibody) versus placebo in rheumatoid arthritis patients receiving concomitant methotrexate: a randomised phase III trial. ATTRACT Study Group. Lancet 1999;354:1932–9.

6. Joseph K, Gershon S, Wise RP, et al. Tuberculosis associated with infliximab, a tumor necrosis factor α–neutralizing agent. N Engl J Med 2001;345:1098–104.

7. Winthrop KL, Baxter R, Liu L, et al. Mycobacterial diseases and antitumor necrosis factor therapy in USA. Ann Rheum Dis 2013;72:37–42.

8. Tubach F, Salmon D, Ravaud P, et al. Risk of tuberculosis is higher with anti-tumor necrosis factor monoclonal antibody therapy than with soluble tumor necrosis factor receptor therapy: the three-year prospective French Research Axed on Tolerance of Biotherapies registry. Arthritis Rheum 2009;60:1884–94.

9. Dixon WG, Hyrich KL, Watson KD, et al. Drug-specific risk of tuberculosis in patients with rheumatoid arthritis treated with anti-TNF therapy: results from the British Society for Rheumatology Biologics Register (BSRBR). Ann Rheum Dis 2010;69:522–8.

10. Seong SS, Choi CB, Woo JH, et al. Incidence of tuberculosis in Korean patients with rheumatoid arthritis (RA): effects of RA itself and of tumor necrosis factor blockers. J Rheumatol 2007;34:706–11.

11. Kim EM, Uhm WS, Bae SC, et al. Incidence of tuberculosis among Korean patients with ankylosing spondylitis who are taking tumor necrosis factor blockers. J Rheumatol 2011;38:2218–23.

12. Baddley JW, Winthrop KL, Chen L. Non-viral opportunistic infections in new users of tumour necrosis factor inhibitor therapy: results of the SAfety assessment of biologic ThERapy (SABER) study. Ann Rheum Dis 2014;73:1942–8.

13. Cantini F, Niccoli L, Goletti D. Adalimumab, etanercept, infliximab, and the risk of tuberculosis: data from clinical trials, national registries, and postmarketing surveillance. J Rheumatol 2014;91:47–55.

14. Wallis RS, Broder MS, Wong JY, et al. Granulomatous infectious diseases associated with tumor necrosis factor antagonists. Clin Infect Dis 2004;38:1261–5.

15. Saliu OY, Sofer C, Stein DS, et al. Tumor-necrosis-factor blockers: differential effects on mycobacterial immunity. J Infect Dis 2006;194:486–92.

16. Plessner HL, Lin PL, Kohno T, et al. Neutralization of tumor necrosis factor (TNF) by antibody but not TNF receptor fusion molecule exacerbates chronic murine tuberculosis. J Infect Dis 2007;195:1643–50.

17. Souto A, Maneiro JR, Salgado E, et al. Risk of tuberculosis in patients with chronic immune-mediated inflammatory diseases treated with biologics and tofacitinib: a systematic review and meta-analysis of randomized controlled trials and long-term extension studies. Rheumatology (Oxford) 2014;53:1872–85.

18. Koike T, Harigai M, Inokuma S, et al. Postmarketing surveillance of tocilizumab for rheumatoid arthritis in Japan: interim analysis of 3881 patients. Ann Rheum Dis 2011;70:2148–51.

19. Maertzdorf J, Ota M, Repsilber D, et al. Functional correlations of pathogenesis-driven gene expression signatures in tuberculosis. PLoS One 2011;6:e26938.
20. Winthrop KL. The emerging safety profile of JAK inhibitors in rheumatic disease. Nat Rev Rheumatol 2017;13:234–43.
21. Winthrop KL, Park SH, Gul A, et al. Tuberculosis and other opportunistic infections in tofacitinib-treated patients with rheumatoid arthritis. Ann Rheum Dis 2016;75(6):1133–8.
22. Weinblatt ME, Moreland LW, Westhovens R, et al. Safety of abatacept administered intravenously in treatment of rheumatoid arthritis: integrated analyses of up to 8 years of treatment from the abatacept clinical trial program. J Rheumatol 2013;40:787–97.
23. Schiff M, Keiserman M, Codding C, et al. Efficacy and safety of abatacept or infliximab vs placebo in ATTEST: a phase III, multi-centre, randomised, double-blind, placebo-controlled study in patients with rheumatoid arthritis and an inadequate response to methotrexate. Ann Rheum Dis 2008;67:1096–103.
24. Winthrop KL, Saag K, Cascino MD, et al. Long-term safety of rituximab in rheumatoid arthritis: analysis from the SUNSTONE registry. Arthritis Care Res (Hoboken) 2018. https://doi.org/10.1002/acr.23781.
25. Buch MH, Smolen JS, Betteridge N, et al. Updated consensus statement on the use of rituximab in patients with rheumatoid arthritis. Ann Rheum Dis 2011;70: 909–20.
26. Maglione PJ, Xu J, Chan JB. Cells moderate inflammatory progression and enhance bacterial containment upon pulmonary challenge with *Mycobacterium tuberculosis*. J Immunol 2007;178:7222–34.
27. Araujo Z, de Waard JH, de Larrea CF, et al. The effect of bacille Calmette-Guérin vaccine on tuberculin reactivity in indigenous children from communities with high prevalence of tuberculosis. Vaccine 2008;26:5575–81.
28. Calabrese C, Overman RA, Dusetzina SB, et al. Evaluating indeterminate interferon-γ-release assay results in patients with chronic inflammatory diseases receiving immunosuppressive therapy. Arthritis Care Res 2015;67:1063–9.
29. Lewinsohn DM, Leonard MK, LoBue PA, et al. Official American Thoracic Society/Infectious Diseases Society of America/Centers for Disease Control and Prevention Clinical Practice Guidelines: diagnosis of tuberculosis in adults and children. Clin Infect Dis 2017;64:111–5.
30. Winthrop KL. The risk and prevention of tuberculosis: screening strategies to detect latent tuberculosis among rheumatoid arthritis patients who use biologic therapy. Int J Adv Rheumatol 2010;8:43–52.
31. Vassilopoulos D, Tsikrika S, Hatzara C, et al. Comparison of two gamma interferon release assays and tuberculin skin testing for tuberculosis screening in a cohort of patients with rheumatic diseases starting anti-tumor necrosis factor therapy. Clin Vaccin Immunol 2011;18:2102–8.
32. Vassilopoulos D, Stamoulis N, Hadziyannis E, et al. Usefulness of enzyme-linked immunospot assay (Elispot) compared to tuberculin skin testing for latent tuberculosis screening in rheumatic patients scheduled for anti-tumor necrosis factor treatment. J Rheumatol 2008;35:1271–6.
33. Ruan Q, Zhang S, Ai J, et al. Screening of latent tuberculosis infection by interferon-γ release assays in rheumatic patients: a systemic review and meta-analysis. Clin Rheumatol 2016;35:417–25.
34. Winthrop KL, Weinblatt ME, Daley CL. You can't always get what you want, but if you try sometimes (with two tests–TST and IGRA–for tuberculosis) you get what you need. Ann Rheum Dis 2012;71:1757–60.

35. Zwerling A, van den Hof S, Scholten J, et al. Interferon-gamma release assays for tuberculosis screening of healthcare workers: a systematic review. Thorax 2012; 67:62–70.
36. Treatment regimens for latent TB infection | Treatment | TB | CDC. Available at: https://www.cdc.gov/tb/topic/treatment/ltbi.htm. Accessed October 24, 2019.
37. Pfizer, Inc. Xeljanz prescribing information. Available at: http://labeling.pfizer. com/ShowLabeling.aspx?id=2191. Accessed October 24, 2019.
38. Swindells S, Ramchandani R, Gupta A, et al. One month of rifapentine plus isoniazid to prevent HIV-related tuberculosis. N Engl J Med 2019;380:1001–11.
39. Winthrop KL, Siegel JN, Jereb J, et al. Tuberculosis associated with therapy against tumor necrosis factor alpha. Arthritis Rheum 2005;52:2968–74.
40. Mariette X, Salmon D. French guidelines for diagnosis and treating latent and active tuberculosis in patients with RA and treated with TNF blockers. Ann Rheum Dis 2003;62:791–2.
41. Ormerod LP, Milburn HJ, Gillespie S, et al. BTS recommendations for assessing risk and for managing *Mycobacterium tuberculosis* infection and disease in patients due to start anti-TNF-a treatment British. Thorax 2005;60:800–5.
42. Rivoisy C, Tubach F, Roy C, et al. Paradoxical anti-TNF-associated TB worsening: frequency and factors associated with IRIS. Joint Bone Spine 2016;83:173–8.
43. I Isu DC, Faldetta KF, Pei L, et al. A paradoxical treatment for a paradoxical condition: infliximab use in three cases of mycobacterial IRIS. Clin Infect Dis 2016;62: 258–61.
44. Yeh JJ, Wang YC, Lin CL, et al. Nontuberculous mycobacterial infection is associated with increased respiratory failure: a nationwide cohort study. PLoS One 2014;9:e99260.
45. Henkle E, Hedberg K, Schafer S, et al. Population-based incidence of pulmonary nontuberculous mycobacterial disease in Oregon 2007 to 2012. Ann Am Thorac Soc 2015;12:642–7.
46. Winthrop KL, Yamashita S, Beekmann SE, et al, Infectious Diseases Society of America Emerging Infections Network. Mycobacterial and other serious infections in patients receiving anti-tumor necrosis factor and other newly approved biologic therapies: case finding through the Emerging Infections Network. Clin Infect Dis 2008;46:1738–40.
47. Liao TL, Lin CF, Chen YM, et al. Risk factors and outcomes of nontuberculous mycobacterial disease among rheumatoid arthritis patients: a case-control study in a TB endemic area. Sci Rep 2016;6:29443.
48. Shim HH, Cai SCS, Chan W, et al. *Mycobacterium abscessus* infection during ustekinumab treatment in Crohn's disease: a case report and review of the literature. J Crohns Colitis 2018;12:1505–7.
49. Winthrop KL, McNelley E, Kendall B, et al. Pulmonary nontuberculous mycobacterial disease prevalence and clinical features: an emerging public health disease. Am J Respir Crit Care Med 2010;182:977–82.

Vaccinations and Biologics

Betty Hsiao, MD[a,b,]*, Aisha Khan, MD[c], Insoo Kang, MD[a,b,]*

KEYWORDS

- Autoimmune diseases • Biologics • Infections • Immunosuppressed
- Rheumatic diseases • Vaccines • Vaccinations

KEY POINTS

- In preparation for initiating biological therapy, vaccination history should be taken carefully and updated annually to maximize benefits while minimizing vaccine-related adverse effects.
- Although biologics can potentially affect different pathways involved in vaccine response, B cell–depleting rituximab seems to have the most suppressive effect on vaccine responses.
- In general, live attenuated vaccines should be given to patients before starting biologics due to the increased concern for vaccine-related infections on immunosuppressive therapies.
- Inactivated and recombinant vaccines can be administered to patients on biologics.

INTRODUCTION

The emergence of biologics over the last few decades has revolutionized the fields of many specialties including rheumatology, gastroenterology, allergy and immunology, pulmonology, dermatology, and neurology. Biologics target cytokines and cell pathways implicated in the pathogenesis of inflammatory conditions such as rheumatoid arthritis (RA), which, if left untreated, may lead to irreversible tissue damage and significant disability. RA is the first disease that was treated with biologics, with the earliest approved biologics being the anticytokine therapies targeting tumor necrosis factor-alpha inhibitors (TNFi) and interleukin (IL) 1 (anakinra), followed by therapies targeting T-cell signaling (abatacept), depleting B cells (rituximab), blocking IL-6 (tocilizumab or sarilumab), and interfering with intracellular signaling through Janus kinase inhibition (JAKis).[1,2] In addition, the same or similar biological agents have been used to treat different inflammatory diseases such as inflammatory bowel disease, psoriasis, psoriatic arthritis, and ankylosing spondylitis.

[a] Section of Rheumatology, Yale University School of Medicine, 300 Cedar Street, TAC Bldg, RM #525 PO Box 208031, New Haven, CT 06520-8031, USA; [b] Department of Internal Medicine, Yale University School of Medicine, New Haven, CT 06520, USA; [c] Department of Internal Medicine, Griffin Hospital, 130 Division Street, Derby, CT 06418, USA
* Corresponding authors
E-mail addresses: betty.hsiao@yale.edu (B.H.); insoo.kang@yale.edu (I.K.)

Infect Dis Clin N Am 34 (2020) 425–450
https://doi.org/10.1016/j.idc.2020.02.012
0891-5520/20/© 2020 Elsevier Inc. All rights reserved.
id.theclinics.com

Although biologics have become a vital component of the treatment approach to many inflammatory diseases, particularly the "Treat-to-Target" approach to RA[3] of establishing either remission or low disease activity through blocking the undesired effects of a dysregulated immune system, these agents may also potentially disrupt the natural immune response against pathogens, thereby increasing the risk for infections.[4] Indeed, it is well known that patients on TNFi have an increased risk of *Mycobacterium tuberculosis* infection.[5] Some infections may be preventable or have a lessened risk through appropriate vaccinations—although unwanted adverse effects have been reported following vaccinations. The concern for the latter can be greater in patients with inflammatory diseases on biologics who have a compromised immune system. Indeed, recommendations for vaccination have been published by the American College of Rheumatology (ACR), the European League Against Rheumatism (EULAR) for adult patients with autoimmune inflammatory rheumatic diseases (AIIRD), the European Society of Clinical Microbiology and Infectious Diseases (ESCMID) Study Group for infections in compromised hosts on targeted and biological therapies, as well as the Center for Disease Control and Protection (CDC). The objective of this review is to summarize recent articles, including guidelines, published on vaccinations among patients who are on biological therapies.

General Principles

Several important points should be considered in terms of vaccinating patients with autoimmune inflammatory rheumatic diseases (AIIRD) on biologics as well as interpreting the results of vaccine studies in this patient population, regardless of the kind of biologic or vaccine type. These include the definitions of vaccine responses, efficacy and immunogenicity, as well as concerns for adverse effects, flaring disease, and timing. The authors discuss these points followed by reviewing vaccinations in individual autoimmune inflammatory diseases.

Vaccine Efficacy, Safety, and Timing

Vaccines are available in different types encompassing recombinant, polysaccharide, toxoid, inactivated, and live attenuated vaccines. Indications and contraindications for individual vaccines may not be the same in individuals taking different biologics, which can affect efficacy and adverse effects of vaccinations. Vaccination efficacy can be defined by the capacity of vaccines to prevent clinical infections, whereas immunogenicity of vaccines indicates the capacity of vaccines to induce humoral and/or cellular immune responses.[6] Although measuring the immune responses to vaccines could be considered as an outcome, such responses may not correlate with clinical efficacy. Thus, the results of studies analyzing vaccine responses based on immunogenicity should be carefully interpreted in assessing vaccine efficacy.

In general, live attenuated vaccines such as vaccine against measles, mumps, and rubella (MMR) can be less safe in patients on biologics compared with recombinant and inactivated vaccines. Different types of vaccines are available for the same infectious disease. For instance, influenza vaccine is available in recombinant, inactivated intramuscular, and live attenuated intranasal types. Similarly, there are two different types of shingles (herpes zoster [HZ]) vaccine, including recombinant and live attenuated ones. Inactivated and recombinant vaccines can be administered to patients on biologics. However, live attenuated vaccines should be given to patients before embarking on biologics due to the increased concern for theoretically causing infections in susceptible hosts on immunosuppressive therapies.

Disease activity of autoimmune inflammatory diseases may affect the vaccine responses. Most studies on this question were done in patients with RA and/or systemic lupus erythematosus (SLE) who received the influenza vaccine. These studies reported mixed results of no change or reduced immunogenicity in patients with active disease. Also, there is a concern of triggering a flare by vaccinations in patients with autoimmune inflammatory diseases. Of interest, a recent case series study reported the development of severe local inflammatory reactions at the injection sites of pneumococcal vaccination in 7 patients with cyropyrin-associated periodic fever syndrome (CAPS) on receiving pneumococcal polysaccharide or conjugate vaccine.[7] CAPS are a group of conditions with mutations in the gene of cryopyrin or NLRP3 (nucleotide-binding domain and leucine-rich repeat containing family, pyrin domain containing 3) that forms a protein platform called NLRP3 inflammasome with caspase 1.[8] The activation of the NLRP3 inflammasome is required to cleave the inflammatory cytokines pro-IL-1β and -IL-18 by caspase 1 into their mature and active forms IL-1β and IL-18, respectively. IL-1β blocking biologics such as canakinumab is used to treat patients with CAPS. Although the exact mechanism for the development of severe local and systemic reactions in abovementioned vaccinated patients with CAPS is unknown, NLRP3 mutations may be involved in developing such a phenomenon. The activation of NLRP3 inflammasome plays a role in the pathogenesis of autoimmune inflammatory diseases such as SLE.[8] Also, mutations in the NLRP3 gene were found in a small number of patients with Behçet disease,[9] and severe local and systemic reactions were reported in 4 patients with Behçet disease who received the 23-valent polysaccharide pneumococcal vaccine.[10] Although these findings from a small number of patients with CAPS and Behçet disease can not be generalized in patients with autoimmune inflammatory diseases, it would be prudent to administer vaccines during quiescent disease. However, this approach should be individualized without precluding patients with active disease who need vaccination.

Biologics can potentially affect different pathways involved in the development of humoral and cellular immune responses to vaccines. Probably, B cell–depleting rituximab has the most suppressive effect on vaccine responses among different classes of biologics. The 2019 update of EULAR recommendations for vaccination in adult patients with AIIRD recommends that vaccinations should be given at least 6 months after or 4 weeks before the next course of B cell–depleting therapy.[6] Compared with B cell–depleting therapy, biologics targeting cytokines and T cells may have less suppressive effect on vaccine responses as determined by antibody measurements. Nonetheless, vaccines should be ideally administered before the initiation of biologics. Thus, vaccination history should be taken carefully in preparation for treatment with biologics and updated annually to maximize benefits while minimizing adverse effects.

METHODS

In this review, the authors summarize recent papers chosen from the list of articles, published between 1 January 2016 and 30 September 2019, generated from Medline searches of the following text words: first, "vaccine" or "vaccination" and "biologic" and "rheumatoid arthritis" or "systemic lupus erythematosus" or "psoriatic arthritis"; then, "vaccine" or "vaccination" and "etanercept" or "adalimumab" or "infliximab" or "golimumab" or "certolizumab" or "anakinra" or "abatacept" or "rituximab" or "tofacitinib" or "upadacitinib" or "baricitinib" or "tocilizumab" or "sarilumab" or "belimumab" or "secukinumab" or "ixekizumab" or "ustekinumab" or "apremilast." Here the authors focus on papers that include adult patients with rheumatic diseases such as RA, psoriasis, and/or psoriatic arthritis, as well as SLE. They refer to biological disease-modifying antirheumatic drugs (DMARDs), including tofacitinib, as bDMARDs and conventional synthetic DMARDs, such as methotrexate, leflunomide, hydroxychloroquine, and/or sulfasalazine, as csDMARDs. A summary of the articles reviewed is provided in **Table 1** and recommendations for vaccinations from the ACR, CDC, ESCMID, and EULAR are outlined in **Table 2**.

HEPATITIS B VACCINE

Reactivation of hepatitis B virus (HBV) infection has been reported in patients on immunosuppressive treatment with csDMARDs or bDMARDs as well as high-dose corticosteroids (CS),[11,12] highlighting the importance of screening and appropriate treatment.[3] Among patients on bDMARDs, the risk of HBV reactivation varies with respect to the status of HBV infection before initiation as well as the degree of immunosuppression. (Please also see Eiichi Ogawa and colleagues' article, "Hepatitis B Virus Reactivation Potentiated by Biologics" in this issue.) Given the risk of HBV reactivation and availability of effective antiviral prophylaxis, screening for HBV infection is recommended in all patients with RA starting bDMARDs.[13] The European Association for the Study of the Liver[14] and the American Association for the Study of the Liver Disease (AASLD)[15] recommend appropriate screening before patients starting chemotherapy or immunotherapy; although the 2015 ACR Guidelines for the treatment of RA include recommendations for treating patients with HBV (and hepatitis C) infection, endorsing the use of immunosuppressive therapy when prophylactic antivirals are also given, there are no specific recommendations for screening. For patients who have no evidence of previous HBV infection, vaccination should be considered before starting bDMARDs based on the CDC and AASLD guidelines[3]; EULAR recommends vaccination in patients with AIIRD at risk.[6]

The hepatitis B vaccine, HepB-CpG, which contains yeast-derived recombinant HepB surface antigen (HBsAg), is prepared by combining purified HBsAg with small synthetic immunostimulatory cytidine-phosphate-guanosine oligodeoxynucleotide motifs, which binds toll-like receptor 9 to stimulate an immune response to HBsAg.[16] The vaccine is administered in 2 to 4 doses depending on vaccine types.[17] Although the hepatitis B vaccination was found to be immunogenic in most patients, high-dose HBV vaccination did not increase the humoral response rate.[18]

The efficacy of the hepatitis B vaccine was evaluated by Intongkam and colleagues[19] among 46 patients with RA receiving csDMARDs (n = 33) and/or bDMARDs (n = 13), as compared with age- and sex-matched control subjects who were vaccinated with 20-μg recombinant hepatitis B vaccine (EuVax B) at weeks 0, 4, and 24. Hepatitis B surface antibody levels were measured 8 weeks after the last dose of vaccination with seroprotection as defined as hepatitis B surface antibody level of 10 mIU/mL or greater; in addition, Disease Activity Score in 28 joints were calculated at weeks 0, 4, and 32. The patients with RA on csDMARDs and bDMARDs were found to have lower levels of seroprotection as compared with the control group. The patients with RA who responded to vaccination were noted to be younger and less likely to be treated with rituximab; overall, hepatitis B vaccination was well tolerated, with no increased rate of RA flare postvaccination.

INFLUENZA VACCINE

Patients with RA have a high risk for influenza and influenza-related complications such as pneumonia, stroke, and myocardial infarction, within 30 days of influenza diagnosis.[20] Similarly, a higher incidence of patients' reports of influenza-like illness was noticed in Italian patients with RA, psoriatic arthritis, ankylosing spondylitis, and spondyloarthropathies who were on biologics compared with the general Italian population (17% vs 9.7%).[21] Clearly, influenza vaccination cannot be overemphasized

Table 1
Summary of discussed articles

Author/Title	Study Population	Objective	Methods	Conclusion
Hepatitis B Virus Vaccination				
Intongkam et al,[19] 2018	46 patients with RA (from Phramongkutklao Hospital recruited from 11/2013–3/2016), 33 on csDMARDs, and 13 on both csDMARDs and bDMARDs, compared with control subjects vaccinated with 20 μg recombinant hepatitis B vaccine (EuVax B) at wk 0, 4, and 24	The aim of this study was to assess efficacy and safety of hepatitis B vaccination in RA patients receiving csDMARDs and/or bDMARDs.	Prospective open-label study	Patients with RA receiving DMARDs had less humoral response to hepatitis B vaccination as compared with control subjects. Aging and rituximab use were associated with impaired response to hepatitis B vaccination. Overall, hepatitis B vaccination is safe and well tolerated in patients with RA.
Herpes Zoster Vaccination				
Calabrese et al,[76] 2019	1146 patients with RA (384 on tofacitinib monotherapy; 376 on tofacitinib + methotrexate; 386 on adalimumab + methotrexate) of which 216 (18.8%) received LZV before study treatment	To explore HZ rates, and LZV safety, in a subset of patients with RA who received LZV before tofacitinib ± methotrexate, or adalimumab and methotrexate.	Randomized triple-dummy, active comparator-controlled study	LZV was well tolerated, and HZ incidence rates were generally similar between treatment groups and vaccinated vsnonvaccinated patients. This study was not powered for comparisons between vaccinated and nonvaccinated patients as <20% of all patients were vaccinated.
Curtis et al,[73] 2016	2526 patients with RA initiating tofacitinib, compared with initiations of other bDMARDs: TNFi, abatacept, rituximab, tocilizumab, identified from Medicare (2006–2013) and Marketscan (2010–2014)	To evaluate the risks of HZ and herpes simplex virus (HSV) infection associated with tofacitinib compared with bDMARDs among patients with RA.	Retrospective cohort study	The rate of HZ associated with tofacitinib was approximately double that observed in patients using bDMARDs.

(continued on next page)

Table 1
(continued)

Author/Title	Study Population	Objective	Methods	Conclusion
Curtis et al,[74] 2019	8030 patients with RA identified in both Medicare (5,369) and MarketScan (2,661) from 2011–2016	To evaluate HZ risk in tofacitinib users with and without methotrexate and glucocorticoids.	Retrospective cohort study	HZ occurred at a rate of approximately 4% per year and was further doubled with glucocorticoid exposure in patients on tofacitinib. Concomitant MTX did not confer additional risk and zoster vaccination may decrease risk.
Winthrop et al,[75] 2017	112 patients were randomized to receive placebo (n = 57) or tofacitinib (n = 55)	To evaluate the effect on the immune response and safety of LZV.	Placebo-controlled trial	Patients who began treatment with tofacitinib 2–3 wk after receiving LZV had VZV-specific humoral and cell-mediated immune responses to LZV as those in placebo-treated patients.
Wu et al,[77] 2019	Randomized clinical trials, review articles, observational studies, case reports, and case series from 1946–2019	To synthesize and evaluate the literature investigating the risk of HZ in patients treated with IL-17 inhibitors, with a focus on patients with psoriasis.	Review article.	To date, IL-17 inhibitors do not seem to increase risk of HZ. However, further long-term data are needed given the recent introduction of these drugs.
Human Papilloma Virus Vaccine				
Dhar et al,[81] 2017	34 women aged 19-50 y with mild to moderate SLE & minimally active or inactive SLE who received quadrivalent HPV vaccine at the standard dosing schedule	To evaluate the safety and immunogenicity of HPV vaccine in SLE.	Open-label clinical trial	In this SLE vaccine study, quadrivalent HPV vaccine was generally safe, well tolerated, and highly immunogenic.

Reference	Sample	Objective	Study Type	Findings
Mok et al,[82] 2018	50 patients with SLE and 50 controls were vaccinated with quadrivalent HPV vaccine	To evaluate the 5-y immunogenicity of a quadrivalent HPV in patients with SLE	Open-label clinical trial	Immunogenicity of the quadrivalent HPV vaccine was retained in a high proportion of SLE patients at 5 y.
Influenza Vaccine				
Huang et al,[27] 2017	13 studies with 886 patients with RA and 685 healthy controls	To compare the humoral immunogenicity and adverse effects of influenza vaccinations between RA patients and healthy controls.	Systemic review and meta-analysis	Immunogenicity was significantly different between patients with RA and healthy controls for the H1N1 strain, but not for the H3N2 or B strains. bDMARDs may play an important role in immunogenicity of inactivated influenza vaccines for patients with RA.
Richi et al,[32] 2019	17 patients with psoriatic arthritis or ankylosing spondylitis and 13 controls	To evaluate whether immunologic response to influenza vaccination is impaired in patients who are receiving IL-17 blocking secukinumab.	Pilot study	In this study, secukinumab has no effect on the immunogenic response to the influenza vaccine.
Pneumococcal Vaccine				
Alten et al,[31] 2016	125 patients (77 from ACQUIRE and 48 from ATTUNE) who received the PPSV23 vaccination; 191 patients from the ACQUIRE study who received the influenza vaccine	To evaluate the antibody response to PPSV23 and the 2011–2012 trivalent seasonal influenza vaccine in adults with RA receiving subcutaneous abatacept and background DMARDs.	Two multicenter, open-label studies	Patients with RA receiving subcutaneous abatacept and background DMARDs were able to mount an appropriate immune response to pneumococcal and influenza vaccines.

(continued on next page)

Table 1
(continued)

Author/Title	Study Population	Objective	Methods	Conclusion
Adawi et al,[55] 2019	18 studies included in analysis with 601 participants	To better understand the efficacy of pneumococcal immunization as well as its safety in patients with SLE.	Systematic review and meta-analysis	Results included 18 studies with 601 participants with vaccine immunogenicity as measured in protective antibody titers ranging from 36% to 97.6%. Overall, no serious adverse events were found.
Broyde et al,[59] 2016	145 consecutive patients treated with csDMARDs and bDMARDs	To estimate the long-term humoral response of PPSV23 in patients with rheumatic diseases and the effect of demographic and clinical factors and treatment on the long-term efficacy of the vaccine.	Prospective observational study	The long-term efficacy of the PPSV23 vaccination seems to be preserved among patients with rheumatic diseases including RA, for at least 10 y. Efficacy is slightly impaired by methotrexate, but it is not affected by bDMARDs.
Chatham et al,[54] 2017	79 patients received pneumococcal vaccination (34 before belimumab, 45 concurrent to belimumab)	To assess the impact of belimumab on immune response to pneumococcal vaccination (PPSV23) in patients with SLE.	Randomized, open-label study.	The proportion of patients generating a response to ≥ 1 and ≥ 2 pneumococcal serotypes did not differ between the pre-belimumab and belimumab-concurrent cohorts.
Gomez et al,[61] 2017	84 participants: 41 on ixekizumab and 43 controls	The objective of this study was to determine the immune response to tetanus and pneumococcal vaccines in healthy subjects administered IL-17 blocking ixekizumab compared with control subjects.	Open-label, parallel-group study	Ixekizumab does not suppress the humoral immune response to nonlive vaccines and was well tolerated in healthy subjects.

Nagel et al,[53] 2017	47 patients with SLE (Department of Rheumatology, Skåne University Hospital in Lund and Malmö) and 21 healthy controls	The objective of this study was to explore the impact of SLE and belimumab given in addition to standard of care therapy on the PCV13 response.	Prospective observational study	Belimumab given in addition to csDMARDs or corticosteroids did not further impair antibody response to PCV13.
Nguyen et al,[49] 2017	Patients with RA, 65 on bDMARDs and 35 on csDMARDs	To evaluate the initial serologic responses to PCV13 followed by PPSV23 among patients with RA on bDMARDs	Investigator-initiated clinical trial	Serologic responses were similar among participants receiving bDMARDs and csDMARDs. However, notable differences in response were observed in patients treated with rituximab. The response for rituximab-treated participants was 25% compared with ≥89% in participants treated with other bDMARD.
Rákóczi et al,[50] 2016	22 patients with RA on etanercept in combination with methotrexate (15) or monotherapy (7) compared to 24 patients with osteoarthritis who were not on csDMARDs or bDMARDs	To prospectively evaluate the immunogenicity of PCV13 in RA patients undergoing etanercept therapy.	Prospective observational study	In RA patients on etanercept, vaccination with PCV13 was effective and safe, resulting in protective antibody response one and 2 months after vaccination.
Rezende et al,[58] 2016	28 patients receiving immunosuppression and 26 controls	To evaluate the immunogenicity of PPSV23 in patients with SLE on immunosuppressive treatment	Prospective open-label study	The vaccine was poorly immunogenic, especially among patients with SLE on immunosuppressive therapy.

(continued on next page)

Table 1
(continued)

Author/Title	Study Population	Objective	Methods	Conclusion
Subesinghe et al,[28] 2018	9 studies were included in the metaanalysis (7 studies investigating antirheumatic drug exposures and influenza humoral response, 2 studies investigating pneumococcal vaccine response).	To evaluate the effect of csDMARDs and bDMARDs on influenza and pneumococcal vaccine immunogenicity.	Systematic review and meta-analysis	DMARDs may limit humoral responses to vaccination as evidenced by pneumococcal responses with methotrexate exposure; however, they are safe and should be considered in all patients with RA and encouraged as part of routine care.
Winthrop et al,[52] 2018	61 patients with psoriasis on tofacitinib received tetanus toxoid and PCV13 vaccinations	To characterize the effect of long-term exposure to tofacitinib 10 mg twice daily on T-cell function in psoriasis patients.	Single-arm, open-label vaccine substudy	Most patients with psoriasis who received tofacitinib could mount satisfactory T cell-dependent responses to PCV13 and tetanus vaccines.
Winthrop et al,[51] 2019	106 patients from the phase 3 long-term extension trial for baricitinib.	To evaluate pneumococcal conjugate and tetanus toxoid vaccine (TTV) responses in patients with RA receiving baricitinib.	Vaccine substudy	Approximately two-thirds of patients on long-term baricitinib achieved satisfactory humoral and functional responses to PCV13 vaccination, whereas TTV responses were less robust. PCV13 response was not diminished in those taking concomitant corticosteroids.

| Croce et al,[86] 2017 | 64 articles were included: 40 on immune-mediated inflammatory diseases (14,427 patients with rheumatic diseases) | To estimate the safety of live vaccinations in patients with immune-mediated inflammatory diseases or solid organ transplantation on immunosuppressive treatment and in patients after bone-marrow transplantation. | Systematic review | Although live vaccinations were safe and sufficiently immunogenic in most studies, some serious reactions and vaccine-related infections were reported in immunosuppressed patients with immune-mediated inflammatory diseases or solid organ transplantation. |

Abbreviations: ACQUIRE, abatacept comparison of sub[QU]cutaneous versus intravenous in inadequate responders to MethotrexatE trial; ATTUNE, abatacept in subjecTs who swiTch from intravenoUs to subcutaNeous therapy trial; bDMARDs, biologic disease modifying anti-rheumatic drugs; csDMARDs, conventional synthetic disease modifying anti-rheumatic drugs; DMARDs, disease modifying anti-rheumatic drugs; HPV, human papillomavirus; HZ, herpes zoster; LZV, live zoster vaccine; PCV13, pneumococcal conjugate vaccine; PPSV23, pneumococcal polysaccharide vaccine; RA, rheumatoid arthritis; SLE, systemic lupus erythematosus; TNFi, tumor necrosis factor-alpha inhibitor(s); TTV, tetanus toxoid vaccine; VZV, varicella-zoster virus.

Table 2
Recommendations for vaccination

Vaccine	ACR Guidelines for RA[88]	CDC Guidelines	ESCMID Guidelines[87,89]	EULAR Guidelines[6]
Hepatitis B	Before initiating and while already taking csDMARDs and/or bDMARDs	All unvaccinated adults at risk for HBV and those requesting protection[17]	Age-appropriate antiviral vaccinations are strongly encouraged	For patients with AIIRD at risk for HBV
Herpes Zoster (live attenuated)	Patients with RA aged ≥50 y before receiving bDMARDs; should be avoided while on bDMARDs	Recommended for immunocompetent adults aged ≥60 y[62]	Live-virus vaccines may be contraindicated due to underlying diseases	May be considered in high-risk patients with AIIRD
Herpes Zoster (recombinant)	Not specified	Adults aged ≥50 y; for those on low-dose immunosuppressive therapy (eg, <20 mg/d of prednisone), anticipating immunosuppression, or recovered from an immunocompromising illness[62]	Not specified	May be considered in high-risk patients with AIIRD
Human Papilloma Virus	Before initiating and while already taking csDMARDs and/or bDMARDs	Recommended at age 11 or 12 y; catch-up vaccination is recommended for all persons through age 26 y[79]	Not specified	Patients with AIIRD, especially those with SLE, should receive vaccination in accordance with general population
Intramuscular Influenza	Before initiating and while already taking csDMARDs and/or bDMARDs	Annual vaccination is recommended for all persons aged ≥6 mo who do not have contraindications; those ≥65 may receive high-dose IIV3; immunocompromised persons should receive an age-appropriate IIV or RIV4[23]	Age-appropriate antiviral vaccinations are strongly encouraged	Vaccination should be strongly considered for majority of patients with AIIRD

Measles, Mumps, Rubella	Live attenuated vaccines should not be used	Not recommended in those with a weakened immune system due to medical treatments (such asradiation, immunotherapy, steroids, or chemotherapy)[40]	Recommended at least 2–4 wk before starting certain bDMARDs (or as soon as possible if therapy is urgent)	Live vaccination should be generally avoided in patients with AIIRD
PCV13	Before initiating and while already taking csDMARDs and/or bDMARDs	Adults aged ≥19 y with immunocompromising conditions, who have not previously received PCV13 or PPSV23, should receive a dose of PCV13 first, followed by a dose of PPSV23 at least 8 wklater[43]	Pneumococcal recommended before starting certain bDMARDs	Vaccination should be strong considered for majority of patients with AIIRD
PPSV23	Before initiating and while already taking csDMARDs and/or bDMARDs	Adults aged ≥19 y with immunocompromising conditions, who previously have received ≥1 doses of PPSV23 should be given a PCV13 dose ≥1 y after the last PPSV23 dose was received[43]	Pneumococcal recommended before starting certain bDMARDs	Vaccination should be strong considered for majority of patients with AIIRD
Tetanus toxoid	Not specified	All persons are recommended to receive routine vaccination[78]	Not specified	Patients with AIIRD should receive tetanus toxoid vaccine in accordance with recommendations for general population

(continued on next page)

Table 2
(continued)

Vaccine	ACR Guidelines for RA[88]	CDC Guidelines	ESCMID Guidelines[87,89]	EULAR Guidelines[6]
Yellow Fever	Not specified	Recommended for persons aged ≥9 mo who are traveling to or living in areas with risk.[90] The vaccine is not recommended for people who are using immunosuppressive and immunomodulatory therapies.	Live-virus vaccines may be contraindicated due to underlying diseases	Live vaccination should be generally avoided in patients with AIIRD

Abbreviations: ACR, American College of Rheumatology; AIIRD, autoimmune inflammatory rheumatic disease; bDMARDs, biologic disease-modifying antirheumatic drugs; CDC, center for disease control and protection; csDMARDs, conventional synthetic disease-modifying antirheumatic drugs; ESCMID, European Society of Clinical Microbiology and Infectious Diseases; EULAR, European League Against Rheumatism; HBV, hepatitis B virus; IIV, inactivated influenza vaccine; IIV3, trivalent inactivated influenza vaccine; PCV13, pneumococcal conjugate vaccine; PPSV23, pneumococcal polysaccharide vaccine; RA, rheumatoid arthritis; RIV4, quadrivalent recombinant influenza vaccine; SLE, systemic lupus erythematosus.

in patients with autoimmune inflammatory diseases. CDC guidelines recommend the yearly administration of an age-appropriate inactivated intramuscular influenza vaccine (IIV) or recombinant influenza vaccine to immunosuppressed patients, with avoidance of the live intranasal attenuated vaccine, given the uncertain but possible risk attributable to the live virus.[22] Currently, all standard-dose IIVs are quadrivalent, thought to provide broader coverage against circulating influenza B strains, and either egg based or cell culture based; high-dose and adjuvanted IIVs are trivalent, licensed for those aged 65 years and older.[23] ACR guidelines include strong recommendations for administering appropriately indicated inactivated vaccines in patients with early or established RA who are currently receiving biologics.[3] Patients on TNFi who received influenza vaccine have been reported to present with fewer influenza-related adverse events over an average of greater than 5 years of follow-up, compared with patients who did not receive the vaccine.[24] Most of the patients on immunosuppressive therapy for the treatment of AIIRD seem to benefit from influenza vaccine, with the seasonal trivalent vaccine shown to reduce overall mortality from influenza as well as pneumonia in this population.[6,25,26]

Using a meta-analysis and systemic review approach, Huang and colleagues[27] compared the humoral immunogenicity of patients with RA and healthy controls by analyzing primary outcome of seroprotection (antibody titers $\geq$1:40 on the hemagglutination inhibition assay after vaccination) and secondary outcome of seroconversion ($\geq$4-fold antibody titer increase after vaccination). Patients with RA were found to have comparable humoral responses as compared with healthy controls for the H3N2 and B strains (even with background bDMARDs) but had a significantly lower seroprotection to the H1N1 strain. Adverse events were reported in patients with RA, with 7 studies that noted a local response after vaccination; although no severe systemic adverse events were reported, one study reported RA flares postvaccination occurring in 6 of 17 patients.

Subesinghe and colleagues[28] conducted a systematic literature review and meta-analysis comparing the humoral response to influenza (pandemic and seasonal trivalent subunit vaccines) among adult patients with RA treated with csDMARDs and bDMARDs. This study with data from 7 studies showed that influenza vaccine responses to all subunit strains (H1N1, H3N2, B strain) were preserved with methotrexate and TNFi. However, a recent study reported that temporary discontinuation of methotrexate improved the immunogenicity of seasonal trivalent influenza vaccination in patients with RA, as compared with either cessation of methotrexate before vaccination or continuing methotrexate unchanged.[29,30] The best results were found when the cessation of methotrexate was done 2 weeks before and 2 weeks after vaccination or 4 weeks following vaccination.

The antibody response to seasonal trivalent influenza vaccine was analyzed in patients with RA who were receiving subcutaneous abatacept and DMARDs.[31] About 61% of the patients (73/119) achieved an immunologic response to influenza vaccine, indicating that patients with RA receiving abatacept and background DMARDs were able to mount an appropriate immune response to influenza vaccines. Richiand colleagues[32] evaluated the immunogenic response to the seasonal inactivated trivalent influenza vaccines in a small number of patients (n = 17) with inflammatory arthropathies on IL-17 blocking secukinumab and 13 controls, showing no significant difference in the proportion of vaccine responders between the 2 groups as determined by antibody fold changes.

Overall, the influenza vaccination should be given annually to all patients with RA regardless of immunosuppressive therapy,[3] as it is relatively unaffected by the presence of bDMARDs, with the exception of rituximab.[33–35] Most patients can have an adequate level of protective antibody following vaccination with no significant adverse effects.[36,37] Given the concern for the suppressive effect of rituximab on humoral response to influenza and pneumococcal vaccinations in patients with RA, spondyloarthropathies, and SLE, the current EULAR guidelines recommend vaccination before the administration of rituximab—ideally, at least 6 months after the administration and at least 4 months before the next course of B cell–depleting therapy.[6]

MEASLES, MUMPS, AND RUBELLA VACCINE

The MMR vaccines available in the United States include a combination of MMR vaccine[38] or a combination of measles, mumps, rubella, and varicella (MMRV) vaccine.[39] Both contain live, attenuated measles, mumps, and rubella virus, with the MMRV containing the attenuated varicella-zoster virus. The CDC warns that patients on systemic immunosuppressive therapy, including oral CS ($\geq$2 mg/kg of body weight or $\geq$20 mg/d of prednisone or equivalent for persons who weigh >10 kg, when administered for $\geq$2 weeks), should not be given the MMR vaccines.[40]

Most data on MMR are from observational studies among pediatric patients with AIIRD. A retrospective study in the Netherlands evaluated immunogenicity among patients with juvenile idiopathic arthritis (JIA) and found long-term seroprotection rates were not affected by concurrent CS or methotrexate use.[41] Also, another study in Germany reported a protective humoral response in patients with JIA who received revaccination while on methotrexate and/or TNFi.[42] Although there is evidence that revaccination may be safe in patients on immunosuppression, live-attenuated vaccines, including MMR, should be generally avoided among patients receiving bDMARDs.[6,40]

PNEUMOCOCCAL VACCINE

Currently, 2 pneumococcal vaccines are licensed for use in the United States: a 13-valent pneumococcal conjugate vaccine (PCV13) and a 23-valent pneumococcal polysaccharide vaccine (PPSV23), which contains 12 of the serotypes in PCV13, with 11 additional serotypes.[43] Pneumococcal polysaccharide vaccine response develops independently of T cells while pneumococcal conjugate vaccine induces T cell-dependent humoral immune response.[44] The CDC recommends PCV13 for all children younger than 5 years of age, all adults $\geq$65 years, and those aged 6 to 64 years with certain medical conditions, as well as a one-time pneumococcal revaccination after 5 years for persons with chronic conditions such as RA.[45] The current ACR guidelines recommend that pneumococcal vaccines should be given before initiation of RA therapy.[3]

The effects of bDMARDs and csDMARDs on pneumococcal vaccine responses are extensively studied in patients with AIIRD including RA, SLE, and ankylosing spondylitis. Subesinghe and colleagues[28] conducted a systematic literature review and meta-analysis comparing the humoral response with pneumococcal vaccines (PCV13 and PPSV23) among patients with RA treated with csDMARDs and bDMARDs by measuring seroprotection rates 3 to 6 weeks postimmunization. Two studies investigating pneumococcal vaccine response showed methotrexate, but not TNFi, exposure was associated with reduced 6B and 23F serotype pneumococcal vaccine response.[46,47] A combination of MTX with tocilizumab or tofacitinib was associated with reduced pneumococcal and influenza vaccine responses.[35,48] These findings suggest the possible detrimental effect of MTX on the immunogenicity of pneumococcal vaccine response. Alten and colleagues[31] evaluated the antibody response among patients with RA on subcutaneous abatacept and DMARDs who received

PPSV23. About 74% of the patients (34/46) were found to achieve an immunologic response to PPSV23.

The initial serologic responses to PCV13 followed by PPSV23 were evaluated in patients with RA on bDMARDs (n = 65) and csDMARDs (n = 35).[49] Participants were randomized (1:1:1) to immunization with single-dose PCV13 followed by PPSV23 after 16 or 24 weeks or double-dose PCV13 followed by PPSV23 after 16 weeks, compared with a cohort of patients with RA on csDMARDs who received a single-dose PCV13 followed by PPSV23 at 16 weeks later. The results showed no significant difference among the 3 arms as determined by the proportion of participants responding to at least 6 of 12 pneumococcal serotypes 4 weeks after both vaccinations. However, notable differences were observed according to individual bDMARDs, with a severely impaired serologic response in patients on rituximab (25%) compared with most of the participants (≥89%) treated with other bDMARDs (including TNFi, anti-IL-6, abatacept, or csDMARD), supporting the possible suppression of pneumococcal vaccine response by rituximab and administration of this vaccine before rituximab if possible.

The immunogenicity of PCV13 was analyzed in a small number of patients (n = 22) with RA on etanercept alone (n = 7) or a combination of etanercept and MTX (n = 15) in comparison to 24 patients with osteoarthritis.[50] The mean protective antibody levels were higher in the osteoarthritis group at 4 and 8 weeks. In the RA group, older age at vaccination was identified as a predictor of impaired protective antibody response, and there were no clinically significant adverse events in any patients. Winthrop and colleagues[51] evaluated PCV13 (and tetanus toxoid vaccine [TTV]) responses in 106 patients with RA receiving baricitinib (30% on CS, 89% on concomitant methotrexate) that blocks signaling of multiple cytokines through inhibiting janus kinase (JAK) 1/2. Approximately two-thirds of patients on long-term baricitinib achieved satisfactory humoral and functional responses to PCV13 vaccination.[51] PCV13 response was not diminished in those taking concomitant CS. These findings indicate that a large number of patients with RA on the JAK inhibitor (JAKi) baricitinib can still develop appropriate antibody response to PCV13. A similar result was observed in patients (n = 60) with psoriasis taking another JAKi, tofacitinib, for more than 3 months when they were vaccinated with PCV13.[52] The results of this study found that most patients who received tofacitinib mounted satisfactory T-cell–dependent responses to PCV13.

The impact of SLE and its treatments was investigated by multiple studies including those using meta-analysis. Nagel and colleagues[53] explored the PCV13 response among 47 patients with SLE (40 on csDMARDs, 11 on concomitant belimumab, and 32 on concomitant prednisone) compared with healthy controls. This study is particularly interesting because the B cell activator factor inhibiting belimumab is the first biologic approved by Food and Drug Administration for the treatment of SLE. In comparing pre- and postvaccination log-transformed antibody levels, patients with SLE patients as a group had lower postvaccination antibody levels and lower fold increase of antibody levels after vaccination compared with controls. However, such levels were not different in patients treated with belimumab in addition to standard of care therapy or hydroxychloroquine compared with controls, whereas the other treatment groups had significantly lower fold increase of postvaccination antibody levels. Also, the effect of belimumab on immune response to PPSV23 was studied in patients with SLE.[54] Patients were randomized (7:9) to receive a PPSV23 vaccination 4 weeks before (pre-belimumab cohort) or 24 weeks after (belimumab-concurrent cohort) commencing 4-weekly belimumab 10 mg/kg intravenous treatment plus standard of care treatment. Analysis included 79 patients who received the vaccine (34 in pre-belimumab cohort and 45 in belimumab-concurrent cohort). At week 4 postvaccination, 97.0% (32/33) and 97.6% (40/41) of patients (pre-belimumab and concurrent belimumab cohorts, respectively) had a positive response to at least 1 of 23 pneumococcal serotypes. More than 85% of patients in both cohorts responded to greater than or equal to 10 of serotypes, approximately 80% responded to greater than or equal to 12 serotypes, and approximately two-thirds responded to greater than or equal to 16 serotypes. A recent meta-analysis evaluated the safety and efficacy of the pneumococcal vaccine in patients with SLE by including 18 studies with a total of 601 participants.[55] Vaccine immunogenicity as measured by protective antibody titers ranged from 36% to 97.6%. Elevated erythrocyte sedimentation rate, older age, earlier SLE onset, high disease activity, and immunosuppressive therapy were predictors of poor immunogenicity. Belimumab was not found to have a significant impact on immunogenicity. No serious adverse events were found. Patients with SLE seem to have impaired antibody response to PPV in general although belimumab may not reduce this response.

Overall, the immunogenicity of PCV13 is reduced among patients with RA on methotrexate[56] as well as those with SLE[53] and systemic vasculitis.[57] The immunogenicity and safety of PPSV23 has been demonstrated in patients with RA and SLE,[55,58] with long-term data that evaluated patients with RA on bDMARDs.[6,59] There were no safety concerns raised except for patients with cryopyrin-associated periodic fever syndromes, who have been reported to develop both local and systemic reactions to PPSV23 as described earlier (see General principles section).[60] In addition, data show variable immune responses to pneumococcal vaccination, with TNFi and tocilizumab having little or no effect on PPSV23 immunogenicity, whereas methotrexate, rituximab, and tofacitinib may negatively affect response to PPSV23.[33] Also, in patients with moderate to severe psoriasis, the IL-17-blockade ixekizumab was found not to suppress the humoral immune response to PPSV23 as compared with control subjects.[61] Therefore, pneumococcal vaccination is recommended before commencement of DMARDs[3,36] and should be considered for most of the patients with AIIRD according to the ACR, CDC, ESCMID, and EULAR guidelines.[6]

HERPES ZOSTER VACCINE

Vaccinations for HZ include a live attenuated version (live zoster vaccine [LZV]) as well as a recombinant adjuvanted version (recombinant zoster vaccine [RZV]). The live vaccine is given as a single dose containing a live attenuated strain of varicella zoster virus (VZV) and used for the prevention of HZ in immunocompetent adults aged 50 years and older. The RZV, which has been shown to have higher levels of efficacy against HZ in clinical trials, contains recombinant glycoprotein E in combination with a novel adjuvant ($AS01_B$) that is given in 2 doses, 2 to 6 months apart.[62] The RZV has also been shown to be more efficacious compared with the live vaccine in elderly adults.[63] The Advisory Committee on Immunization Practices (ACIP) recommends administration of the RZV in immunocompromised patients on low-dose immunosuppressive therapy (eg, <20 mg/d of prednisone or equivalent or using inhaled or topical steroids) and those initiating immunosuppression or who have recovered from an immunocompromising illness.[62] Of note, immunocompromised persons and those on moderate to high doses of immunosuppressive therapy were not included in the efficacy studies (Zoster Efficacy Study in Adults 50 Years of Age or Older [ZOE-50] and Zoster Efficacy Study in Adults 70 Years of Age or Older [ZOE-70]).[62,64] The medical board of the National Psoriasis Foundation made consensus recommendations that the recombinant zoster vaccine should be given to all patients with psoriasis and psoriatic arthritis older than 50 years and patients younger than 50 years on tofacitinib, systemic glucocorticoids, or combination systemic treatment.[65]

Previous studies showed conflicting data on the risk of HZ among bDMARDs. Several studies demonstrated an increased risk of HZ among patients with RA on TNFi compared with others, whereas other studies did not show increased risk of HZ with TNFi as compared with csDMARDs.[66–71] Among the TNFi, infliximab may confer a greater risk of HZ but a retrospective study did not show differences among patients starting TNFi, abatacept, rituximab, or tocilizumab.[72] In a study in the United States, the risk for HZ in patients with RA on tofacitinib was approximately double as compared with patients on other bDMARDs (TNFi, abatacept, rituximab, tocilizumab).[73] Using the same health plan data from Medicare and Marketscan, Curtis and colleagues[74] found the occurrence of HZ in patients with RA on tofacitinib almost doubled with concomitant glucocorticoid use (median dose of prednisone-equivalent 5–6.7 mg/d) but was not affected by concomitant methotrexate exposure.

Winthrop and colleagues[75] evaluated the effect on the immune response and safety of LZV among patients with RA on background methotrexate who were given LZV and randomized to receive tofacitinib 5 mg twice daily or placebo. The results of this study showed patients who began treatment with tofacitinib after receiving LZV had VZV-specific humoral and cell-mediated immune responses to LZV similar to those in placebo-treated patients at 2 to 3 weeks postvaccination. Vaccination seemed to be safe in all of the patients except one patient who lacked preexisting VZV immunity and subsequently developed disseminated primary varicella. The safety of LZV was assessed in ORAL Strategy, a 1-year, global Phase 3b/4 study evaluating the efficacy and safety of tofacitinibmonotherapy, tofacitinib with methotrexate, and adalimumab with methotrexate in RA.[76] Among a total of 1146 patients, 18 patients (1.6%), of whom 3 were vaccinated, developed HZ. HZ incidence rates (events per 100 patient-years) were 1.1, 2.3, and 1.7 for tofacitinib monotherapy, tofacitinib with methotrexate, and adalimumab with methotrexate, respectively.

IL-17 inhibitors, including secukinumab and ixekizumab, may not seem to increase the risk of HZ as compared with controls, with few to no reported cases of HZ in those treated with IL-17 inhibitors for rheumatologic and dermatologic diseases.[77] However, long-term data would be needed, as anti-IL-17 targeting therapy is relatively new.

Overall, HZ vaccination should be considered for patients with rheumatic diseases, ideally before commencement of immunosuppression; although live vaccines should be avoided for those on immunosuppressive therapy, additional research is needed to assess long-term safety of RZV in immunocompromised patients on bDMARDs.[62,64]

TETANUS TOXOID VACCINE

Tetanus vaccines for adult can be given as tetanus and diphtheria (Td) or tetanus, diphtheria, and pertussis (Tdap) vaccines, which are both inactivated. Winthrop and colleagues[52] evaluated the response to T-cell–dependent vaccine (monovalent TTV and PCV13) among 60 patients with psoriasis who were completing at least 3 months of continuous treatment with tofacitinib 10 mg twice daily. The results showed that 51 (88%) patients had greater than or equal to 2-fold and 35 (60%) patients had greater than or equal to 4-fold increase in antibody concentration at 4 weeks postvaccination. The same group evaluated the TTV (and pneumococcal conjugate) responses in 106 patients with RA receiving baricitinib (30% on corticosteroids, 89% on concomitant methotrexate).[51] In this study, 43% and 74% of the patients achieved a greater than or equal to 4-fold increase and a greater than or equal to 2-fold increase in anti-tetanus concentrations, respectively. Gomez and colleagues[61] determined whether the immune response to tetanus and pneumococcal vaccines in healthy subjects administered ixekizumab was noninferior to control. The results showed that healthy subjects on ixekizumab were able to respond to tetanus vaccine administered 2 weeks after the ixekizumab 160-mg dose (week 0) and on the same day as the 80-mg dose of ixekizumab (week 2),[61] with the proportion of responders comparable to control subjects. Generally, patients with AIIRD are recommended to receive TTV in accordance with the recommendations for general population.[78]

HUMAN PAPILLOMA VIRUS VACCINATION

The ACIP currently recommends the routine administration of the quadrivalent HPV vaccine to women aged 11 or 12 years, with catch-up vaccination for women aged 13 years through 26 years.[79] Most of the research on HPV vaccination is based on studies involving female patients with SLE who have an especially increased risk for high-risk serotypes for cervical cancer at baseline.[80] Studies have shown similar immunogenicity of quadrivalent HPV vaccine among patients with SLE as compared with controls,[81,82] although there is some concern regarding the potential flare or onset of SLE following vaccination.[83] However, population-based studies demonstrate overall safety.[84] The current EULAR guidelines recommend HPV vaccination be given among patients with AIIRD.[6]

YELLOW FEVER VACCINE

The yellow fever vaccine available in the United States is the 17D-204, YF-VAX, which is a freeze-dried supernatant of centrifuged embryo homogenate. The CDC and EULAR recommend avoiding this vaccine in patients on bDMARDs regardless of a prior history of vaccination.[6,33] Of note, Oliveira and colleagues[85] evaluated the effects of inadvertent revaccination of 31 Brazilian patients with rheumatic diseases who were treated with methotrexate (n = 16), leflunomide (n = 16), infliximab (n = 3), or rituximab (n = 3). Four patients reported mild adverse events up to 30 days after vaccination. Twenty-four patients reported no reactions, and 3 did not recall the occurrence of any adverse reaction. Although the titers of neutralizing antibodies were lower among the patients with rheumatic disease as compared with healthy controls, the titers were still high enough to confer seroprotection. However, these observations should be interpreted carefully. A systematic review of the safety of live vaccinations in immunosuppressed patients, including those with immune-mediated inflammatory diseases, found a fatal case of yellow fever vaccine–associated viscerotropic disease.[86] Overall, live yellow fever vaccination is not recommended for patients on immunosuppressive therapy.[6,87]

SUMMARY

Although bDMARDs have revolutionized the way physicians treat AIIRD, appropriate evaluations and vaccinations before initiating biologics should be undertaken to prevent infectious complications in this vulnerable patient population.

DISCLOSURE

The authors have no conflict of interest related to this article.

REFERENCES

1. McInnes IB, Schett G. The pathogenesis of rheumatoid arthritis. N Engl J Med 2011;365(23):2205–19.

2. Singh JA. Infections with biologics in rheumatoid arthritis and related conditions: a scoping review of serious or hospitalized infections in observational studies. Curr Rheumatol Rep 2016;18(10):61.

3. Singh JA, Saag KG, Bridges SL Jr, et al. 2015 American College of Rheumatology guideline for the treatment of rheumatoid arthritis. ArthritisRheumatol 2016; 68(1):1–26.

4. Ramiro S, Sepriano A, Chatzidionysiou K, et al. Safety of synthetic and biological dmards: a systematic literature review informing the 2016 update of the eular recommendations for management of rheumatoid arthritis. Ann Rheum Dis 2017; 76(6):1101–36.

5. Handa R, Upadhyaya S, Kapoor S, et al. Tuberculosis and biologics in rheumatology: a special situation. Int J Rheum Dis 2017;20(10):1313–25.

6. Furer V, Rondaan C, Heijstek MW, et al. 2019 update of eular recommendations for vaccination in adult patients with autoimmune inflammatory rheumatic diseases. Ann Rheum Dis 2019;79(1):39–52.

7. Walker U, Hoffman H, Williams R, et al. Severe inflammation following vaccination against streptococcus pneumoniae in patients with cryopyrin-associated periodic syndromes (caps). ArthritisRheumatol 2016;68(2):516–20.

8. Kahlenberg JM, Kang I. The clinicopathologic significance of inflammasome activation in autoimmune diseases. ArthritisRheumatol 2020;72(3):386–95.

9. Yuksel S, Eren E, Hatemi G, et al. Novel nlrp3/cryopyrin mutations and pro-inflammatory cytokine profiles in behcet's syndrome patients. IntImmunol 2014; 26(2):71–81.

10. Hugle T, Bircher A, Walker UA. Streptococcal hypersensitivity reloaded: Severe inflammatory syndrome in behcet's disease following 23-valent polysaccharide streptococcus pneumoniae vaccine. Rheumatology (Oxford) 2012;51(4):761–2.

11. Tan J, Zhou J, Zhao P, et al. Prospective study of HBV reactivation risk in rheumatoid arthritis patients who received conventional disease-modifying antirheumatic drugs. ClinRheumatol 2012;31(8):1169–75.

12. Cheng J, Li JB, Sun QL, et al. Reactivation of hepatitis b virus after steroid treatment in rheumatic diseases. J Rheumatol 2011;38(1):181–2.

13. Sebastiani M, Atzeni F, Milazzo L, et al. Italian consensus guidelines for the management of hepatitis b virus infections in patients with rheumatoid arthritis. Joint Bone Spine 2017;84(5):525–30.

14. European Association for the Study of the Liver. Electronic address eee and European Association for the Study of the L. Easl 2017 clinical practice guidelines on the management of hepatitis b virus infection. J Hepatol 2017;67(2):370–98.

15. Terrault NA, Bzowej NH, Chang KM, et al. Aasld guidelines for treatment of chronic hepatitis b. Hepatology 2016;63(1):261–83.

16. Administration FaD. Product approval information: Package Insert. Heplisav-b, vol. 2019. Silver Spring (MD): US Department of Health and Human Services, Food and Drug Administration; 2018.

17. Schillie S, Vellozzi C, Reingold A, et al. Prevention of hepatitis b virus infection in the united states: Recommendations of the advisory committee on immunization practices. MMWR Recomm Rep 2018;67(1):1–31.

18. HaykirSolay A, Eser F. High dose hepatitis b vaccine is not effective in patients using immunomodulatory drugs: A pilot study. Hum Vaccin Immunother 2019; 15(5):1177–82.

19. Intongkam S, Samakarnthai P, Pakchotanon R, et al. Efficacy and safety of hepatitis b vaccination in rheumatoid arthritis patients receiving disease-modifying

antirheumatic drugs and/or biologics therapy. J ClinRheumatol 2019;25(8): 329–34.

20. Furer V, Rondaan C, Heijstek M, et al. Incidence and prevalence of vaccine preventable infections in adult patients with autoimmune inflammatory rheumatic diseases (aiird): A systemic literature review informing the 2019 update of the eular recommendations for vaccination in adult patients with aiird. RMD Open 2019; 5(2):e001041.

21. Bello SL, Serafino L, Bonali C, et al. Incidence of influenza-like illness into a cohort of patients affected by chronic inflammatory rheumatism and treated with biological agents. Reumatismo 2012;64(5):299–306.

22. Rubin LG, Levin MJ, Ljungman P, et al. 2013 idsa clinical practice guideline for vaccination of the immunocompromised host. Clin Infect Dis 2014;58(3):309–18.

23. Grohskopf LA, Alyanak E, Broder KR, et al. Prevention and control of seasonal influenza with vaccines: recommendations of the advisory committee on immunization practices - united states, 2019-20 influenza season. MMWR Recomm Rep 2019;68(3):1–21.

24. Burmester GR, Landewe R, Genovese MC, et al. Adalimumab long-term safety: Infections, vaccination response and pregnancy outcomes in patients with rheumatoid arthritis. Ann Rheum Dis 2017;76(2):414–7.

25. Chen CM, Chen HJ, Chen WS, et al. Clinical effectiveness of influenza vaccination in patients with rheumatoid arthritis. Int J Rheum Dis 2018;21(6):1246–53.

26. Chang CC, Chang YS, Chen WS, et al. Effects of annual influenza vaccination on morbidity and mortality in patients with systemic lupus erythematosus: a nationwide cohort study. Sci Rep 2016;6:37817.

27. Huang Y, Wang H, Tam WWS. Is rheumatoid arthritis associated with reduced immunogenicity of the influenza vaccination? A systematic review and meta-analysis. Curr Med Res Opin 2017;33(10):1901–8.

28. Subesinghe S, Bechman K, Rutherford AI, et al. A systematic review and meta-analysis of antirheumatic drugs and vaccine immunogenicity in rheumatoid arthritis. J Rheumatol 2018;45(6):733–44.

29. Park JK, Lee MA, Lee EY, et al. Effect of methotrexate discontinuation on efficacy of seasonal influenza vaccination in patients with rheumatoid arthritis: a randomised clinical trial. Ann Rheum Dis 2017;76(9):1559–65.

30. Park JK, Lee YJ, Shin K, et al. Impact of temporary methotrexate discontinuation for 2 weeks on immunogenicity of seasonal influenza vaccination in patients with rheumatoid arthritis: a randomised clinical trial. Ann Rheum Dis 2018;77(6): 898–904.

31. Alten R, Bingham CO 3rd, Cohen SB, et al. Antibody response to pneumococcal and influenza vaccination in patients with rheumatoid arthritis receiving abatacept. BMCMusculoskeletDisord 2016;17:231.

32. Richi P, Martin MD, de Ory F, et al. Secukinumab does not impair the immunogenic response to the influenza vaccine in patients. RMD Open 2019;5(2): e001018.

33. Friedman MA, Winthrop K. Vaccinations for rheumatoid arthritis. CurrOpinRheumatol 2016;28(3):330–6.

34. Friedman MA, Winthrop KL. Vaccines and disease-modifying antirheumatic drugs: Practical implications for the rheumatologist. Rheum Dis Clin North Am 2017;43(1):1–13.

35. Winthrop KL, Silverfield J, Racewicz A, et al. The effect of tofacitinib on pneumococcal and influenza vaccine responses in rheumatoid arthritis. Ann Rheum Dis 2016;75(4):687–95.

36. Wong PKK, Hanrahan P. Management of vaccination in rheumatic disease. Best-Pract Res ClinRheumatol 2018;32(6):720–34.
37. Caso F, Ramonda R, Del Puente A, et al. Influenza vaccine with adjuvant on disease activity in psoriatic arthritis patients under anti-tnf-alpha therapy. ClinExpRheumatol 2016;34(3):507–12.
38. Merck & Co. Inc. M-M-R II (Measles, mumps, and rubella virus vaccine live); 2009.
39. Merck & Co. Inc. ProQuad (measles, mumps, rubella and varicella virus vaccine live lyophilized preparation for subcutaneous injection). 2011.
40. Marin M, Broder KR, Temte JL, et al. Use of combination measles, mumps, rubella, and varicella vaccine: Recommendations of the advisory committee on immunization practices (acip). MMWRRecomm Rep 2010;59(RR-3):1–12.
41. Heijstek MW, van Gageldonk PG, Berbers GA, et al. Differences in persistence of measles, mumps, rubella, diphtheria and tetanus antibodies between children with rheumatic disease and healthy controls: a retrospective cross-sectional study. Ann Rheum Dis 2012;71(6):948–54.
42. Borte S, Liebert UG, Borte M, et al. Efficacy of measles, mumps and rubella revaccination in children with juvenile idiopathic arthritis treated with methotrexate and etanercept. Rheumatology (Oxford) 2009;48(2):144–8.
43. Matanock ALG, Gierke R, Kobayashi M, et al. Use of 13-valent pneumococcal conjugate vaccine and 23-valent pneumococcal polysaccharide vaccine among adults aged ≥65 years: updated recommendations of the advisory committee on immunization practices. MMWRMorbMortalWkly Rep 2019;68:1069–75.
44. Westerink MA, Schroeder HW Jr, Nahm MH. Immune responses to pneumococcal vaccines in children and adults: Rationale for age-specific vaccination. Aging Dis 2012;3(1):51–67.
45. Centers for Disease Control and Prevention (CDC). Use of 13-valent pneumococcal conjugate vaccine and 23-valent pneumococcal polysaccharide vaccine among children aged 6–18 years with immunocompromising conditions: Recommendations of the advisory committee on immunization practices (ACIP). MMWRMorbMortalWkly Rep 2013;62(25):521–4.
46. Kapetanovic MC, Saxne T, Sjoholm A, et al. Influence of methotrexate, tnf blockers and prednisolone on antibody responses to pneumococcal polysaccharide vaccine in patients with rheumatoid arthritis. Rheumatology (Oxford) 2006;45(1):106–11.
47. Kapetanovic MC, Roseman C, Jonsson G, et al. Antibody response is reduced following vaccination with 7-valent conjugate pneumococcal vaccine in adult methotrexate-treated patients with established arthritis, but not those treated with tumor necrosis factor inhibitors. Arthritis Rheum 2011;63(12):3723–32.
48. Mori S, Ueki Y, Hirakata N, et al. Impact of tocilizumab therapy on antibody response to influenza vaccine in patients with rheumatoid arthritis. Ann Rheum Dis 2012;71(12):2006–10.
49. Nguyen MTT, Lindegaard H, Hendricks O, et al. Initial serological response after prime-boost pneumococcal vaccination in rheumatoid arthritis patients: Results of a randomized controlled trial. J Rheumatol 2017;44(12):1794–803.
50. Rákóczi É, Perge B, Vegh E, et al. Evaluation of the immunogenicity of the 13-valent conjugated pneumococcal vaccine in rheumatoid arthritis patients treated with etanercept. Joint Bone Spine 2016;83(6):675–9.
51. Winthrop KL, Bingham CO 3rd, Komocsar WJ, et al. Evaluation of pneumococcal and tetanus vaccine responses in patients with rheumatoid arthritis receiving

baricitinib: results from a long-term extension trial substudy. Arthritis Res Ther 2019;21(1):102.

52. Winthrop KL, Korman N, Abramovits W, et al. T-cell-mediated immune response to pneumococcal conjugate vaccine (pcv-13) and tetanus toxoid vaccine in patients with moderate-to-severe psoriasis during tofacitinib treatment. J Am Acad-Dermatol 2018;78(6):1149–55.e1.

53. Nagel J, Saxne T, Geborek P, et al. Treatment with belimumab in systemic lupus erythematosus does not impair antibody response to 13-valent pneumococcal conjugate vaccine. Lupus 2017;26(10):1072–81.

54. Chatham W, Chadha A, Fettiplace J, et al. A randomized, open-label study to investigate the effect of belimumab on pneumococcal vaccination in patients with active, autoantibody-positive systemic lupus erythematosus. Lupus 2017; 26(14):1483–90.

55. Adawi M, Bragazzi NL, McGonagle D, et al. Immunogenicity, safety and tolerability of anti-pneumococcal vaccination in systemic lupus erythematosus patients: an evidence-informed and prisma compliant systematic review and meta-analysis. Autoimmun Rev 2019;18(1):73–92.

56. Kapetanovic MC, Nagel J, Nordstrom I, et al. Methotrexate reduces vaccine-specific immunoglobulin levels but not numbers of circulating antibody-producing b cells in rheumatoid arthritis after vaccination with a conjugate pneumococcal vaccine. Vaccine 2017;35(6):903–8.

57. Nived P, Nagel J, Saxne T, et al. Immune response to pneumococcal conjugate vaccine in patients with systemic vasculitis receiving standard of care therapy. Vaccine 2017;35(29):3639–46.

58. Rezende RP, Ribeiro FM, Albuquerque EM, et al. Immunogenicity of pneumococcal polysaccharide vaccine in adult systemic lupus erythematosus patients undergoing immunosuppressive treatment. Lupus 2016;25(11):1254–9.

59. Broyde A, Arad U, Madar-Balakirski N, et al. Longterm efficacy of an antipneumococcal polysaccharide vaccine among patients with autoimmune inflammatory rheumatic diseases. J Rheumatol 2016;43(2):267–72.

60. Walker UA, Hoffman HM, Williams R, et al. Brief report: Severe inflammation following vaccination against streptococcus pneumoniae in patients with cryopyrin-associated periodic syndromes. ArthritisRheumatol 2016;68(2): 516–20.

61. Gomez EV, Bishop JL, Jackson K, et al. Response to tetanus and pneumococcal vaccination following administration of ixekizumab in healthy participants. Bio-Drugs 2017;31(6):545–54.

62. Dooling KL, Guo A, Patel M, et al. Recommendations of the advisory committee on immunization practices for use of herpes zoster vaccines. MMWRMorbMortalWkly Rep 2018;67(3):103–8.

63. Cunningham AL, Lal H, Kovac M, et al. Efficacy of the herpes zoster subunit vaccine in adults 70 years of age or older. N Engl J Med 2016;375(11):1019–32.

64. Harpaz R, Ortega-Sanchez IR, Seward JF, Advisory Committee on Immunization Practices Centers for Disease C and Prevention. Prevention of herpes zoster: recommendations of the advisory committee on immunization practices (acip). MMWRRecomm Rep 2008;57(RR-5):1–30 [quiz: CE2–4].

65. Baumrin E, Van Voorhees A, Garg A, et al. A systematic review of herpes zoster incidence and consensus recommendations on vaccination in adult patients on systemic therapy for psoriasis or psoriatic arthritis: From the medical board of the national psoriasis foundation. J Am AcadDermatol 2019;81(1):102–10.

66. Smitten AL, Choi HK, Hochberg MC, et al. The risk of herpes zoster in patients with rheumatoid arthritis in the united states and the united kingdom. Arthritis Rheum 2007;57(8):1431–8.
67. Strangfeld A, Listing J, Herzer P, et al. Risk of herpes zoster in patients with rheumatoid arthritis treated with anti-tnf-alpha agents. JAMA 2009;301(7):737–44.
68. Galloway JB, Mercer LK, Moseley A, et al. Risk of skin and soft tissue infections (including shingles) in patients exposed to anti-tumour necrosis factor therapy: Results from the british society for rheumatology biologics register. Ann Rheum Dis 2013;72(2):229–34.
69. Che H, Lukas C, Morel J, et al. Risk of herpes/herpes zoster during anti-tumor necrosis factor therapy in patients with rheumatoid arthritis.Systematic review and meta-analysis. Joint Bone Spine 2014;81(3):215–21.
70. Dewedar AM, Shalaby MA, Al-Homaid S, et al. Lack of adverse effect of anti-tumor necrosis factor-alpha biologics in treatment of rheumatoid arthritis: 5 years follow-up. Int J Rheum Dis 2012;15(3):330–5.
71. McDonald JR, Zeringue AL, Caplan L, et al. Herpes zoster risk factors in a national cohort of veterans with rheumatoid arthritis. Clin Infect Dis 2009;48(10): 1364–71.
72. Tran CT, Ducancelle A, Masson C, et al. Herpes zoster: Risk and prevention during immunomodulating therapy. Joint Bone Spine 2017;84(1):21–7.
73. Curtis JR, Xie F, Yun H, et al. Real-world comparative risks of herpes virus infections in tofacitinib and biologic-treated patients with rheumatoid arthritis. Ann Rheum Dis 2016;75(10):1843–7.
74. Curtis JR, Xie F, Yang S, et al. Risk for herpes zoster in tofacitinib-treated rheumatoid arthritis patients with and without concomitant methotrexate and glucocorticoids. ArthritisCare Res (Hoboken) 2019;71(9):1249–54.
75. Winthrop KL, Wouters AG, Choy EH, et al. The safety and immunogenicity of live zoster vaccination in patients with rheumatoid arthritis before starting tofacitinib: a randomized phase II trial. ArthritisRheumatol 2017;69(10):1969–77.
76. Calabrese LH, Abud-Mendoza C, Lindsey SM, et al. Live zoster vaccine in patients with rheumatoid arthritis treated with tofacitinib with or without methotrexate, or adalimumab with methotrexate. ArthritisCare Res (Hoboken) 2020; 72(3):353–9.
77. Wu KK, Lee MP, Lee EB, et al. Risk of herpes zoster with il-17 inhibitor therapy for psoriasis and other inflammatory conditions. J Dermatolog Treat 2019;1–7.
78. Liang JL, Tiwari T, Moro P, et al. Prevention of pertussis, tetanus, and diphtheria with vaccines in the united states: recommendations of the advisory committee on immunization practices (acip). MMWRRecomm Rep 2018;67(2):1–44.
79. Meites E, Szilagyi PG, Chesson HW, et al. Human papillomavirus vaccination for adults: Updated recommendations of the advisory committee on immunization practices. Am J Transplant 2019;19(11):3202–6.
80. Lyrio LD, Grassi MF, Santana IU, et al. Prevalence of cervical human papillomavirus infection in women with systemic lupus erythematosus. Rheumatol Int 2013; 33(2):335–40.
81. Dhar JP, Essenmacher L, Dhar R, et al. The safety and immunogenicity of quadrivalenthpv (qhpv) vaccine in systemic lupus erythematosus. Vaccine 2017; 35(20):2642–6.
82. Mok CC, Ho LY, To CH. Long-term immunogenicity of a quadrivalent human papillomavirus vaccine in systemic lupus erythematosus. Vaccine 2018;36(23): 3301–7.

83. Ito H, Noda K, Hirai K, et al. A case of systemic lupus erythematosus (sle) following human papillomavirus (hpv) vaccination. Nihon Rinsho Meneki Gakkai Kaishi 2016;39(2):145–9.

84. Gronlund O, Herweijer E, Sundstrom K, et al. Incidence of new-onset autoimmune disease in girls and women with pre-existing autoimmune disease after quadrivalent human papillomavirus vaccination: A cohort study. J Intern Med 2016;280(6): 618–26.

85. Oliveira AC, Mota LM, Santos-Neto LL, et al. Seroconversion in patients with rheumatic diseases treated with immunomodulators or immunosuppressants, who were inadvertently revaccinated against yellow fever. ArthritisRheumatol 2015; 67(2):582–3.

86. Croce E, Hatz C, Jonker EF, et al. Safety of live vaccinations on immunosuppressive therapy in patients with immune-mediated inflammatory diseases, solid organ transplantation or after bone-marrow transplantation - a systematic review of randomized trials, observational studies and case reports. Vaccine 2017; 35(9):1216–26.

87. Winthrop KL, Mariette X, Silva JT, et al. Escmid study group for infections in compromised hosts (esgich) consensus document on the safety of targeted and biological therapies: An infectious diseases perspective (soluble immune effector molecules [ii]: Agents targeting interleukins, immunoglobulins and complement factors). ClinMicrobiol Infect 2018;24(Suppl 2):S21–40.

88. Singh JA, Wells GA, Christensen R, et al. Adverse effects of biologics: A network meta-analysis and cochrane overview. Cochrane Database Syst Rev 2011;(2):CD008794.

89. Esposito S, Bonanni P, Maggi S, et al. Recommended immunization schedules for adults: Clinical practice guidelines by the escmid vaccine study group (evasg), european geriatric medicine society (eugms) and the world association for infectious diseases and immunological disorders (waidid). Hum VaccinImmunother 2016;12(7):1777–94.

90. Staples JE, Bocchini JA Jr, Rubin L, et al, Centers for Disease Control and Prevention (CDC). Yellow fever vaccine booster doses: Recommendations of the advisory committee on immunization practices, 2015. MMWR Morb Mortal Wkly Rep 2015;64(23):647–50.

Moving?

Make sure your subscription moves with you!

To notify us of your new address, find your **Clinics Account Number** (located on your mailing label above your name), and contact customer service at:

Email: journalscustomerservice-usa@elsevier.com

800-654-2452 (subscribers in the U.S. & Canada)
314-447-8871 (subscribers outside of the U.S. & Canada)

Fax number: 314-447-8029

Elsevier Health Sciences Division
Subscription Customer Service
3251 Riverport Lane
Maryland Heights, MO 63043

To ensure uninterrupted delivery of your subscription, please notify us at least 4 weeks in advance of move.

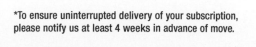